Health Care Reform:
A Human Rights Approach

Contributors

Mary Ann Baily, Ph.D., Adjunct Associate Professor of Economics and Public Policy, George Washington University.

Dan W. Brock, Ph.D., Professor of Philosophy and Biomedical Ethics, Brown University.

Audrey R. Chapman, Ph.D., Program Director, Science and Human Rights, American Association for the Advancement of Science.

Larry Churchill, Ph.D., Professor and Chair, Department of Social Medicine, School of Medicine, University of North Carolina-Chapel Hill.

Jack Donnelly, Ph.D., Andrew W. Mellon Professor, Graduate School of International Studies, University of Denver.

Michael Garland, D.Sc.Rel., Associate Professor, Department of Public Health and Preventive Medicine, Oregon Health Sciences University-Portland.

Tom Jabine, Statistical Consultant and former Chair of the Committee on Scientific Freedom and Human Rights, American Statistical Association.

Virginia A. Leary, Ph.D., Professor of Law, State University of New York-Buffalo.

James L. Nelson, Ph.D., Associate for Ethical Studies, The Hastings Center.

Janet O'Keeffe, Dr.P.H., Assistant Director for Public Interest Policy, American Psychological Association.

Robert M. Veatch, Ph.D., Professor of Medical Ethics, Kennedy Institute of Ethics, Georgetown University.

Janet Weiner, M.P.H., Research Associate, American College of Physicians.

Daniel Wikler, Ph.D., Professor of Medical Ethics, University of Wisconsin-Madison.

Health Care Reform:
A Human Rights Approach

Edited by
AUDREY R. CHAPMAN

GEORGETOWN UNIVERSITY PRESS / WASHINGTON, D.C.

Georgetown University Press, Washington, D.C. 20007-1079
© 1994 by Georgetown University Press. All rights reserved.
Printed in the United States of America
10 9 8 7 6 5 4 3 2 1   1994
THIS VOLUME IS PRINTED ON ACID-FREE OFFSET BOOK PAPER.

Library of Congress Cataloging-in-Publication Data

Health care reform : a human rights approach / Audrey R. Chapman,
    editor.
        p.   cm.
    Includes bibliographical references.
    1. Health care reform—United States.   2. Right to health care—
United States.   I. Chapman, Audrey R.
RA395.A3H4137   1994
362.1'0973—dc20
ISBN 0-87840-554-2 — ISBN 0-87840-555-0 (pbk.)   94-2311

Contents

v

Preface

Health care reform has found its way to the top of the American policy agenda. The reasons for this priority are not hard to find. Over thirty million citizens lack health insurance while many more are a pink slip away from the possibility of financial ruin. For those with coverage, the costs of health care have risen much faster than incomes creating pressure on the living standards of the middle class. For the next year or more, the health care reform proposals from President Clinton and others will be debated in Congress and throughout the United States. *Health Care Reform: A Human Rights Approach* seeks to inform that debate by examining the neglected ethical dimension of this issue.

Two years ago the Science and Human Rights Program of the American Association for the Advancement of Science (AAAS), with the assistance of The Robert Wood Johnson Foundation, initiated a project to explore a human rights approach to health care reform in the United States. Unlike previous work on human rights, the project decided to focus on concrete issues for establishing the scope and limitations of a right to health care. In particular, we sought to translate an abstract right to health care into specific obligations and commitments consistent with available resources. Such obligations could then be translated into criteria which served as a kind of "human rights report card" to shape health care reforms and to evaluate whether specific proposals are consistent with human rights requirements.

Between September 1992 and May 1993, the project sponsored four consultations which brought together a wide range of health care specialists to discuss health care as a human right. In selecting participants an effort was made to have a variety of perspectives and positions as well as disciplines represented. The project sought to mix human rights specialists with health care providers, health policy analysts, bioethicists, and health care economists. Speakers and participants were drawn from the fields of medicine, biology, genetics, law, philosophy, statistics, economics, political science, theology, and ethics. Health care providers participating in the project represented the fields of nursing, primary care and internal medicine, psychiatry, psychology, public health, forensic pathology, and occupational therapy. *Health Care Reform: A Human Rights Approach* grew out of these exciting and fruitful sessions. Because of the nature of the AAAS project, the essays in this volume present a sustained a coherent argument about health care reform.

This book is organized into four parts. The essays in the first part, "The Framework for Health Care Reform", examine the evolution of the American medical system and the concomitant debate about a right to health care. Contributors to the second part "Health Care as a Human Right" conceptualize the content and limitations of a right to health care. International perspectives as well as human rights theory are used to lay an ethical foundation for current reform efforts and set out criteria for evaluating health care reform efforts. The third section "Defining a Basic Standard of Health Care" provides answers to an essential question of health care reform: what level of care should be guaranteed to all citizens? The fourth section raises some fundamental questions about managed competition and its stepchild, the Clinton health care reform proposal. Speaking directly to current debates, the final article recommends changes in the Health Security Act to make it more consistent with a human rights approach.

The criteria developed in this volume can play a major role in monitoring and evaluating health care reform measures over time. To be effective and just, reform of the health care system should be understood as an ongoing process of assessment and revision, not a one time decision. In view of the complexity and scope of the various health care reform proposals and the fact that many of them, particularly the managed competition model, have not been implemented elsewhere, there will be a long period of trial and error. Thus these criteria and the underlying vision of a human rights approach will be relevant even if the articulated rationale of the specific legislation that is adopted is not explicitly based on recognition of a right to health care. A human rights approach provides the standard, the goals, for the present and future evolution of the health care system.

In publishing this volume, we hope to contribute an ethical and human rights perspective to the debate on health care reform which has been largely absent. Most of the claims and arguments for specific proposals have focussed on the economics rather than the ethics of health care reform. In contrast, the contributors to this volume believe cost containment is a necessary but not sufficient basis for reshaping the health care system. Health care is a social good, not a commodity, and principles of justice, equity, and social obligation need to be at the foundation of health care reform.

A human rights approach also sets a higher standard of universality and equality. Although most of the health care proposals currently put forward are ostensibly committed to universal coverage, none advocate recognition of a right to health care. Yet a putative commitment to universality in the absence of a guaranteed right may not achieve this goal. With a phase in of coverage to those currently without health care insurance implicitly or explicitly contingent on cost containment measures, it is very probable that universal coverage may be indefinitely delayed or even dropped if such savings do not materialize. Moreover, many of the proposals appear to be predicated on a nominal rather than a meaningful or effective form of universality. A human rights approach mandates that health care reform go beyond the provision of some form of health insurance to rectify inadequacies and structural deficiencies in the health care system.

By stressing the social foundations of health care reform this volume will help counter the tendency of individuals and special interests to view issues and proposals through the exclusive prism of private benefit. Health care is first and foremost a social good dedicated to the improvement of the health and well-being of the entire community, not a private commodity. A great deal more than individual needs and advantage is at stake. Health care reform involves the renegotiation of the social covenant defining social obligations and commitments between the government and the society and between members of the society. The nature and humaneness of the society in which current and future generations will live will depend on decisions made regarding the structure and standards of the health care system. A determinant will be whether the reform process primarily protects the insurance coverage and benefits of groups that are amongst the "haves" or, consistent with a human rights approach, accords priority to improving the health status of "have nots." Another major question is whether a commitment to the common good can outweigh the influence of the "medical-industrial" complex in setting the agenda for reform.

A volume which is the outgrowth of a two year multi-consultation project could not have been possible without the assistance and cooperation of a large number of persons and organizations. Just as a human rights approach acknowledges that health care is first and foremost a social good, the exploration of a right to health care in this volume represents a community effort. I would like to express particular appreciation to The Robert Wood Johnson Foundation for its willingness to support a pioneering effort to develop a human rights approach to health care reform. I would like also to thank the contributors to the volume for the time spent in preparing and revising their articles. This volume became a reality through the hard work of two other AAAS staff members, Alexandra Allen, who edited most of the articles, and Elisa Munoz, who handled the logistics for the consultations and for the preparation of this volume. Many of the participants in the four consultations, too numerous to name, also contributed valuable ideas, now incorporated in this volume.

Health Care Reform:
A Human Rights Approach

AUDREY R. CHAPMAN

Introduction

The United States stands before the most important and extensive reform of its health care system in a generation. Given the scope of this undertaking, citizens and policymakers should examine fundamental assumptions about the changes to come. The contributors to this volume believe that a right to a basic and adequate standard of health care should be adopted as the fundamental premise of a reformed health care system for the United States. Currently the United States is the only western democracy that does not recognize a right to health care. Other industrialized nations like Canada, Great Britain, France, Germany, the Netherlands, and Japan have long provided a legal entitlement to health care. By way of introducing our argument, the following pages will examine the problems of our health care system and the solutions suggested by a human rights approach to health care reform.

The Impetus for Health Care Reform

Four disturbing trends account for much of the momentum toward change of the health care system in the United States. The first is escalating health costs. ¡With spending on health care now rising at an annual rate of twelve to fifteen percent and consuming more than fourteen percent of the nation's total economic output, the cost of health care is straining the economy and state and federal budgets. These figures stand in marked contrast with such countries as Canada, Britain, Germany, Sweden, France, and Japan, whose health care spending in 1990 ranged between six percent and nine percent while providing universal health insurance for their population. An aging population, leading to a growing demand for health care and a need for more care for the chronically ill, and the increasing use of sophisticated and expensive equipment have created pressures on financial resources in virtually all industrialized countries. In the United States, these factors are further compounded by the commercialization of health care and the comparatively high earnings of many people in the health-care sector.[1] In the absence of significant policy changes, estimates are that health spending will reach 18.1 percent of the GNP in the year 2000 and almost twenty percent of state and local spending. The figure for 2030 is even more ominous - thirty two percent of GNP, most of it paid by government.[2]

The second trend is increasing gaps in health insurance coverage and persistent inequities in access to health care. Despite the highest levels of health spending in the world, the number of Americans without basic health insurance rose to 38.9 million in 1992, an increase of some 2.3 million over the previous year.[3] As many as seventy million people may be substantially underinsured. No other industrialized country has comparable gaps in coverage. A majority of those without insurance are full time employees and their dependents whose employers do not provide medical insurance benefits.[4]

Moreover, low-income Americans and ethnic minorities, particularly blacks, Hispanics, and native Americans, are far more likely than other groups to have inadequate health insurance. Latinos have the worst health insurance coverage of any ethnic group in the country; approximately 39 percent of Latinos are uninsured. Some 24 percent of the black population lack health insurance as compared with just under 14 percent of whites.[5] Lack of health insurance for minority groups translates into the failure to obtain timely and appropriate health care. A recent study by the Institute of Medicine of access to health care in America documented inequities for blacks and other ethnic minorities in the timely receipt of ambulatory care, immunizations, dental visits, and some sophisticated procedures.[6] Death rates among low-income populations are twice the rates of the highest income groups.[7]

The third trend accounting for the momentum toward change is a lack of security about obtaining health insurance. Currently, access to medical care is a top concern of the nation's poor, ranking ahead of basic needs like food and shelter and problems like crime, drug abuse, and violence in their neighborhoods.[8] Nevertheless, the catalyst for health care reform has been the fears of the middle class, not the plight of the poor. Perhaps for the first time, anxieties about the scope, security, and cost of health insurance coverage have become a major preoccupation of the middle class. As health care has become more and more expensive, insurance premiums have escalated, with the result that increasing numbers of Americans cannot afford to buy insurance. During the 1980s the first-ever drop in the percentage of the population with private health insurance occurred. Depending on assumptions made about multiple coverage, the total share of the population with private coverage in 1990 as compared with 1980 dropped five to ten percentage points.[9]

Even if individuals are able to afford insurance, there is no assurance that they will be able to secure coverage. To cope with financial pressures and, in the case of for-profit companies, to maintain profits, health insurers have decreased the availability of community-rated insurance, under which anyone who applies for coverage is accepted, and instituted experience ratings, which exclude those deemed high risk from coverage. Rising health costs have also led many large firms to self-insure in order to save the cost of insurance company commissions, overhead, and profits and to obtain the benefits of investing large reserves. Because such employee health plans are exempted from state insurance regulations, employers have the flexibility of limiting liability for chronic and expensive conditions. These policies have made many people hostage to their current jobs in order to retain their health insurance and left others "medically uninsurable" as insurers deny coverage both for numerous pre-existing conditions and for those considered likely to develop such conditions, no matter how minimal the risk.[10]

Fourth, there is evidence of serious inadequacies in the American model of health care, with its reliance on treatment rather than prevention and its investment in high technology rather than basic health care. Although the United States has the most advanced medical technology, the largest ratio of doctors to population in the world, and the highest hospital bills, the country fares worse than other developed countries on many health indicators. For example, the United States ranks (from best to worst) nineteenth in infant mortality, twenty eighth in the rate of infants born at low birth weights, fifteenth in the rate of maternal mortality, and ninth in life expectancy, worse in some cases than Hong Kong, Singapore, Jordan, or Costa Rica.[11] The American Public Health Association describes this situation as a "public health crisis."[12] Incentives in the American health care system that encourage physicians to specialize rather than enter primary health care practices, perform as many specialty procedures as possible, and over-use expensive technologies also contribute to the high cost of health care.[13]

As a consequence of these trends, a consensus has finally emerged that the country needs to change its health care system. Many questions remain, however, about the direction and scope of health care reform. The contributors to this book agree that policymakers should conceptualize health care as a human right while reforming our system. Providing some specifics to this argument is our next task.

Health Care as a Human Right

Rights in moral philosophy and political theory are understood as justified claims.[14] A right is an entitlement a person possesses to some good, service, or liberty. As entitlements, rights are contrasted with privileges, group ideals, societal obligations, or acts of charity. A moral right is an entitlement which appeals to moral principles as its foundation. Legal rights are claims justified by the laws of a state. A right creates correlative obligations or duties to secure, or not interfere with the enjoyment of, that entitlement. Human rights are a special class of rights, the rights one has by virtue of being a human being. Human rights are predicated on the recognition of the intrinsic value and worth of all human beings. As such, human rights are considered to be universal, vested equally in all persons regardless of their gender, race, nationality, economic status, or social position. Like other moral rights, human rights exist independently of legal recognition. Human rights are also characterized as inalienable or not separable from right-holders. While human rights are high priority norms, they do not confer absolute claims.

Modern conceptions of human rights formulated at the end of World War II assume a very different conception of the nature of rights and the role of governments than the eighteenth century liberal interpretation still current in the United States. Much of this is implicit rather than explicit. To achieve the widest possible consensus, the drafters of the Universal Declaration of Human Rights avoided philosophical discussions of the grounding of human rights. The preamble roots human rights in the "inherent dignity" and equality of all human beings and "the foundations of freedom, justice, and peace in the world."[15] Neither the Universal Declaration nor the human rights instruments based on the Declaration, however, explain how the inherent dignity of the human being gives rise to these rights.

The text of the Universal Declaration of Human Rights replaces generic rights to life, liberty, and property with nearly two dozen specific rights. Among the civil and political rights enumerated are rights to freedom from discrimination, to life, liberty, the security of the person, to freedom of religion, thought, expression, movement, and assembly, freedom from torture and cruel punishment, from arbitrary arrest, to protections of privacy, and of a fair trial. Social and economic rights recognized in the Declaration include rights to education, availability of a job, marriage and founding a family, freedom from forced marriage, adequate standard of living, security during illness and disability, participation in the cultural life of the community. Together these rights are considered to establish minimal standards of decent social and government practice.[16]

Any consideration of human rights, particularly in support of a positive right not yet recognized in the United States, bears the burden of providing a satisfactory theoretical framework. The following sketch of the foundations and interpretation of human rights in this section is based on the author's unpublished paper.[17]

Human rights, which are expressions of each person's intrinsic value and dignity, are recognized and given practical form and content through membership in a community.[18] Rights are defined, shaped, implemented and limited by relationships of mutual commitment and responsibility within and to that community. They are an embodiment of the ongoing social covenant linking members of the society to each other. Cumulatively human rights represent "the minimum conditions for life in community."[19] Thus a viable community or society with relatively effective institutions is a prerequisite for upholding and implementing human rights. One need only consider the situation in countries like the former Yugoslavia or Somalia where civil society has broken down and political institutions no longer function to affirm the social character of rights.

Human rights serve as positive instruments of human and community development. In designating a human or social attribute as a right, a society underscores that it is regarded as essential to the adequate functioning of the human being within the context of community and accepts responsibility for its promotion and protection.[20] In using rights language a society assigns priority to a particular human attribute or social good. While rights claims are not absolute, they impose *prima facie* duties or obligations on the community. Because the fulfillment of specific rights is so central to human and community welfare, the failure to do so can only be justified by a competing moral and/or legal claim.

While human rights are based on moral universals, their formulation is historically contingent and reflects societal understandings at particular points in history.[21] Human rights are universal because they are understood to derive from the inherent dignity of the human person. Because all human beings have the same nature and dignity by virtue of their humanity, they have the same rights. Nevertheless the delineation and interpretation of those rights reflect a particular political conception of what it means to be a human being. Over time the "standard threats" against human dignity also change:[22] in the eighteenth century rights were interpreted as fences or protection for the individual from the unfettered authoritarian governments that were considered the greatest threat to human welfare. In late twentieth century democratic governments do not pose the same problems and there are many new kinds of threats to the right to life and well-being. Moreover, varying resource levels historically and contemporarily amongst societies at different levels of development translate into different capabilities for promoting human and societal development; a commitment to providing basic and adequate health care or other types of positive entitlements is far more appropriate and possible for a late twentieth century advanced industrial economy than for an eighteenth century agrarian economy. Thus the list of universal rights enumerated in the Universal Declaration of Human Rights in the middle of the twentieth century would be expected to be different than the human rights incorporated in a late eighteenth century Bill of Rights.

To be able to protect and promote rights effectively, a community requires a consensus interpreting human rights standards amongst its members and institutions through which to express this agreement. Human rights can be translated into norms or criteria by which to shape and evaluate institutional arrangements. Fundamental rights serve as constraints on communities, ruling out certain kinds of structures as unacceptable because they violate rights or cannot effectively protect or promote rights. Rights can also provide a positive agenda establishing needed institutional capabilities for their secure implementation. The major means by which the social covenant becomes institutionalized is through translating moral norms into laws. Government or political institutions serve a positive role, serving as a major, but not sole guarantor of rights.

All members, particularly in a democratic society, can be seen both as rights-holders and duty-bearers. As rights-holders, individual members of society are entitled to make claims. As duty-bearers, each person is responsible individually and collectively for respecting and protecting the rights of others and promoting conditions conducive to the implementation of human rights. Since realization of human rights rests on the integrity and viability of the community, all members have both the right and duty to participate in the life and activity of the community's social and political institutions. The system of reciprocal rights and responsibilities also places a high premium on shared commitments to work toward the evolution of a just society and political system better able to guarantee the rights of all members individually and collectively and to adjudicate conflicting claims in ways that are considered fair and balanced.

The litmus test in this model of human rights is the extent to which the rights of the most vulnerable and disadvantaged individuals and groups within the community are assured by these arrangements. A human rights standard assumes a special obligation or bias in favor of the needs and rights of the poor, the disadvantaged, the powerless, and those at the periphery of society. If human rights are conceptualized as instruments to protect and promote human dignity in the context of community, it follows that their implementation can only be considered effective when those in greatest need of protection and development are benefitted.

How should a human right encompassing access to basic health care be defined and formulated? Can a right to health care be achieved independently of broader efforts to improve the health status and health protection of the population? The contributors to this volume define a right to health care as "a right to a basic and adequate standard of health care consistent with societal resources." This wording approximates the definition given elsewhere by contributor Larry Churchill that "a right to health care based on need means a right to equitable access based on need alone to all effective care society can reasonably afford."[23] Health care thus encompasses a comprehensive range of services—prevention and health protection, curative and therapeutic services, rehabilitative measures, mental health, and auxiliary social services.

This definition of a right to basic and adequate health care differs from the comprehensive language of the Universal Declaration of Human Rights and the covenants based on the Universal Declaration, as well as the formulation of the World Health Organization. The International Covenant on Economic, Social and Cultural Rights, which is based on the Universal Declaration of Human Rights, incorporates a right to health care as a component of a broader right to health. It recognizes (article 12) "the right of everyone to the enjoyment of the highest attainable standard of physical and mental health."[24] To that end, it identifies that state parties to the Covenant (which now number 122 countries) undertake the following steps to achieve the full realization of this right:

(a) The provision for the reduction of the stillbirth-rate and of infant mortality and for the healthy development of the child;

(b) The improvement of all aspects of environmental and industrial hygiene;

(c) The prevention, treatment and control of epidemic, endemic, occupational and other diseases;

(d) The creation of conditions which would assure medical service and medical attention to all in the event of sickness.[25]

Constitutions of a number of countries enumerate a right to health protection.[26] While not as broad as a right to health, the right to health protection encompasses attention to the public health context of curative medicine. Thus a right to health protection goes beyond medical interventions to include preventive measures, such as the provision of potable water and improvement of environmental conditions. Sometimes the distinction is that the right to health care applies when one is sick and the right to health protection seeks to prevent the population from becoming sick.

A narrow definition of a right to basic and adequate health care has three advantages over a more inclusive right to health or right to health protection. First, it is difficult to determine the scope and limits of a right to health.[27] The World Health Organization (WHO) formulation that links the right to health with a definition of health as a "state of complete physical, mental and social well-being and not merely the absence of disease or infirmity"[28] has been seen as particularly problematic. This is because the WHO definition turns health into a norm virtually synonymous with human well-being. If the right to health is understood as a positive right, it implies that a government has the duty to promote complete physical, mental, and social well-being for its citizens, an impossible goal. Critics argue that these formulations mistakenly imply that good health is an end rather than a limited means to a fruitful and meaningful life.[29]

Second, the narrow definition of a right to health care is more relevant to public policy. While the Clinton administration has stated a commitment to ratification of all remaining international human rights instruments, including the International Covenant on Economic, Social and Cultural Rights with its recognition of a right to health, the issue of health rights has reentered the American political arena phrased in terms of a right to health care. Proponents of a human rights approach to health care reform are identifying their goal as a right to health care rather than as a right to health.

Third, a right to health care seems logical. Delineating the scope and limitations of the narrower right to basic health care seemed to be a helpful step before attempting to conceptualize the broader right to health, of which a right to health care is a component. Conversely, it did not seem possible to conceptualize a right to health without having a clearer delineation of the appropriate scope and limitations of a right to health care.

For all that, a narrow definition of a right to health care has significant limitations. Clearly there are regions of the world in which the most valuable steps toward improvement of health are not medical services but public health protection. Poor countries with limited resources would better improve health standards by investing scarce resources in clean water and environmental clean-up rather than by offering curative health care to a small fraction of the population. Moreover, even within an advanced industrialized country, health status will continue to deteriorate and health care costs will continue to escalate unless there is greater attention to promoting more favorable health conditions.

Accordingly, it is reasonable to conclude that a basic standard of health care cannot be achieved, even in a more affluent society, apart from a commitment to health protection. As a recent publication of the American Public Health Association (APHA) points out, improvements in the standard of health depend on preventing health problems before they arise. Investments in curative health care make little sense unless they are accompanied by policies that deal with the roots of public health problems. Moreover, the failure to do so contributes to the escalating cost of health care.

There are many examples of how the lack of a consistent commitment to health protection undermines health status and contributes to the escalating costs of curative health care. Federal crop subsidies for the cultivation of tobacco persist despite the fact that cigarettes are estimated to be responsible for a high incidence of lung cancer and 419,000 premature deaths in this country each year.[30] Despite estimates by the Environmental Protection Agency and the Centers for Disease Control that inhaling secondhand smoke causes 3,000 deaths from lung cancer, 150,000 to 300,000 cases of bronchitis and pneumonia in youngsters, and asthma attacks in more than twice that number,[31] there are not laws banning smoking in public buildings. The epidemic of violence claims a toll of 37,000 people shot and killed each year and hundreds of thousands wounded yet this country lacks effective gun control laws.[32] At least $140 billion of the $1 trillion Americans will spend on health care next year will be attributable to substance abuse and addiction, but the National Institutes of Health invest less than $8 million a year on research dealing with the causes, cures and prevention of substance abuse and addiction.[33] Although scientific evidence linking pesticides to breast cancer and other human health problems is growing, the Environmental Protection Agency has been reluctant to tighten control of pesticides used in food production.[34] Low birth weight infants require expensive neonatal care, and even with that care, often sustain lifelong neurological disabilities. Investments in family planning, nutrition education, and comprehensive prenatal care would significantly reduce the frequency of low weight births. Current government practices that disproportionately site municipal and hazardous waste disposal facilities in low-income and minority neighborhoods burden groups with the least access to quality health care with the greatest exposure to toxic substances.[35]

The American Public Health Association identifies five basic determinants of health: medical care access, a healthy environment, healthy neighborhoods, healthy behaviors, and community health service. Components of a health environment include clean air, safe drinking water, fluoridation of the water supply, and reducing avoidable workplace accidents. Healthy neighborhoods refer to places where young people can grow up well-educated and free from crime and drugs, where governments provide basic services for all of their constituents, and where families have resources to care for their children. Healthy behaviors mean lifestyles and conduct calculated to reduce or eliminate unnecessary risk to one's own health and that of others—proper eating habits, regular exercise, use of a seat belt, avoiding drugs, tobacco, and alcohol. Community health service incorporates basic health and sanitary programs.[36] In addition to these determinants, health status also reflects exposure to toxic substances. Healthy neighborhoods and work places require that toxic waste sites be cleaned up and exposure to asbestos, lead, and other toxics be significantly reduced or eliminated.

So where does that take us? Do broader concerns with the factors affecting health status and outcomes mandate dropping a right to health care in favor of a broader right to health protection or health? The American Public Health Association's list of health determinants suggests a reformulation of a right very similar to the International Covenant on Economic, Social and Cultural Rights, if not in terminology then at least in the obligations it imposes. The participants in the discussions that led to this volume have come to believe that a right to health care should be placed in the wider context of commitments to improve the public's health. A right to health care then becomes a component of a broader effort at improving public health. As important as securing the right to health care is, it can only be part of a larger strategy which acknowledges the dynamic relationship between health conditions and health status on the one hand and investments in public health as a meaningful and effective strategy to reduce the bill for health services.

A Basic and Adequate Standard of Care

To be meaningful and effectively implemented, the right to health care must be translated into specific obligations and commitments consistent with the resources of a society. This is a difficult and complex task. Many appeals to a right to health care are little more than rhetorical exercises. A right to health care can often imply quite different things, both with regard to the scope of what is being claimed and to the types of justification it requires.[37] Some critics of rights-based approaches therefore argue that the concept of individual rights in general and a right to health care in particular are overloaded to the point of meaninglessness.[38]

Moreover, most advocates of this approach have not specified either a methodology to set or the content of such an entitlement.

The few proposals that have become more concrete, such as the Oregon Plan, have engendered a great deal of controversy. Moreover, Americans tend to resist discussions of the topic of rationing health care. They seem reluctant both to acknowledge the prevalence of *de facto* rationing based on financial considerations or a proposed formula reflecting more equitable and rational criteria. Surveys suggest that Americans want universal access to affordable health care but resist the imposition of limits on the care they themselves can receive.[39]

More broadly, enumeration of a basic human right to health care in key international human rights instruments has not been paralleled by a conceptual development specifying the content of this right. In contrast with civil and political rights, international standards for economic, social, and cultural rights do not rest on foundations of extensive domestic jurisprudence. Moreover, there have not been effective international mechanisms to promote the intellectual development of these rights.[40] The United Nations body responsible for oversight of the International Covenant on Economic, Social and Cultural Rights, the Committee on Economic, Social and Cultural Rights, has not had either the resources commensurate with this task or the effective cooperation of states parties to this treaty. The United Nations Human Rights Centre, the secretariat body for all human rights activities of the United Nations, including the treaty monitoring bodies, did not convene an expert seminar on developing indicators for economic, social and cultural rights until January 1993, and the conclusions and recommendations of that seminar, for which this author served as rapporteur, stressed the need to clarify the content of specific rights and the nature of the parties's obligations in order to improve evaluation and monitoring of progressive realization.[41] Difficulties notwithstanding, a major goal of the project that produced this book has been to give concrete content to the idea of health care as a human right.

Operatively a basic and adequate standard of health care is the minimum level of care, the core entitlement, that should be guaranteed to all members of society. As conceptualized in this study, basic health care covers a wide range of common health services needed to maintain, restore, or provide functional equivalents (where possible) to adequate species functioning. It includes at least some preventive, curative, mental health, and rehabilitative personal medical services. Because basic health care includes preventive health services offered at predictable intervals, it goes beyond traditional notions of "insurance" for costly, unpredictable events.

The right to basic health care is society specific, defined in relationship to the level and type of resources available. In an affluent industrialized society, like our own, resources are sufficient to provide more than a minimal level of care. The basic standard of health care envisioned here is quite comprehensive. Nevertheless, in view of finite levels of resources, basic health care does not include all beneficial services. This means addressing the necessity of withholding beneficial health care in some instances or rationing.[42] Just as the legitimate scope of basic health services depends on resources available in a society, the types of limitations and the manner by which they are determined are also society-specific. At the very least it involves the identification and elimination of medically useless/non-cost effective procedures/treatments (something easier to agree on than to identify and implement). It is also likely to entail more stringent and controversial limitations on health care entitlements.

There are three different approaches to elucidating the notion of a basic standard of health care: (1) the articulation of general criteria by which to determine whether services are within the basic standard or beyond it; (2) the description of a fair procedure for determining the minimum; and (3) the simple listing of the types of services to be included.[43] Articles in this volume address the possibilities and problems with all three approaches.

Recognition of a right to a basic standard of health care or of a decent minimum requires a means to define the scope and limitations of this proposed entitlement on an ongoing basis. This is a very complex and difficult task. Tom Beauchamp and James Childress comment, for example, that

> Despite its attractions, the proposal of a decent minimum has proved difficult to explicate and to implement. It raises problems of whether society can fairly, consistently, and unambiguously structure a public policy that recognizes a right to care for primary needs without creating a right to exotic and expensive forms of treatment, such as liver transplants. More important, the model is purely programmatic unless one is able to define what "decent minimum" means in concrete operational terms. This task is, we believe, the major problem confronting health policy in the United States today.[44]

The task of defining a basic and adequate standard of health care is challenging for a variety of reasons. Such a standard varies from one society to another because of the availability of resources and the structure of the health care system. Priorities also differ across and within societies reflecting the distribution of health conditions and their impact on individuals. The claims of other social goals on society's resources are also likely to be evaluated differently over time and by population subgroups.

As James Nelson notes in his article in this volume, defining a basic and adequate standard of health care also involves reconciling or compromising three antagonistic moral values: fair access to health care, prudent husbandry of social resources or cost control, and excellence in health care. Moreover, to be able to do so requires both factual knowledge about the costs and outcomes of medical interventions and ethical insights into what it is that citizens in a just society owe one another, neither of which is available. Outcomes research is in its infancy, and theories of ethical knowledge do not offer definitive insights around which there is likely to be broad agreement. Given this situation, top-down determinations of the content of a basic package by policy makers do not seem either feasible or appropriate. The alternative is to use a bottom-up approach that elicits the input of those who will ultimately bear the cost, enjoy the benefits, and suffer the limitations of the basic package.[45]

The ability to use a bottom-up approach is complicated, however, by the contradictory views about health care reform that American people hold. Based on survey results, an overwhelming majority of Americans favor universal access and consider basic health care to be a fundamental right. Yet until now they have been reluctant to make the necessary societal financial commitment or to accept the personal trade-offs that a national health care system would entail. Moreover the public does not really understand why beneficial health care must be limited. In her article in this volume Mary Ann Baily characterizes current attitudes as follows: "They want universal access to health care at an affordable cost but without limits on the care they themselves receive. They give lip service to the desirability of a single-tier system with guaranteed access to quality care for everyone, yet are reluctant to vote the funds to pay for it."[46] Resolution of these contradictions is a prerequisite for moving ahead with health care reform.

Moreover, the definition of a basic standard of care or a "decent minimum" is an ongoing rather than a one time decision. Mary Ann Baily, for example, argues that the "decent minimum" should not be seen as a list of conditions and treatments to be developed once and for all and imposed on the health care system. Instead, defining adequacy requires an continuous process capable of defining a standard of care that evolves over time to incorporate changes in technology, preferences, and resources available.[47]

It is very difficult for both health care professionals and the public to address the topic of limiting beneficial health services. The notion of rationing contradicts the presumptions (although not the actuality) of the current model of health care on demand. As one health care analyst noted, "Few words in medicine evoke stronger emotions than rationing. Images are conjured up of children dying of liver disease while administrators give lectures on economic theories to grieving parents and angry reporters."[48] Health care professionals are not trained to be cost conscious. Indeed in this country many physicians believe it is unethical to consider cost in their clinical decisions.[49] Moreover, in a market-oriented health care system based on a fee for service arrangement, there is a bias in the other direction. This is further exacerbated by entrepreneurial arrangements whereby many practitioners hold limited partnerships in for-profit diagnostic-laboratory facilities, for-profit ambulatory surgery facilities, and shares in free-standing imaging units where they refer their own patients.[50]

That there is extensive *de facto* rationing in our health care system is an incontrovertible but conveniently ignored reality. It is not rationing by a central authority with regulatory ceilings on the prices of health care goods and services or global expenditure limits, as in some national health care systems, but instead rationing by income, insurance coverage, geographic location, and in some instances by disease. Allowing market forces to determine access to health care somehow has seemed consistent with basic economic philosophy and therefore has absolved any particular person from assuming responsibility for the results.[51] Implicit or covert rationing is apparently considered acceptable, but explicit rationing has been quite another matter.

Reactions to the Oregon health care experiment are indicative of this denial. The public outcry suggests that cruder but covert *de facto* rationing through decreasing the number of individuals eligible for Medicaid services is more acceptable, at least to people outside of Oregon, than an arrangement that trades some limits on beneficial services in order to provide universal coverage. The Oregon Basic Health Services Act was passed by the Oregon legislature in 1989 in response to the fact that eighteen percent of the Oregon population, some 400,000 people, were without health insurance. The package of legislation approached coverage of the uninsured from three avenues. One bill required employers to provide insurance to uninsured employees either directly or through a state-run pool. A second piece of legislation assured coverage for individuals with pre-existing conditions who are often denied commercial coverage. A third dimension of the program increased eligibility for Medicaid coverage to 100 percent of the federal poverty level from sixty seven percent by limiting the number of health services the state would provide. To determine what health services would be covered, the Oregon Health Services Commission was given a mandate to develop "a list of health services ranked by priority from the most important to the least important, representing the comparative benefits of each service to the entire population to be served." The methodology employed is described in Michael Garland's article in this section.[52]

While there have been a variety of criticisms of the Oregon Plan, four have been most frequent. First, many people argue that there are alternatives to rationing, and that such alternatives, particularly the elimination of administrative waste and nonbeneficial services, should precede any initiatives to limit access to services. Second, there are claims that the prioritization process and the resultant list are flawed methodologically. Third, it is considered unfair to single out the Medicaid population, which is composed of particularly vulnerable groups like poor women and children, to bear the brunt of rationing.[53] Fourth, the ground on which the Medicaid waiver, which was required from the federal government, was initially denied was that the Oregon Plan methodology discriminated against persons with disabilities.

In other industrialized countries, when national health care systems were established, there was not explicit debate on what *not* to provide. Instead, universal access was introduced together with financial structures that incorporated a variety of methods to restrain utilization and reduce costs. In the Canadian system, for example, where ostensibly all "medically necessary" care is provided, there are waiting times for certain types of services. There are also constraints on the diffusion of medical technology.[54]

Although many of these cost-controlling measures may be very difficult to implement in a population used to health care services on demand, it is necessary to do so. Regulating the introduction of high technology innovations and the use of expensive technology is one potential area of cost savings. Another is to limit tertiary care services covered in the basic package, such as excluding cosmetic surgery, experimental techniques, many transplants, and some expensive diagnostic procedures. There also needs to be open debate and public consensus leading to reduction or elimination of futile care. Futile care includes that which prolongs biological processes in unconscious or nonsentient patients, imposes treatment on patients who prefer a nonmedicalized death with dignity, or invests in treatment procedures unlikely to improve the quality of life or comfort of terminally ill patients.

By linking limits to an entitlement, a rights based approach to health care reform may offer a framework through which to seek a national consensus on a cost-conscious standard of medical care that can be provided to all Americans. The political system would provide the security of an entitlement to basic health care that does not depend on financial or employment status and that cannot be lost because of health disabilities or loss of a job. In exchange, individuals would accept limits on the scope of the health care benefits that would be publicly provided. The principle underlying this arrangement would be that persons not demand a standard of care for themselves that would not also be available to all other members of society and affordable within the specific, agreed upon budgetary levels.

Efforts to incorporate a cost-conscious standard of health care through a human rights approach would be more palatable than rationing has hitherto been for three reasons: (1) it would be a component of an explicit reformulation of a new social covenant in which there is a trade-off between benefits and limits; (2) it would be accompanied by initiatives to make the entire structure of the health care system more equitable and affordable through a new paradigm of health care emphasizing preventive and primary health care services, both of which would be fully covered, and (3) the basic health package would be based on a comprehensive and uniform standard determined through meaningful public input.

Once a comprehensive and uniform standard is defined, monitoring the implementation of a right to health care and using these data to revise public policies is also an important obligation of governments. Because a human rights approach requires ongoing citizen involvement, public interest groups should also evaluate the impact of health care reforms. Effective monitoring has at least three requirements: (1) the development of appropriate standards and indicators through which to assess the achievement of the right to basic health care; (2) the use of a database that permits disaggregation into appropriate categories, particularly one that facilitates the assessment of the health status of minorities and disadvantaged groups; and (3) ongoing and regular data collection so as to have time series data. Some of this monitoring could be accomplished through national health care surveys. It would also require the design of special research projects, particularly to monitor the status of the homeless, migrant workers, and some ethnic minorities. Tom Jabine's article in this volume provides a way to measure the realization of a right to health care.

American Realities

Although Americans typically frame claims in the language of rights, the United States is the only major democracy that fails to recognize a universal entitlement to health care. Why? That there is no mention in the Constitution or the Bill of Rights is not surprising. Modern concepts of human rights, particularly of economic and social rights, emerged in response to World War II, particularly the Holocaust. Moreover, until the development of modern medicine and public health measures in the late nineteenth and early twentieth centuries, there was little that governments could do to improve health or health outcomes.

American political culture is built upon a rather narrow conception of rights which has affected both ideological alignments and public policy debates. Ian Shapiro argues that there is a distinctive way of conceiving individual rights that has been central to the Anglo-American tradition of political theory since the mid-seventeenth century.[55] The Anglo-American liberal tradition can be characterized as follows: (1) rights are predicated on a highly individualistic and atomistic view of human nature; (2) rights are conceptualized as negative in character, as fences or barriers protecting the individual from intrusions; (3) freedom is considered to be the most important goal or social good; and (4) the primary (or sole) role of government is to protect the liberty of the individual.

This liberal tradition, particularly its libertarian stream, has been inimical to the recognition of a right to health care understood as an entitlement that requires positive public action. Many libertarian theorists interpret the provision of such an entitlement through public financing as amounting to an unwarranted seizure of private property and/or an intrusion on a property owner's freedom to dispose of his own goods. Given this ideological framework, it is not surprising that ethicists dealing with rights issues have focused primarily on "rights in" rather than "rights to" medical care. Issues related to the individual, both the rights of the patient and the prerogatives/responsibilities of the health care provider, have been at the center of bioethics. Questions of distributive justice in the allocation of resources or access to health care have received less attention.

The consequences of such liberal commitments are not hard to detect. Whereas other societies tend to consider health care to be a social or public good, in this country health care has usually been treated more as a private good or a commodity.[56] Beginning at the end of the nineteenth century with reforms in Germany, other western countries developed a consensus that health care is a social good that should be collectively financed and available to all citizens on the basis of need, regardless of the individual recipient's ability to pay for that care. In the period following World War II, these countries translated this consensus into the recognition of a right to health care. In contrast, health care in the United States has usually been considered to be a private consumption good, whose financing is the responsibility of the individual. The application of market principles to health care enabled individual practitioners and health oriented corporations to treat health care as a for-profit commodity.

While professional ethics emphasize that physicians' responsibility to their patients takes precedence over their own economic interests, most physicians in the United States have functioned much like business owners. Until recently virtually all doctors practiced almost exclusively as solo or small group practitioners on a fee-for-service basis. Initially patients paid doctors' fees directly. More recently private insurance, financed either by employers or by individuals retrospectively, have reimbursed provider-set charges or costs under the assumption that physicians are acting in the best interests of patients. Potential conflict of interest was minimized because economic pressures were relatively weak and the tradition of professionalism strong.

In the past two decades, however, health care has become increasingly commercialized and a "medical-industrial complex" developed. The expansion of health care has engendered a great increase in specialization and technological sophistication, raising the price of services and providing greater economic rewards for the practice of medicine. With insurance available to pay bills, physicians have powerful economic incentives to prescribe a multitude of tests and procedures to earn extra income. Generous fee-for-service reimbursement and the lack of government regulation have encouraged ever more utilization of services, without built-in controls or government regulation to limit prices or dictate utilization patterns.[57]

Groups benefiting from the expansion and commercialization of the health sector in the United States have had strong incentives to resist government regulation and structural changes. Physicians' incomes have been substantially higher in the United States than elsewhere, making doctors one of the highest income groups in society. According to data compiled by the American Medical Association, the average net income among all doctors was $171,000 in 1991. Other data sources have shown that some specialists earn substantially more. Cardiac surgeons, for example, made an average of $575,000 in 1992, and neurosurgeons an average of $449,000.[58] Attracted by opportunities for profit from the expansion of private and public health insurance, new investor-owned for-profit health care businesses have emerged, including chains of hospitals, clinics, nursing homes, and diagnostic hospitals, and a growing number of doctors have become limited partners in such enterprises. As health care has become big business, health related corporations, including pharmaceutical companies, instrument and device manufacturers, health maintenance corporations, and insurance companies have also tended to earn consistently high profits. The pharmaceutical industry, for example, is the nation's most lucrative legal industry with profit margins that routinely average at least three times those of other Fortune 500 companies.[59] Major actors in this profit-driven "medical-industrial complex" have opposed public financing of health care and related reforms that would regulate and potentially reduce their incomes and profits.[60]

Moreover, the juxtaposition of a market ideology with the American tradition of individualistic and negative rights has enabled actors in the health care industry to appropriate the language of rights for their private benefit: many physicians assume that they have the "right" to practice free of government regulation and interference; companies typically claim that they have the "right" to sell their products and secure high rates of profit. Affluent individuals and groups who either have comprehensive health care benefits or can afford to pay for their care also argue that they have the "right" to all the health care services they desire on demand.

Conversely, the absence of lobbies representing public interests and needs has meant that the right of citizens to affordable and appropriate health care has not been sufficiently voiced in policy debates.

The failure to treat health care as a social good rather than as a commodity or a private consumption good has discouraged the formation of citizens lobbies or other groups representing the public interest. Professional medical associations whose mandate is broader and less self-interested than the American Medical Association, like the American Public Health Association, have not played an active role in attempting to influence policy formation. Even though national health insurance is not equivalent to the establishment of a government owned and operated health care system, the American Medical Association has associated such a system with socialized medicine.

For these reasons, previous legislation did not recognize a right to health care. One of the first public programs enacted was the Emergency Maternal and Infant Care Act in 1943 to ensure that the spouses and children of low-ranking servicemen would be able to receive health care. In 1948, the Hospital Survey and Construction Act furnished federal funds to build hospitals in underserved communities, with the requirement that hospitals built with these funds had to offer a certain amount of charity care. In 1956, Congress extended federal health care benefits to dependents of military servicemen and women through the Civilian Health and Medical Program of the Uniformed Services.[61] The Indian Health Service, a distinct federally funded health care service, was created in 1955 on the basis of federal treaty obligations.[62]

These programs paved the way for the enactment of Medicare and Medicaid, the two most comprehensive medical services entitlements. In 1965, the Social Security Act was amended to create Medicare as a federal health insurance program with a uniform eligibility and benefit package for those over sixty five years old. In 1972, coverage was extended to people with chronic renal disease and to the disabled under sixty five years old who had received disability benefits for two or more years. Although Medicare is often considered an entitlement to comprehensive health care for all persons over sixty five years old, the Part A entitlement portion only covers acute hospital costs. Physician and other outpatient services are supplied only if a premium is paid for Part B. This approach, and the inclusion of life-saving dialysis and kidney transplants into the program, provides Medicare with an acute care focus.

The 1965 amendment of the Social Security Act that created Medicare also established Medicaid, but the latter was more a consolidation and expansion of federally financed state programs for certain broad "categories" of needy recipients than a uniform or comprehensive entitlement. Medicaid, while limited in its coverage, provides a more comprehensive array of benefits than Medicare, including early periodic screening and treatment services for children and long-term care services for persons who are functionally impaired. Eligibility criteria and benefits vary among the states and even within a particular state over time.[63] Low reimbursement rates limit access to health care by discouraging participation by health care providers. Moreover, Medicaid has been more vulnerable to budget cuts and an erosion in coverage than Medicare. To contain Medicare costs, states have made eligibility requirements increasingly stringent: in 1989, thirty two states have set the maximum income level for public assistance eligibility at less than fifty percent of the federal poverty level standard.[64]

Court decisions have recognized a limited right to life-saving treatment. Hospitals are legally obligated to provide care to the underserved if the condition is life-threatening. Anti-dumping laws have also been enacted in response to egregious cases of hospitals denying care in emergency situations. The rulings and legislation, however, stem primarily from a sense that there is an obligation to act when an individual's life is at stake and not from a recognition of a right to health care. Moreover, this recognition of a limited right to emergency care, combined with a failure to provide access to preventive and primary care, has led to higher overall costs for the health system. Persons who are denied appropriate and cost-conscious treatment are then admitted to more expensive emergency room facilities when their health status has deteriorated sufficiently to make them eligible for emergency treatment.[65]

While the United States has gradually legislated a substantial role for the government in financing health care, particularly during the mid 1960s, it has done so with little clarity about the underlying rationale. Debates over extending entitlements have usually focused on the needs of specific groups, avoiding broader ethical issues about government responsibility in the health care sector. Policies and programs that provide a legal right to limited health care services through public programs were enacted from a recognition that society in general and hospitals in particular have a responsibility to provide health care for certain categories of vulnerable persons and to all individuals in particular emergency circumstances.[66] Advocates have been reluctant to employ rights language or to try to generalize these obligations. This has impoverished political debate and left a legacy of uncertainty about the grounds for the government's role in the financing of health services.[67]

The Prospects for Health Care Reform

The United States has not lacked proposals for fundamental health care reform. Social reformers inspired by the compulsory system of health insurance instituted by Germany in 1883 sought to create social financing for medical care in this country through a national health insurance or state level plans. While organized medicine was at first receptive, by 1920 the American Medical Association took a position against any form of compulsory insurance. The AMA's opposition, in combination with the waning of Progressive influence and anti-German sentiment from the war, undermined these initial efforts to introduce national health insurance.[68]

As in many other industrial democracies, the issue of national health insurance reemerged in the United States in the years following World War II. In 1948, President Harry S. Truman introduced proposals for national insurance. A United States President's Commission on the Health Needs of the Nation reporting in 1953 concluded that "access to the means for the attainment and preservation of health is a basic human right."[69] Despite the example of Great Britain's National Health Service, started in 1948, political opposition undermined these proposals for national health insurance. The Truman administration cut back the proposals to limit assistance to the elderly, but after extensive legislative consideration, the plan was not enacted. Moreover, the impetus for health care reform declined because during the 1950s a combination of private action and tax subsidy brought private health coverage to much of the middle class.[70]

While health care reform was not a policy priority of President Dwight Eisenhower, the decade of the 1960s began with John F. Kennedy's "New Frontier," one provision of which was federal medical coverage, at least for the elderly. As with earlier reform initiatives, strong opposition came from medical interest groups, spearheaded by the AMA, and from conservatives. Opponents argued that an expanded federal role would allow federal bureaucrats to control clinical decisions in medicine and labeled reform initiatives as constituting "socialized medicine," contrary to the American tradition. This opposition prevented enactment of system-wide changes and delayed expansion of coverage to the elderly until after President Lyndon

Johnson's landslide victory in 1964. In 1965 amendment of the Social Security Act created Medicare to provide conventional third-party coverage for those past retirement age and the disabled. Almost as an after thought, a state-federal Medicaid program was also established to cover basically the poor. Under Medicaid, the federal government reimbursed state spending on a sliding scale from fifty percent to eighty three percent, with more aid going to the poorer states. However, to contain costs few states have opted for the maximum available coverage, and most states have set the maximum income level for eligibility at less than fifty percent of the federal poverty standard.[71]

In the early 1970s, the cost of medical care renewed discussions of national health insurance for all. In 1971, President Richard M. Nixon, who two years earlier had diagnosed the health system as in "massive crisis," submitted a legislative proposal. Senator Edward Kennedy, ever the proponent of reform, introduced two bills, and Representative Wilbur Mills also offered plans for universal coverage. Although a compromise national plan, based on mandatory private coverage supported by federal gap-filling, came close to enactment, it was ultimately a victim of the political aftermath of Watergate and Chappaquiddick and the opposition of providers and insurers. During 1976, Jimmy Carter campaigned on a promise of national health insurance, but once in office he decided that hospital costs had to be controlled before universal coverage would be affordable. President Carter twice requested Congress to enact national hospital cost controls, but strong industry resistance undermined these proposals.[72]

In 1980, a President's Commission for the Study of Ethical Problems in Medicine and Biomedical Research was given a mandate by Congress to study the "ethical and legal implications of differences in the availability of health services as determined by the income or residence of the person receiving the service."[73] Perhaps the most influential public study and report on access that focused on ethical issues, *Securing Access to Health Care for All*, concludes that (1) society has an ethical obligation to ensure equitable access to health care for all; (2) individuals have an obligation to pay a fair share of the cost of their own care; (3) equitable access to health care requires that citizens be able to secure an adequate level of care without excessive burdens; (4) when private forces produce equitable access there is no need for government involvement, though ultimate responsibility for ensuring that society's obligation is met, through a combination of public and private sector arrangements, rests with the federal government; and (5) the goal of cost containment should not focus on limiting the attainment of equitable access for those least well-served by the current arrangements.[74]

An important feature of *Securing Access to Health Care for All* is that the Commission explicitly chose not to frame its conclusions in terms of the human rights of individuals to health care. Although the initial draft of the ethics chapter of the access report included an endorsement of a right to health care, the final version of the report shifted to the formulation of a societal obligation. As Dan Brock's article in this volume explains, political factors, and not the philosophical rationale given in the report, apparently determined the Commissioner's position on the right to health care. Brock, the staff philosopher at the Commission for the first year of its work, attributes their position first and foremost to the conservative political climate of the early years of the Reagan administration when the Commission was finalizing its report. Although the Commissioners were initially appointed by President Carter, Reagan appointees, who shared his conservative political ideology, were a clear majority when the Commission was shaping its conclusions and recommendations. Recognition of a right would have entailed recommendations for major and costly new social programs, something very difficult to support in an administration committed to reducing the federal government's role and budget.[75] The conservative ideological tilt during the Reagan and Bush administrations blocked implementation of the Commission's recommendations and instead placed an emphasis on the more thorough application of market principles to the health care sector.

Recently the language of rights has reemerged in the American health care reform debate, albeit in a very muted tone. President George Bush spoke about a right to health care in his 1991 State of the Union Address, and the 1992 Democratic platform had a provision advocating a right to health care. In January 1993, Rep.Ed Pastor (D-Ariz.) introduced a non-binding concurrent resolution stating that it is the sense of Congress that "access to health care services is a fundamental human right" and that all legislative proposals by the President and Congress concerning national health care reform should be based upon recognition of this fundamental right.[76]

Like the 1983 President's Commission, the Health Security Plan developed by President Bill Clinton's Task Force on Health Reform refrains from using a rights formulation. The American Health Security Act proposes to guarantee comprehensive health coverage for all

Americans regardless of health, employment status, or geographic location. Stated ethical foundations echo many of the refrains of rights language. The values and principles it cites include universal access, comprehensive benefits, quality of care, fair distribution of costs, and personal responsibility.[77] The failure to propose recognition of an explicit right to health care appears to have resulted from the reluctance to provide a legal entitlement, as well as political decisions to avoid controversy and reach out to the broadest potential political constituency.

Will the Clinton administration finally achieve the elusive goal of universal health care? There is currently broader support for health care reform than at any other point in American history. Rather than resisting change, medical professionals are advocating comprehensive reforms to achieve universal coverage. Editorials, articles, and even special issues of the *Journal of the American Medical Association* (JAMA) regularly address health care reform issues. In a May 1993 editorial, George Lundberg, the editor, stated that it would be "immoral and very costly to the economy" if President Clinton's health care reform plan did not include rapid coverage of the nation's uninsured. It goes on that "we should bite the bullet right away and not delay universal coverage."[78] The American College of Physicians, which is a professional society for physicians specializing in internal medicine and is second only to the American Medical Association in membership, has been even more forthright in supporting health care reform. A position paper approved by their Board of Regents in February 1990 states that "A nationwide program is needed to assure access to health care for all Americans, and we recommend that such a program be adopted as a policy goal for the nation. The College believes that health insurance coverage for all persons is needed to minimize financial barriers and assure access to appropriate health care services."[79]

Yet this consensus may not create a willingness to make fundamental tradeoffs, to sacrifice self-interest for the sake of the wider community, or to accept fundamental changes in the delivery of health care. Opinion polls suggest that the American people want the security and entitlement of a right to health care but are not willing to make any sacrifices in the form of higher taxes, reduced choices, or changes in coverage. Medical Political Action Committees representing physicians, dentists, hospital associations, pharmaceutical corporations, and the insurance industry, are increasing in number, influence, and giving to politicians so as to have a major role in the shaping of health care reform. To maintain influence, the health care industry is estimated to have donated $8.4 million to members of Congress during the first ten months of 1993, an increase of twenty seven percent over the previous year.[80] Moreover, a study by Citizen Action shows that members of the Senate Finance Committee averaged nearly $393,000 each in donations by the health and insurance industry from 1987 through 1993, compared with $232,553, on average for other Senators.[81] Many of these interest groups have also begun media advertising campaigns reminiscent of presidential races. Furthermore, the proliferation of proposals being put forward, by fragmenting support, does not improve prospects for consensus.

Against these intrigues of narrow interests, policymakers may yet find the courage to realize a strong right to health care for Americans. It may well turn out that a right to health care will emerge only over time as a result of a series of incremental measures designed to improve our health care system. If so, the conception of a health care right elucidated in this book provides a way to measure and judge ongoing reforms. Whether genuine changes comes now or later, the moral force of a right to health care should sustain continuing efforts to provide equitable health care for all for only then will our nation have achieved true health care reform.

NOTES

   1. Robert Pear, "Health-Care Costs Up Sharply Again, Posing New Threat," *The New York Times*, January 5, 1993, p. A1.

   2. Randall R. Bovbjerg, Charles C. Griffin, Caitline E. Carroll, "U.S. Health Care Coverage and Costs: Historical Development and Choices for the 1990s," *The Journal of Law, Medicine & Ethics* 212 (Summer 1993): 141, 155–156.

   3. Robert Pear, "Fewer Now Have Health Insurance", *The New York Times*, December 15, 1993, p. A24.

   4. Guy Gugliotta, "Number of Poor Americans Rises for 3rd Year," *The Washington Post*, October 5, 1993, p. A6.

   5. R. Burciaga Valdez, Hal Morgenstern, Richard Brown, Robert Wyn, Chao Wang, and William Cumberland, "Insuring Latinos Against the Costs of Illness," *Journal of the American Medical Association* 269 (February 17, 1993): 889.

   6. Michael Millman, ed., *Access to Health Care in America* (Washington, D.C.: National Academy Press, 1993), p. 3.

7. American Public Health Association, *America's Public Health Report Card: A State-by-State Report on the Health of the Public* (Washington, D.C.: American Public Health Association, 1992).

8. "Medical Bills Are Top Concern of Nation's Poor, Report Says," *The New York Times*, January 4, 1993, p. 13.

9. Rovbjerg, Griffin, and Carroll, p. 154.

10. See Janet O'Keefe's contribution to this volume.

11. American Public Health Association, p. 2

12. *Ibid.*, p. 1.

13. Generalist physicians make up 50% to 70% of the medical cadres in other developed countries but only 30% in the United States. Dr. Steven Schroeder, the President of the Robert Wood Johnson Foundation, estimates that anywhere from 20% to 50% of the commonly performed specialty procedures in this United States could be avoided without harming the health of the public. See Steven A Schroeder, "Medicine's Glut of 'Fighter Pilots,' " *Los Angeles Times*, March 4, 1992.

14. The characterization of rights here makes use of three sources: James W. Nickel, *Making Sense of Human Rights: Philosophical Reflections on the Universal Declaration of Human Rights* (Berkeley: University of California Press, 1987); Tom L. Beauchamp and Ruth R. Faden, "The Right to Health and the Right to Health Care," *The Journal of Medicine and Philosophy* 4, 2 (1979), pp. 118–131; and Caroline Whitbeck, "Moral Rights and Obligations: Self Instructional Units on Ethical Concepts," (Massachusetts institute of Technology, Unpublished, February 1993).

15. Universal Declaration of Human Rights, in *The International Bill of Human Rights* (New York: United Nations, 1985), p. 4.

16. On this point see Nickel, p. 4. While the U.S. government initially endorsed the broad conception of human rights contained in the United Nations Universal Declaration of Human Rights, U.S. support for economic, social, and cultural rights became a casualty of the Cold War. Eleanor Roosevelt chaired the committee which drafted the Universal Declaration, and the U.S. delegation voted in favor of this international bill of rights in the General Assembly on December 10, 1948. As Cold War hostilities increased, however, the U.S. government began to identify the rights to economic and social benefits such as social security, an adequate standard of living, and education, enumerated in articles 22 through 27 of the Universal Declaration, with socialism, and the more traditional civil and political rights as a product of capitalist democracy. Viewing all international treaties with suspicion as an unacceptable infringement on U.S. sovereignty, the Senate was reluctant to provide its advice and consent for international human rights instruments during the Cold War. Although President Jimmy Carter signed four of these treaties including the International Covenant on Economic, Social and Cultural Rights, they were not ratified by the Senate. Under the Reagan administration human rights were explicitly defined for purposes of U.S. foreign policy as individual political rights and civil liberties and economic, social and cultural rights were described as goals, and not valid rights. See Philip Alston, "U.S. Ratification of the Covenant on Economic, Social and Cultural Rights: The Need for an

Entirely New Strategy," *American Journal of International Law*, 84 (April 1990): 365–393. With the end of the Cold War, the Senate has given its advice and consent to the International Covenant on Civil and Political Rights and the Clinton administration has indicated its intention of ratifying all major international human rights instruments. It is also willing to acknowledge certain economic, social, and cultural rights, even though they are not accorded the same status as political and civil rights under U.S. domestic law, including the right to work, social security, health care, and education. See Nancy Ely-Raphael, Deputy Assistant Secretary of State, "Democracy and Human Rights in a Clinton Foreign Policy," Speech to the World Conference NGO Briefing, American Academy for the Advancement of Science Headquarters, Washington, D.C., September 23, 1993, p. 9.

17. The author's views have been enriched by Larry R. Churchill's *Rationing Health Care in America: Perceptions and Principles of Justice* (Notre Dame, Indiana: University of Notre Dame Press, 1987) and Annette C. Baier's paper, "Claims, Rights, Responsibilities," to appear in *Prospects for a Common Morality*, J.P. Reeder and Gene Outka, eds. (Princeton: Princeton University Press, forthcoming) and a collection of her essays titled *Passions of the Mind*, forthcoming from Harvard University Press.

18. Mary Ann Baily's comments on an earlier draft were helpful in clarifying that the role of the community is in recognizing and giving practical form and content to the right rather than in creating rights.

19. On this point see National Conference of Catholic Bishops, *Economic Justice for All* (Washington, D.C.: United States Catholic Conference, 1986), p. ix.

20. This borrows from and adapts Michael Freeden's definition. According to Freeden, "a human right is a conceptual device expressed in linguistic form, that assigns priority to certain human or social attributes regarded as essential to the adequate functioning of a human being that is intended to serve as a protective capsule for those attributes and then appeals for deliberate action to ensure such protection." See his *Rights* (Minneapolis: University of Minnesota Press, 1991), p. 7.

21. See Jack Donnelly's article in this volume.

22. The concept of "standard threats" is from Henry Shue, *Basic Rights: Subsistence, Affluence, and U.S. Foreign Policy* (Princeton: Princeton University Press, 1980), pp. 29–34.

23. Churchill, p. 94.

24. International Covenant on Economic, Social and Cultural Rights, G.A. Res. 2200A, U.N. GAOR, 21st Sess., Supp. No. 16, At Art. 25, U.N. Doc. A/6316.

25. *Idem.*

26. A constitutional right to health or to health protection is rarely an individual, immediately enforceable right. It is more likely to be a programmatic or policy right that articulates goals. See for example, Hernan Fuenzalida-Puelma and Susan Scholle Connor, eds., *The Right to Health in the Americas: A Comparative Constitutional Study*, (Washington, D.C.: Pan American Health Organization, 1989), p. 608.

27. For critiques of the right to health see Daniel Callahan, *What Kind of Life* (New York, Touchstone Books, 1990), pp. 34–40 and Joseph M. Boyle, Jr., "The Concept of Health and the Right to Health Care," *Social Thought* 3 (Summer 1977), pp. 5–17.

28. World Health Organization, "Preamble to the Constitution," in *The First Ten Years of the World Health Organization* (Geneva: World Health Organization, 1958), p. II.

29. On this point, see the discussion in Callahan, pp. 36–40.

30. "Substance Abuse is Blamed for 500,000 Deaths," *The New York Times*, October 24, 1993, p. 20.

31. "Snuffing Out Secondhand Smoke," *The New York Times*, November 7, 1993, p. E14.

32. Jane Gross, "Joining War Over Guns, New Voices: Physicians," *The New York Times*, November 16, 1993, p. 18.

33. Joseph A. Califano, Jr., "America in Denial," *The Washington Post*, November 14, 1993, p. C7.

34. Gary Lee, "Studies Give Pesticides Role in Breast Cancer," *The Washington Post*, October 22, 1993, p. A20.

35. Robert D. Bullard, "Race and Environmental Justice in the United States," *The Yale Journal of International Law*, 18(Winter 1993) 319–336.

36. *Ibid.*, 3–4.

37. On this point, see Normal Daniels, *Just Health Care* (Cambridge and New York, Cambridge University Press, 1985), p. 8.

38. Daniel Callahan, *What Kind of Life: A Challenging Exploration of the Goals of Medicine* (New York, Touchstone Books, 1990), p. 56.

39. See for example, Mary Ann Baily, "Defining the Decent Minimum," paper prepared for the AAAS Right to Health Care Project.

40. On these points, see Philip Alston, "The Committee on Economic, Social and Cultural Rights," in Philip Alston, ed., *The United Nations and Human Rights: A Critical Appraisal* (Oxford, Clarendon Press, 1992), pp. 490–91.

41. *Report of the Seminar on Appropriate Indicators to Measure Achievements in the Progressive Realization of Economic, Social and Cultural Rights*, Geneva, 25–29 January, A/CONF.157/PC/73/20 April 1993.

42. This definition is taken from Kenneth F. Schaffner, M.D., "Health Care Rationing: Major Forms and Alternatives," Unpublished paper, March 1991.

43. Norman Daniels, *Just Health Care* (Cambridge: Cambridge University Press, 1985), p. 73.

44. Tom Beauchamp and James Childress, *Principles of Biomedical Ethics*, Third Edition (New York: Oxford University Press, 1989).

45. See James Nelson's contribution to this volume.

46. See Mary Ann Baily's contribution to this volume.

47. *Ibid.*

48. David Eddy, M.D., "Rationing by Patient Choice," *Journal of the American Medical Association*, 265 (January 2, 1991) 105.

49. Mary Ann Baily, "Rationing Medical Care: Processes for Defining Adequacy," J. Agich and C.E. Begley, eds. *The Price of Health* (Dordrecht: Reidel Publishing Company, 1986), p. 165.

50. For a discussion of the economic and ethical implications of such arrangements, see Arnold S. Relman, M.D., "Shattuck Lecture—The Health Care Industry: Where Is It Taking Us," *The New England Journal of Medicine*, 325 (September 19, 1991) 854–859.

51. On this point see Churchill.

52. See Michael Garland's contribution to this volume.

53. On these points see, for example, Martin A. Strosberg, "Introduction," in *America's Medical Care: The Oregon Plan and Beyond*, Martin A. Strosberg, Joshua M. Wiener, Robert Baker and I. Alan Fein, eds., (Washington, D.C.: The Brookings Institution, 1993), pp. 5–10.

54. Schaffner.

55. Ian Shapiro, *The Evolution of Rights in Liberal Theory* (Cambridge: Cambridge University Press, 1986).

56. Uwe E. Reinhardt, "Reforming the Health Care System: The Universal Dilemma, *American Journal of Law & Medicine*, XIX, 1&2 (1993), p. 47.

57. Arnold S. Relman, "What Market Values Are Doing to Medicine," *National Forum* LXXIII (Summer 1993): 117–21.

58. Erik Eckholm, "Health Plan Is Toughest on Doctors Making Most," *The New York Times*, November 7, 1993, pp. 1, 26.

59. Art Levine and Ken Silverstein, "How the Drug Lobby Cut Cost Control" *The Nation*, December 13, 1993, p. 730.

60. On these developments, see Arnold S. Relman, M.D., "The Shattuck Lecture — The Health Care Industry: Where Is It Taking Us," *The New England Journal of Medicine*, 325 (September 19, 1991), pp. 854–859.

61. See Janet O'Keefe's contribution to this volume.

62. Timothy Taylor, "The Needs of Native Americans," presentation at the AAAS Right to Health Care Consultation, November 13, 1992.

63. Securing Access, pp. 146–154.

64. *Including the Poor*, Health Policy Agenda for the American People: The Final Report of the Ad Hoc Committee on Medicaid, February 1989. Cited in Bioethics Consultation Group, "Health Care Crisis in America Fact Sheet," Minneapolis, October 1989.

65. O'Keeffe.

66. O'Keeffe.

67. Theodore R. Marmor, "History and Politics of Health Care," In Thomas J. Bole III and William B. Bondeson, eds., *Rights to Health Care* (Dordrecht: Kluwer Academic Publishers, 1991), pp. 26–27.

68. Bovbjerg, Griffin, and Carroll, p. 142.

69. President's Commission on the Health Needs of the Nation (Washington, D.C.: U.S. Government Printing Office, 1953), p. 3.

70. By 1960, over two-thirds of Americans had private coverage, but more than half of personal health spending still came from patients' own resources. *Ibid.*, 146.

71. Bovbjerg, Griffin, and Carroll, p. 148.

72. *Ibid.*, p. 152; Marmor, pp. 32–33.

73. Securing Access, p. 6.

74. Securing Access, pp. 3–5.

75.   See Dan W. Brock's contribution to this volume.

76.   House Concurrent Resolution No. 56, 103rd Cong., 1st Session.

77.   The White House Domestic Policy Council, *The President's Health Security Plan: The Clinton Blueprint* (New York: Times Books, 1993), pp. 11–12.

78.   George S. Lundberg, "American Health Care System Management Objectives: The Aura of Inevitability Becomes Incarnate," *Journal of the American Medical Association*, 269 (May 19, 1993) 2554.

79.   American College of Physicians, "Access to Health Care," *Annals of Internal Medicine* 112 (May 1990) 643.

80.   Neil A. Lewis, "Medical Industry Showers Congress with Heavy Money", *The New York Times*, December 13, 1993, p. A1.

81.   Charles R. Babcock, "Health Interests and Lawmakers", *The Washington Post*, December 30, 1993, p. A21.

PART ONE

The Framework for Health Care Reform

Janet O'Keeffe

The Right to Health Care and Health Care Reform

There is broad agreement that our current health care system is simultaneously expensive, inequitable, and wasteful, and that escalating health care costs and the erosion of private insurance coverage are seriously undermining the health and economic security of all Americans. There is also agreement that, as a society, we can provide affordable health care to all our citizens—as all other Western industrialized democracies do—and many believe that this fact alone supports the moral argument that we ought to do so. This volume focuses on the importance of establishing a right to health care as a necessary step in assuring universal access.

The language of rights is useful in highlighting the inequities and inadequacies of our current system, and in organizing public support for reform in general. It is also useful in helping to define the broad parameters of a system that can assure a right to health care. However, in determining the myriad details in the design of this system, it may not prove useful as an operational guide, for it raises as many questions as it answers. How much health care? What quality health care? What is the responsibility of individuals for their own health?[1] Just as importantly, it is unlikely that the language of rights will be helpful in reaching consensus among the many players in the health care reform debate, consensus that is essential if comprehensive reform is to be enacted. This is seen clearly in a telling exchange between two physicians at a discussion on health care during a meeting of a physician's association in the 1970's. While one physician stated that every person in the country had an "inalienable right to the very best in health care", the response from another was, "they may have that right, but they don't necessarily have the right to get it from me."[2]

In the United States today there is already a limited—albeit insecure—right to some health care for the majority of the population. There is also an absolute entitlement to some health care through government programs for particular categories of persons. The central dilemma of health care reform is how to restructure our nation's health care system to extend and ensure an entitlement for all our citizens to the most comprehensive health care that our society can afford. While there are compelling reasons to do so—irrespective of the establishment of a human right to health care—there is also formidable opposition to doing so.

This paper will review existing, limited rights to health care under public law and programs, and public and private health insurance. This overview of the limitations of existing rights will provide a background for understanding the financing and other system reforms that are needed to assure universal access to comprehensive health care. It will then discuss the necessary features of a health care system that will assure such access. Finally, it will discuss the economic and political factors that impede reform, and the need to go beyond the concept of an individual right to health care to a more communitarian ethic in order to overcome the opposition to reform.

Rights to Health Care through Public Program and Policies

In the United States today there is a legal right to limited health care services through public hospitals and programs. There is also a legal right to life-saving hospital care in emergencies for people who have neither public nor private health insurance. However, the establishment of these public programs and policies did not evolve from a recognition of a universal right to health care, but rather, from a recognition that government and health providers have a responsibility to provide health care for certain categories of vulnerable persons, and to all individuals in life-threatening situations. They have also evolved from concerns about the detrimental impact of specific communicable diseases—e.g. tuberculosis and sexually transmitted disease—on society as a whole, as well as pragmatic economic interests. One historical example of such societal concern comes from the late 1790's when recruitment of merchant seamen became difficult because port hospitals did not want to provide care to seamen from other towns. In response, the United States government began garnishing seamen's wages to fund a system of merchant marine hospitals which later evolved into the United States Public Health Service.[3]

The Government has always assumed responsibility for the health care of members of the armed forces and veterans with service-connected health conditions and disabilities, groups it could not afford to leave to the uncertain coverage of the private market.[4] The Department of Defense and Veterans Administration health programs are "socialized medicine," with all health facilities owned and operated by the government, and all health personnel, including doctors, salaried by the government. The responsibility to provide health care to the armed forces was incrementally expanded to the dependents of military servicemen and women; first through the Emergency Maternal and Infant Care Act of 1943, which ensured that spouses and children of low-ranking servicemen would be able to obtain health care, and then in 1956, when Congress permanently extended federal health care benefits to spouses and dependents through the Civilian Health and Medical Program of the Uniformed Services (CHAMPUS).[5]

Thus, a variety of health programs were established incrementally over several decades, as federal and state governments gradually assumed responsibility for ensuring access to health care for some groups. These public programs paved the way for the enactment of Medicare and Medicaid in 1965. Medicare is a single-payer, national health insurance program that was originally intended to cover only persons over age 65.[6] At the time of its enactment, only 56 percent of the elderly had hospital insurance.[7] In 1973, Medicare was expanded to cover permanently disabled persons receiving Social Security Disability Insurance (SSDI) benefits for at least two years (and their dependents), and persons with end-stage renal disease. In 1990, Medicare covered 13 percent of the United States population, but paid 17 percent of the nation's health care bill.[8] This is due to the fact that the Medicare population—the elderly, persons with disabilities, and those with end-stage renal disease—has higher health care expenditures on average than the rest of the population.

While Medicare is often viewed as a program that guarantees a right to comprehensive health care, in fact, the program guarantees only a limited right to hospital services through the Medicare Hospital Trust Fund—Part A. Because enrollment in Part A is mandatory and requires no premiums, it establishes an entitlement to most hospital services, hospice care, and a very limited post-acute nursing home and home health benefit. Coverage for physician and other outpatient services is obtained by purchasing Medicare Supplementary Medical Insurance—Part B. The $382 annual premium is heavily subsidized from general revenues regardless of a person's income. Approximately 89 percent of Medicare's revenue is obtained from payroll and income taxes levied on persons under age 65.[9] For persons who are near the poverty level and who have less than $4000 in assets, Medicaid is required to pay the Part B premium, the deductible, and any copayments incurred. However, only a third of the poor elderly are eligible for this Medicaid coverage.[10] For the near-poor elderly who can't afford the Part B premium and who are ineligible for Medicaid, their entitlement to health care is limited to hospital coverage.

Medicare does not assure access to comprehensive health care because its limited package of benefits pays primarily for acute care. Most notably, Medicare does not pay for prescription drugs, many preventive and early diagnostic services, and long-term care. Additionally, the program requires considerable cost-sharing. Hospital coverage is subject to a $652 annual deductible and there is substantial cost sharing for hospital stays over 60 days, no cap on out-of-pocket liability, and no coverage for persons needing more than 150 days of hospital care. Deficiencies in coverage for expensive items such as prescription drugs and extensive cost-sharing impoverish one third of the near poor elderly each year, and lead 72 percent of persons over age 65 to purchase supplementary coverage through private "Medi-Gap" policies that generally pay all of Medicare's cost sharing requirements. However, most do not pay for any benefits that Medicare doesn't cover, specifically prescription drugs and long-term care. The few policies that cover prescription drugs are medically underwritten, thereby excluding many persons who want to purchase such coverage. Forty-two percent of the poor elderly pay as much as 10 percent of their income to purchase Medi-Gap policies.[11]

Medicaid is a combined federal and state funded, means-tested health care program for targeted categories of the poor, such as mothers with children who are enrolled in the Aid to Families with Dependent Children Program (AFDC), and recipients of the Supplemental Security Income Program (SSI), which provides cash benefits to disabled persons under age 65 and the elderly poor. Strict categorical eligibility and unrealistically low income requirements greatly reduce the number of poor persons eligible for Medicaid. Medicaid income eligibility for a family of three averages $5,100 nationwide, an amount equal to 44 percent of the federal poverty level. In the state of Alabama, a family of three is not eligible for Medicaid if their income exceeds $1788 annually, which is 16 percent of poverty.[12] Thirty-six states have a "medically needy" standard that allows persons who are categorically eligible for Medicaid, but whose income and assets exceed eligibility guidelines, to "spend down" to the state determined poverty level to become eligible for Medicaid. In states without this standard, persons are not eligible for Medicaid even if their medical expenses exceed their income. The failure of the program to cover the poor is evident in the fact that 25 percent of poor children, and 40 percent of poor adults are not covered by Medicaid and have no other source of health insurance.[13]

While limited in its coverage of the poor, Medicaid does provide a more comprehensive array of benefits than Medicare, including preventive, diagnostic, acute, rehabilitative, and long-term care for the elderly and persons with disabilities who are poor enough to qualify. However, while those eligible for Medicaid have a statutory right to certain health benefits, it is a very limited right. Low reimbursement rates restrict access to health care by discouraging program participation by health care providers. Additionally, since some services, such as long-term care, are generally covered only when delivered in institutions, families with long-term care needs are generally required to institutionalize their disabled parents or children in order to receive care. Because they are reluctant to do so, most families assume the personal and financial costs of long-term care until they are either impoverished or no longer physically or mentally able to provide the level of care required.

Finally, while federal Medicaid mandates require states to offer certain services and prohibit them from arbitrarily limiting services based on diagnosis, states are permitted to place limits on the duration and amount of services provided. For example, when a lawsuit was brought against the state of Tennessee for reducing Medicaid coverage of hospital days from 20 to 14 per year, the Supreme Court ruled that it was permissible for states to place a limit on the number of hospital days that Medicaid would cover. In its ruling, the Court stated that Medicaid's purpose is to assure the delivery of necessary medical care, "not adequate health care."[14] As a result of this interpretation, when denial of life-saving treatment is challenged, the courts are often predisposed to rule differently. In a recent case, a federal court in Florida ruled that the Florida Department of Health and Rehabilitation Services was required to use Medicaid funds to pay for a life-saving liver small bowel transplant for an infant, even though the state argued that the procedure was experimental and therefore not covered under Medicaid.[15]

This orientation to guaranteeing health care only for life threatening conditions is also found in the legal obligation imposed on hospitals to provide care for the uninsured if they present with a medically unstable or life-threatening condition. Historically, many hospitals were founded by religious or charitable groups whose major purpose was to provide free care for the poor and destitute. However, the particular statutory obligation of hospitals to provide charity care had its origins with the passage of the Hospital Survey and Construction Act in 1948, more widely known as the Hill Burton Act. The Act provided federal funds to build hospitals, and in return required the hospitals to provide a defined amount of free and below-cost care to uninsured, low income persons, each year for twenty years. A right to emergency care is also ensured through a variety of state and federal statutes, including hospital licensing laws and tax-exempt status standards. Under the tax code, non-profit hospitals are required to provide some charity care to their communities in exchange for their exemption from federal and state taxes. More recently, in response to egregious cases of hospitals denying care in emergency situations, an anti-dumping law was enacted in 1986 that prohibits hospitals from refusing to treat persons with life-threatening conditions, medically unstable conditions, and pregnant women in active labor.[16]

This legal requirement and court rulings such as the one cited above in the Florida case, stem less from a recognized right to health care than from a sense that there is an obligation to act when individuals' lives are at stake. This is due to a generally accepted sense that the refusal to save a life when resources are available is morally indefensible. Given this limited notion of society's obligation to provide health care, it is understandable that the emergency room has become a major source of care for many of the uninsured. However, a right to emergency care does little to meet the ongoing health needs of the general population, particularly those with chronic conditions. Approximately 85 percent of the American population utilize health care in a given year, and the overwhelming majority of health care provided is not of an emergency nature.[17]

The recognition of a limited right to services for acute medical needs, combined with the failure to assure access to preventive and primary care, has led to higher overall costs for the health system. People with health care needs are unable to obtain preventive, early diagnostic, and primary care, but are admitted to the most expensive institutions when their health status has deteriorated sufficiently to require emergency treatment. The recognition of a moral obligation to save life, but not to provide a comprehensive array of health services, has led to the current situation where uninsured women cannot obtain prenatal care costing about $800, but hospitals will provide neonatal intensive care—often costing over $100,000—to save the life of an uninsured infant born prematurely. Similarly, Medicare will pay for hospital care for a person who has had a stroke, but not for the medication to treat the hypertension that caused the stroke. A recent study found that Medicaid and uninsured patients are hospitalized at much higher rates for preventable complications of diabetes and asthma than are patients with private insurance.[18]

Clearly, as the cost of technologically advanced interventions continues to climb, it is irrational to require treatment at the acute end of the health care continuum for health conditions which, if not totally preventable, could be treated at a far lower cost in a system designed to provide comprehensive primary health care to all its citizens. However, the continuing escalation of costs in both Medicare and Medicaid have made federal and state governments wary of expanding coverage under these programs because of fears that significant costs would be incurred before cost-savings would be realized.

In sum, while Medicare and Medicaid provide an entitlement to some health care for eligible individuals, the right to health care guaranteed through these public programs is a limited one that is oriented primarily to acute medical needs, and in addition, under Medicaid, the provision of long-term care to the impoverished severely disabled population of all ages.

Private Contractual Rights

For persons with private health insurance, there is a limited contractual right to some health care. However, there is no assurance that individuals will be able to buy insurance, even if they can afford it. This situation is a major change from the late 1930's when the non-profit Blue Cross and Blue Shield first began to market their policies. At that time, health insurance was community rated, and anyone who applied for coverage was accepted. The number of people with private coverage increased because the preferential tax treatment of employee health benefits provided an incentive for employers to offer health benefits to their workers. This incentive was increased during World War II when employer-provided health benefits were exempted from the wartime freeze on wages.[19] As more employers began to offer insurance, an increasing number of for-profit insurers entered the market and competition for low-risk groups intensified, thereby changing the principles under which health insurance was sold. Experience rating increasingly replaced community rating and the health insurance market became increasingly segmented, thereby reducing the ability to spread risk over a large population.

From the 1950's through the 1990's, increases in health care costs have affected the availability of health insurance in two major ways. First, as health care has become more and more expensive, insurance premiums have likewise escalated, thereby excluding a large number of Americans who cannot afford to buy insurance. Second, in an effort to maintain their profits, health insurers have instituted more intensive medical underwriting. The competition for low-risk groups has led, not only to numerous pre-existing condition exclusions and an increase in the number of individuals deemed "medically uninsurable," but also to the exclusion of those who are judged likely to develop such conditions no matter how minimal the risk. As a result, entire occupations, industries, and geographic areas are routinely excluded from coverage by health insurers on the grounds that individuals in these areas and groups are at high risk for needing health care.

As rising health care costs have pushed premiums even higher, an increasing number of large firms have chosen to self-insure, thereby saving themselves the cost of insurance company commissions, overhead and profits, and allowing them to obtain the benefits of investing large reserves. The Employee Retirement Income Security Act (ERISA), which governs employer health benefit plans, also exempts employer health plans from state insurance regulations and taxes, thereby providing another financial incentive to self-insure. By 1990, approximately half of all Americans with employer-provided insurance were covered by plans that were to some extent self-insured.[20] As a result, the market that remains for private insurance consists primarily of small companies and organizations, and the self-employed. And as the market has shrunk, the competition to screen out bad risks has intensified, with many insurers going to extremes to avoid rather than manage risk.[21]

As a result, from 1980 through 1991, the number of the uninsured grew by 30 percent. In 1991 alone, 3.3 million people lost coverage, and only 61.6 percent of the civilian non-institutionalized United States population had health insurance through private coverage.[22]

In this same period, public programs covered an increasing portion of the population, although this increase did not offset the decline in the proportion with coverage through private insurance. As a result, the percentage of the nation's uninsured rose to 13.9 percent in 1991.[23] Since there is virtually universal coverage for persons over age 65, if we look only at those under age 65, the percentage of uninsured in 1991 was even higher—18 percent.[24] However, since this figure is derived from cross-sectional data, it underestimates the scope of the problem. If we look at the percentage of the population uninsured over a longer period of time an even higher percentage is without insurance for significant periods. In a Census Bureau study over a 28 month period, 28 percent of the population—63 million Americans—lacked insurance for months at a time.[25]

While it is increasingly difficult to obtain and retain private health insurance, the majority of the population under age 65 is covered by health insurance available through employment. In 1991, employers covered 55.8 percent of the population and approximately 17 percent of the population has individually purchased private coverage.[26] However, while insured individuals have a limited contractual right to the health benefits in their policies, this right is not secure, nor are the benefits comprehensive. While a great deal of attention has been given to the 37 million Americans without insurance, there are also millions who are under-insured. This is related to several factors: (1) lack of coverage for pre-existing conditions, (2) exclusion from coverage of certain categories of health care and related services, including preventive and diagnostic services, prescription drugs, extended rehabilitation, durable medical equipment, and long-term care, (3) exclusions for "experimental" drugs, treatments, and procedures,[27] (4) annual and lifetime caps and high copayments for certain conditions or treatments, most usually for mental health and substance abuse services, (5) no limits on out-of-pocket payments for covered services,[28] (6) no limits on expenses that exceed "usual, customary and reasonable" charges for covered benefits, and (7) a host of other exclusions based on restricted definitions of "medical necessity," or arbitrary limitations on services, such as physical therapy. As a result, many families **with insurance** are faced with financial ruin in the event of a catastrophic illness or accident. In one study of uncompensated hospital care, 47 percent of the 1689 patients who incurred uncompensated costs, **had** health insurance.[29]

These limitations in coverage are often not apparent until a person becomes seriously ill. Consequently, most Americans report high levels of satisfaction with their current health insurance coverage. It is only when persons suffer catastrophic illness or accidents that require a wide range of ongoing medical, rehabilitative and support services, that they discover just how few services their policies cover. They also find out that hospital and physician charges which the insurer determines are above "usual, customary, and reasonable" charges, are neither paid by the insurer nor applied to the out-of-pocket limits. Thus, actual out-of-pocket expenses are often far higher than stated limits. Additionally, many insurance plans nominally include a particular benefit, but the services covered are so limited that they are often insufficient. As an example, a plan may provide only 60 days of rehabilitation, but a person with a severe stroke, a spinal cord injury, or a traumatic brain injury may require intensive rehabilitation for six months or longer, and intermittent rehabilitation services for another six to twelve months. Persons with multiple sclerosis or severe rheumatoid arthritis often find that their insurer will not pay for their physical therapy—even though it's a covered benefit—because it is being used only to "maintain" and not to "improve" their function. Persons with serious mental illness generally exhaust their inpatient lifetime mental health benefit within a year. Health insurance also rarely, if ever, covers long-term care, services and supports for persons who are disabled as a result of a congenital condition, a chronic disease, or an injury. The rationale often given for not covering these services is that they are not "acute", not "medically necessary" or not "health-related".

Insurers also deny access to covered diagnostic procedures. In a recent case, an insurer denied approval for a Magnetic Resonance Imaging (MRI) test for a women whose headaches were increasing in severity and intensity. Subsequently, an aneurism, which the MRI could have detected, ruptured, leaving her with severe neurological impairment, partial paralysis, and visual impairment.[30] If persons in a self-insured plan have been denied covered benefits and suffered negative effects as a result, the Employment and Retirement Income Security Act (ERISA) does not permit them to sue for damages. At best, they can sue to have the insurer pay for the covered benefit.

Insurers attempt to deny coverage for covered benefits through a number of practices, including the use of ambiguous policy exclusions and elaborate rules for validating claims.[31] For example, a person with a pre-existing condition exclusion for diabetes develops heart disease after many years and finds that his insurer will not cover the costs of treatment because the insurer claims the heart disease was "caused" by the diabetes. In another case, a woman undergoing a biopsy for possible breast cancer forgets to call her insurer within 24 hours of the surgery as the company required, and as a result, the insurer refuses to pay her bills.[32]

Perhaps the most troubling aspect of our system of private health insurance is that it provides no security over time. Policies issued to small groups often are non-renewable. Thus, many individuals are at risk of having their coverage terminated when they, or someone in their group, becomes ill. Once a member of the group has a serious illness, finding insurance to cover the group becomes much more difficult and expensive, and coverage usually cannot be obtained without pre-existing condition exclusions. In testimony offered to the United States Bipartisan Commission on Comprehensive Health Care Reform in 1990, a couple with a group policy for their family business recounted how they where forced to drop coverage for their employees when their premiums rose from $198 per person to $766 per person per month after their child was born with a birth defect. The couple was forced to drop their own coverage the following year when the monthly premium was further increased to $1375 per month.[33]

Even employees in large groups are not guaranteed a contractual right to health care because so many are covered by self-insured plans and are not protected by the limited state regulations that govern commercial insurers. As noted above, ERISA protects employers from lawsuits by employees for damages when covered benefits are denied. ERISA also permits employers to cut benefits for specific conditions, even after an employee has become ill. In a recent highly publicized case, McMann *v.* H & H Music, the Supreme Court ruled that a self-insured plan could cut benefits for AIDS treatment from $1 million to $5000, even though it left a current employee with AIDS without any coverage for his condition.[34]

The lack of security in the private insurance market has recently become even more acute for retired workers under the age of 65, some of whom retire due to poor health. As of 1993, the Federal Accounting Standards Board requires companies to include the cost of retiree health benefits as liabilities on their balance sheets. As a result, many employers are cutting back or entirely eliminating retiree health benefits. Recent Congressional hearings highlighted the problems faced by retired persons with serious health conditions who are unable to purchase private insurance because they are considered "medically uninsurable," and who will not be eligible for Medicare for many years. Even for those retirees who may not be excluded for health reasons, the cost of health insurance is often prohibitive, amounting sometimes to one half of their annual pension. Some retirees have had to re-enter the labor force, solely to obtain health insurance.[35]

This brief overview of private insurance coverage highlights the limitations of a contractual right to health care for persons who currently have private health insurance. Not only is there no guarantee that an individual will always be covered by insurance, there is no guarantee that the insurance company will continue to offer the benefits an individual needs, or that they will even pay for the benefits covered under the contract. In sum, there is a limited right to health care in the United States, but the circumstances under which this right is guaranteed are increasingly tenuous and the benefits provided are often inadequate to meet the health care needs of those covered.

Extending a Right to Comprehensive Health Care

If a right to health care is to become a reality for all Americans, our nation must reach a consensus on the purpose, the financing, and the control of our nation's health care system. This section will outline the social context of the American health care system—its purpose and financial support—and will discuss the fundamental features of a system that are needed to guarantee access to health care. It will then discuss the obstacles to creating such a system in the United States, and the need to go beyond the language of rights in order to overcome these obstacles.

The President's Commission for the Study of Ethical Problems in Medicine and Biomedical and Behavioral Research concluded that "health care is a social product requiring the investment, skills, and efforts of many individuals."[36] While discrete aspects of health care are delivered by individual health care providers to individual patients, all health care is delivered within a highly complex, interdependent system that is financed *collectively* by millions of individuals through the payment of premiums, through general and earmarked taxes, and through direct out-of-pocket payments. These payments comprise 81 percent of our nation's expenditures on health care. While employers pay a significant portion of health care costs—19 percent—they recoup these expenses by charging higher prices to the public for goods and services, and through lowered compensation to employees and lower returns to investors.[37]

The private insurance sector, including for-profit and non-profit insurers as well as self-insured plans, frequently refers to its coverage of the majority of Americans as a major justification for its continued role in the financing and delivery of health care. However, in 1992, private insurers paid only 30.7 percent of the nation's health care bill.[38] The low proportion paid by private insurance is due to the fact that it primarily covers younger, employed people who have lower health expenses on average, and also because the industry works assiduously to exclude both those who need health care and those they deem to be at high risk for needing health care.

In the same year, federal, state and local government—i.e. the taxpaying public—paid 45.9 percent of the nation's annual health care bill through a variety of health programs: Medicare, Medicaid, the Department of Defense, CHAMPUS, the Veterans Administration, federal and state employee and retiree programs, and other discrete health programs such as Community Mental Health Centers. If we take account of the federal tax subsidy for employer provided insurance—estimated at over $56 billion in 1990[39] —taxpayer financing contributes well over 50 percent of total payments, a share that will increase as the "Baby Boom" cohort ages and becomes eligible for Medicare. Thus, the public sector is currently the largest single financier of health care in this country. Clearly, the characterization of our current financing as predominately private is inaccurate. It ignores the extent of public financing and the fact that the current health care system would not exist without the payments of millions of citizens acting *communally* for a common purpose.

The design of a health care system—its financing and delivery— should be based on its purposes and goals. In order to reach consensus on how to reform our system, it is essential that the public, those with a financial interest in the current system and the elected officials who will enact reform, all understand that a health care system has a single social purpose: to meet the health care needs of the public in order to ensure a healthy population and a productive society. This simple fact is often lost in the policy debate, where some would have our elected officials believe that the purpose of the system is to assure a satisfactory income for health care providers, and employment and profits for those who organize the financing and delivery of health services. The financial interests of the private health sector that comprise over thirteen percent of our nation's economy cannot be ignored. However, since the public provides both the mandate for a health system and its financial support, it is the public that the system should serve and be accountable to.[40] The American public pays enough money into our current system to guarantee universal coverage to a high quality of health care. What is needed is a system to distribute it more equitably and efficiently.

To ensure a meaningful and secure right to health care, a health care system must have the following features: (1) mandatory universal coverage, (2) equitable financing, (3) a mandated comprehensive benefits package, (4) an efficient delivery system that provides coordinated, comprehensive health care in accessible settings, and (5) appropriate and adequate mechanisms to contain overall health care spending. Each of these features will be discussed in turn.

(1) Mandatory Universal Coverage. A meaningful and secure right to health care can only be assured through the establishment of a system of health insurance that provides continuous coverage for everyone regardless of age, health status, disability, employment, income, or any other factor. Since it is highly unlikely that the United States will enact a public, single-payer system of national insurance, it is expected that the majority of the population under age 65 will continue to receive coverage through non-profit and commercial insurers.[41] The goal of universal coverage through a multi-payer system will require not only that private insurers accept all applicants, but that every American enroll in a health plan. Mandating that insurers must accept all applicants while permitting the purchase of insurance to be voluntary would lead to adverse selection and would perpetuate the current situation where "free riders" incur uncompensated costs that are then shifted to those Americans who are already contributing. Leaving anyone out of the system also undermines the central premise of insurance that makes it work: everyone is at risk for needing health care and everyone must contribute.

(2) Equitable Financing. An equitable financing mechanism is needed to assure universal coverage. Health insurance is unaffordable

for many individuals and families with low incomes and so the financing mechanism will need to be progressive, with those who are better off financially subsidizing those who are less well off. This would be a marked change from the current system of financing which is extremely regressive, providing the greatest subsidy for health insurance to high-income groups through the tax exclusion for employer-provided insurance. Currently, those with the highest incomes pay the lowest percentage for their health insurance. In 1987, families with incomes between $16,000 and $21,000 spent 15 percent of their income on health insurance premiums, out-of-pocket health costs and taxes to support government health programs, while families with incomes between $72,000 and $93,000 spent only 11 percent of their income.[42] This regressivity is also found in the Medicare program, which subsidizes middle and high income elderly with the taxes of low-income workers, many of whom have no insurance for themselves and their families.

The simplest and most progressive form of financing would be a payroll tax, an approach utilized by both single-payer and multi-payer systems in other countries.[43] A recent study by the Economic and Social Research Institute found that the elimination of employer-provided insurance and the imposition of a 7.75 percent payroll tax could save up to $3.1 trillion in health spending over the next ten years.[44] However, there is powerful opposition to a payroll tax from businesses, particularly small businesses and those with low profit margins and a large number of employees who work for low wages. This opposition is strongest from those businesses who currently do not provide insurance. For those who currently provide insurance, a payroll tax in the range of 7 to 9 percent on annual earnings of $25,000 (United States median earnings) would be far less than the average cost of a health insurance premium, which for small businesses can range as high as $4000 to $6000 per person.

If the United States does not enact a payroll tax to finance health care, financing will most likely continue to be provided through the payment of premiums. In this event, premiums will need to be community rated so that everyone is charged the same irrespective of their health condition or risk of illness. This basic tenet of social insurance ensures that the healthy subsidize the sick and that those with large out-of-pocket costs due to illness or injury are not also burdened by higher premiums. Community rating also has the potential to reduce the overall cost of health care by providing incentives to all purchasers to work together to control aggregate costs.[45]

However, financing through community-rated premiums rather than a payroll tax will necessitate a subsidy for low income persons who otherwise could not afford to pay a community-rated premium. Financing through premiums paid to a private system of multiple, competing, for-profit insurers will also necessitate some form of risk adjustment and/or reinsurance, since such a system will not spread risk as well as a system with a single insurer, or a few dominant insurers, and, as a result, there will be a greater chance for each plan to become insolvent if they incur catastrophic costs. Clearly, financing universal coverage through a multi-payer system will be more administratively complex and costly than financing through a single-payer system.[46]

(3) Mandated Comprehensive Benefits. A health system should provide the full range of services needed to prevent and treat illness, and to maintain optimal physical and mental health and functioning. To do so, the current system's acute care bias must be altered to eliminate the incentives that have led to the neglect of preventive, primary, rehabilitative, and long-term services. To ensure that these services are covered, a comprehensive health benefits package must be mandated to cover primary and secondary preventive services, diagnostic services, primary care for acute and chronic illnesses and conditions, and rehabilitation, transitional, and long-term services for persons with functional impairments. Decisions regarding which services to include in a mandated standard benefits package should be based on a consideration of their effectiveness and their cost effectiveness.

(4) An Efficient Delivery System. In order to assure timely access to quality health care, we need to correct the inefficiencies, duplications, inadequacies and inequities in our current health care delivery system. To assure that individuals receive the services they need, and to assure the continuing affordability of health insurance, a health care delivery system must efficiently provide coordinated, comprehensive health care in accessible settings. This does not require that the full range of specialized services be located in every geographic area. Rather, it requires that persons in underserved areas be provided primary care in accessible locations, and the means to access specialty

services that are not located in their immediate geographic area. Without the assurance of accessible health services, a right to health care through universal insurance will be rendered meaningless.

(5) Cost Containment. A health care system must include appropriate and effective mechanisms for cost containment. The rate of increase in health care costs over the past two decades is clearly unsustainable and must be reduced to keep health insurance both affordable and comprehensive. The debate over the best way to contain costs is likely to be divisive and contentious. However, without adequate cost containment mechanisms, the cost of insurance will continue to climb, taking scarce resources away from other areas of our economy. Additionally, if the health care industry and health care providers are successful in blocking cost containment mechanisms that affect their charges for products and services, it is virtually inevitable that both benefit coverage and financial protections for consumers will be reduced.

While these five features of a health care system are fundamental to assuring a right to health care, they are not sufficient. There are many other factors that affect the availability and cost of health services that must also be addressed. For example, it is generally recognized that the shortage of primary care physicians and the oversupply of specialists and sub-specialists in the United States is a major factor contributing to excessive health care costs, without a measurable improvement in health status indicators.[47] Therefore, a coherent health policy must also address this imbalance and provide incentives to increase the number of primary care physicians relative to specialists.[48] Additionally, health care delivery systems will need to have mechanisms to control the inappropriate utilization of specialists for health problems that could be handled by lower cost primary care health providers.

Another factor contributing to health care cost inflation is the uncontrolled proliferation of both proven and unproven technology. The overabundance of technology simultaneously increases cost and decreases access. As one analyst noted, it is ironic that many women in the United States can't afford to have a mammogram because there are too many under-utilized mammography machines driving up the average cost of the procedure.[49] A rational and coherent national health policy would either regulate the dissemination of technology to more appropriately meet the needs of the population, or design a system which provides incentives to purchase only that technology that will be utilized appropriately and to full capacity.

In the area of health research, while the public provides $10 billion each year to fund research at the National Institutes of Health (NIH), very little of this research is focused on the prevention of illness. In addition, little is focused on the care of people with functional impairments that remain after technologically advanced treatment is provided under the assumption that we must save and extend life whatever the personal or societal cost. It is essential that research priorities be altered to give equal attention to the prevention of accidents and illnesses, the maintenance of health and functioning, and the rehabilitation of persons with functional impairments.

Finally, we need to invest a greater proportion of our resources in the public health infrastructure, particularly in the area of infectious disease prevention and control. The recent re-emergence of tuberculosis, and in particular, multiple drug resistant tuberculosis, which can cost $400,000 per case to treat, underscores the importance of public health services in controlling our nation's health care expenditures.

Obstacles to Reform

There is widespread recognition of the need for comprehensive reform of our health care system and strong public support for universal coverage and comprehensive benefits. However, there are many factors that attenuate the strength of that support. Most importantly, there is strong opposition to needed changes from those who financially benefit from the current health care system and those who are ideologically opposed to expanding the government's role in the financing of health care. There is also opposition from the public to increased taxes—even if those taxes were to replace premiums—primarily because the public does not understand the full cost of employer-provided insurance and the extent to which it is currently subsidized through the tax system. Thus, any attempt to enact reforms to ensure universal comprehensive health care will confront a wide range of obstacles that have the potential to seriously undermine, if not totally prevent, fundamental reform of our health care system.

Even among those who accept the need for fundamental reforms and who are not opposed to government financing, there are major disagreements about how to assure universal access and how to control costs. These disputes are also based on ideological positions, such as the "right" of business to be free from government mandates in a free market economy and the right to contract freely with labor. They are also due to a fundamental lack of understanding by the American public of what is wrong with our health care system and what is needed to fix it.

Opposition to a national system of health insurance has a long history. Opposition based on political ideology and economic self-interest have been closely linked and many times the latter has been couched in terms of the former. Rhetoric about the dangers of "government medicine" reached new heights of hyperbole in the 1992 presidential election when then President Bush proclaimed that Gov. Clinton's health proposals would give Americans a system with the "compassion of the KGB". As one commentator noted, as far as compassion is concerned, we can hardly do worse than we're doing now.[50] Much conservative rhetoric is aimed at the segment of the United States population that holds similar views, but also affects those who are ambivalent about government action in the area of health care, either because they are concerned about additional taxes or because they have a general mistrust of government. Perfectly capturing this ambivalence—as well as a lack of understanding about the health system—is the statement of one man: "I'm for national health care, but I don't want the government involved".[51]

That political ideology and economic interests are closely linked in opposition to comprehensive health care reform is no surprise. Conservatives have long opposed government interference in the "free market," and in particular, mandates and regulations for both small businesses and large corporations. And the business interests in the health care sector contribute generously to conservative members of the United States Congress. The special interest groups with the biggest financial stake in maintaining the current health care system—the medical, insurance and pharmaceutical industries—together have contributed more than $60 million to congressional candidates since 1980.[52] However, having seen the proverbial "writing on the wall," many of these groups now support universal coverage and other reforms, but only so far as they judge these reforms to minimally affect their own financial interests. Simply put, each player wants to shift the "costs" of reform to someone else. For example, the American Medical Association supports increased government spending on health care for the poor, but strongly opposes any measures to constrain overall cost increases that might limit physician incomes. In contrast, the small business lobby supports cost-containment mechanisms that don't directly affect them, including increased regulation of the insurance industry and limits on physician charges, which the general public also supports.

Special interest groups often attempt to garner public support for their position by reframing their economic self interest as concern for the wellbeing of patients and the public good. Thus, the American Medical Association reframes government attempts to slow the growth in Medicare physician reimbursement rates as a government attempt to limit services to senior citizens. The pharmaceutical industry reframes proposals to limit the increase in prescription drug costs as a threat to the development of new drugs. Such obfuscation contributes to the general confusion of the American public about the problems in our health care system, and what is needed to correct them.

Opposition in the past has been effective in impeding health care reform, but the 1992 election of an Administration committed to comprehensive health care reform has raised hopes that the United States will finally enact a system to provide secure health insurance coverage for all Americans. Despite this commitment, there are major concerns that even if a system of universal insurance is enacted, the political influence of special interests will prevent the institution of effective cost-containment measures, which over time will undermine the goal of comprehensive coverage. Powerful opposition to cost-containment mechanisms that would limit the rate of increase in provider payments—all-payer rate setting, price controls, and global budget— leave only two areas to reduce costs to the insurance system: the mandated benefits package and cost sharing provisions. As a result, there are major concerns among consumer groups that a mandated standard benefits package will be limited, and that cost-sharing requirements will be increased in order to reduce the cost of premiums and the necessary subsidies for persons with low incomes.

Concerns about the affordability of premiums and the extent of subsidies required are certainly legitimate. However, there are serious concerns about the legitimacy of limiting beneficial health services in order to assure unlimited incomes for health care suppliers and providers, and profits for private insurers and investors in a health sector with excess capacity. It is difficult to justify limitations on coverage for items like electric wheelchairs for persons with quadriplegia on the grounds that society can't "afford" such extensive coverage of durable medical equipment, when the 1992 total *annual* compensation for the CEO of the Hospital Corporation of American—a for-profit hospital chain—was $127 million. [53]

The Potential for Public Opposition to Reform

While the American public generally supports a right to health care for all Americans and recognizes the need to reform the health care system, it is also alarmingly uninformed and misinformed about the causes and consequences of the current health care crisis, and does not understand how health insurance must be structured and financed in order to provide universal coverage.[54] Additionally, the public has evidenced a general reluctance to equitably share the cost of financing a universal health care system. Thus, the American public clamoring for health care reform is by no means united in its views of what is wrong with the health care system, and what needs to be done to fix it.

Many, if not most Americans do not understand the fundamental principle of universal health insurance: that the healthy subsidize the sick. In the past several decades, the combination of rapidly rising health care costs, the shift from community rating to experience rating, and an increasingly segmented insurance market, have all led to a climate in which the young are pitted against the old, and the healthy against the sick; where individuals resent having to pay for "other's" care, and spreading the cost of health care as broadly as possible is viewed as "unfair." Many groups purchasing insurance believe that if they are a young, lower-risk group, they should not have to subsidize the care of an older, higher-risk group. During a television program on the health care crisis, a young man asked angrily why he should have to pay for "old people."[55] On a recent radio call-in show on health care, one caller asked why someone like herself, who hadn't been sick in 20 years, shouldn't receive a large rebate from her insurance company. And in a recent magazine article, a twenty-six year old woman who said she didn't need health insurance because she was young and healthy, stated that it wasn't fair that she should have buy insurance in order to subsidize people with "bad health habits."[56]

Such attitudes reflect a lack of understanding not only of how health insurance is supposed to work, but also, of the risk for major illness and catastrophic accidents for people of all ages. The simplistic application of experience rating to "unhealthy" behaviors also ignores the complexity of disease etiology and the many other factors that affect health outcomes. In assigning individual responsibility for one's health, this view also assumes an exaggerated notion of control over behaviors that are rooted in culture and factors associated with one's socio-economic status, not in personal decision-making.[57] In its consideration of the notion of personal responsibility for one's health, the President's Committee on Bioethics concluded that it is inappropriate, and in most cases not feasible to apply the notion of personal responsibility for one's health status and one's need for health care in a fair way.[58]

Many Americans concerned about the high cost of their own insurance also do not believe they should have to subsidize insurance for those who can't afford it. In response to media reports that the Clinton Administration health plan will necessitate increased taxes, one Republican Senator stated, that reform shouldn't call for new taxes "to pay for *someone else's* health insurance" (emphasis added).[59] While Americans support the idea of universal coverage, they appear unwilling to recognize that by definition, it will require that those with higher incomes subsidize those with low incomes or no income.

Surprisingly, when Americans express discontent about costs, they are referring to their own out-of-pocket costs for premiums and cost sharing. Many are astounded and even skeptical when confronted with figures on United States health care spending and how much of their taxes are going to health care.[60] The public does not realize the amount they are currently paying for a system that provides them neither the comprehensive coverage nor the economic security they want. Neither does it realize that if health care financing and delivery were restructured to provide universal coverage and effective cost containment, the amount we are currently paying would be sufficient to provide universal coverage. Few Americans understand the reasons underlying the continuing escalation of health care costs to levels of unaffordability: the uncontrolled proliferation of costly and duplicative technology; fee-for-service medicine with financial incentives to increase the volume and intensity of services, whether needed or not; the tax subsidy for employer-provided insurance; the dominance of for-profit industries in the health sector; and other factors that have resulted in a system in which both providers and patients are, in one analyst's words, "cost unconscious." The public, on the other hand, cite greed, fraud, waste and abuse as the major causes of out-of-control costs.[61] As a result, the majority of Americans with insurance do not understand that unless the factors that are driving costs are altered and universal coverage is required, they too may one day be either priced out of the market altogether, or they will have to pay an increasing proportion of their income for their own and others' health care.

Another potential obstacle to reform is public concern about cost containment strategies that rely on delivery systems that restrict choice. For many Americans, choice of health plans and choice of doctors is increasingly curtailed by their employers. Despite this, or perhaps because of this, many Americans are concerned that any health reform proposal allow them to freely choose their own doctor. Thus, they are unlikely to support any cost containment measures that restrict their ability to choose their own doctors and hospitals, and yet some of the proposals to contain costs—e.g. managed care systems—would do just that. It is ironic that many of the features of managed care systems espoused by some conservatives as an acceptable way to contain costs in a free market system, have features similar to the British National Health Service, which is so often maligned by conservatives as "socialized medicine": responsibility for a defined population in a geographic area, salaried physicians, and the use of a primary care gate keeper to control access to specialists. However, a fundamental difference between the two systems is that British physicians don't have financial incentives to underserve their patients, whereas physicians in the United States in many HMOs do.[62]

The Future of Health Care Reform

If, as is likely, health care reform requires the enactment of new taxes but does not meet the needs and expectations of the American public, the power of public opposition to reform should not be underestimated. The public outcry which led to the repeal of the Medicare Catastrophic Act is ample evidence of the need to ensure an informed and educated public during enactment of health care legislation. In order for comprehensive health care reform to succeed, the public must be educated so they will clearly understand how they are at risk in the current system, why certain structural reforms are needed, and what the necessary trade-offs will be. If they have a more accurate understanding of the problems, they will likely be more accepting of real reform and more critical of solutions which are aimed at maintaining the status quo. Most importantly, they must see that the only way for social insurance to work is that the healthy subsidize the sick and the well off subsidize those less well off. Finally, the public needs to understand that since we are all at risk of needing health care and we are all at risk of losing our health insurance, the only way each individual can have a secure right to health care is for all Americans to have that right. To bring about this awareness, the federal government must assume an unprecedented role in educating the public about the causes and consequences of our health care crisis, and the need to support—and pay for—comprehensive change.

If efforts to reform our health care system are to succeed, it is essential that the American public, our elected representatives and those with a financial stake in the current system reach a consensus about how to restructure our health care system. Most importantly, we must reach agreement regarding the elements of a fair system of reimbursement for health services that will bring the current rate of increase in health expenditures in line with the rest of the economy. Without effective cost containment, it will be impossible to sustain the affordability and therefore, the comprehensiveness of the coverage. Unless we find a common language to achieve this consensus, there is a real possibility that the structural reforms needed will be blocked by a multitude of competing interests.

The language of rights in the public rhetoric accompanying health care reform efforts is a very effective tool for organizing general public support for health care reform. The unexpected victory of Pennsylvania Senator Harris Wofford in 1992 is attributed in part to his focus on health care reform during the campaign, and television ads stating that "if a criminal has a right to a lawyer, every American family should have the right to see a doctor." With the election of an Administration committed to comprehensive health care reform, reform efforts are intensifying and various slogans are being heard more frequently, including the now familiar "health care is a right, not a privilege," and, more to the point, "health care is a right, not a business."

However, at the policy level, where decisions about health care reform will be made, the issue of rights is rarely mentioned. The major factor driving state and federal reform efforts is concern about the continuing escalation of health care costs for employers and households, and the increasing proportion of tax revenues going to health care. Concerns about equity and fairness are frequently expressed, not in abstract philosophical terms related to theories of justice, but in very concrete financial terms, e.g. cost shifting from businesses that don't provide insurance to those who do is unfair; higher premiums for small businesses than for large businesses are unfair; requiring small businesses to provide insurance is unfair; community rating is unfair; and so on. The public also express their concerns in economic terms. While the uninsured worry that they will not be able to afford necessary health services, the insured worry not only that they will lose their insurance, but that a major illness or accident could destroy the economic security that they have worked hard all their lives to attain.

Since the concerns driving health care reform are primarily economic, approaches to health care reform that rely on the language of rights often find the right to health care pitted against the rights of health service providers and others with a financial stake in the health care system to profit from the delivery of health care. Similarly, small businesses generally oppose an employer mandate to provide insurance to their employees because it interferes with their "right" to freely contract with labor. Many companies also believe they have the "right" to sell products—be they health insurance or prescription drugs—in a market free of government intervention. [63] Thus, it is unlikely that the language of rights alone will be sufficient to bring about the necessary consensus.

To reach the consensus needed to enact comprehensive health care reform, we must go beyond the language of individual rights to a language of community and a recognition of the social context of the health care system in which a right to health care must operate. A debate about individual rights will tend to obscure the fundamental social nature of health care financing and delivery and the needs of the larger society. What is needed instead is a discussion of the moral justification for the social obligation to establish an equitable system to finance and deliver universal health care. It is the social obligation to ensure the public good that necessitates mandated participation in a universal health insurance system, whether it is financed through the public or the private sector. And it is the language of community and social obligation that is needed to overcome the opposition to government action to assure access to health care for all.

All of the Western industrialized democracies have defined health care as a public good, and have recognized that government has an obligation to assure the public good. When Theodore Roosevelt signed the legislation authorizing the creation of the Food and Drug Administration to protect consumers from unscrupulous marketing, he stated, "There are times when the public good must outweigh the right to private gain." This is the crux of the current health care reform debate and the outcome will not depend on the establishment of a right to health care, but on a moral decision that the public good in this case must take precedence over the right to private gain.

NOTES

1. Paul R. Torrens, *The American Health Care System: Issues and Problems* (St. Louis: C.V. Mosby Company, 1978), p. 74.

2. *Ibid.*, p. 70.

3. Laura Shefler, "No Easy Cure," *Pitt Magazine* (March 1993): 12–18.

4. The federal government also provides health care for Native Americans through the Indian Health Service. This program was enacted in 1955 based on federal treaty obligations. Timothy Taylor, "The Needs of Native Americans" (Paper presented at the AAAS Right to Health Care Consultation November 13, 1992).

5. For a brief overview of the history of American health policy, see Emily Friedman, "Fifty Years of U.S. Health Care Policy," *Hospitals* (May 5, 1986): 95–96, 98, 100, 102, 104.

6. One percent of persons over 65 are not insured through Medicare because they are not eligible for Social Security or Railroad Retirement benefits. However, they are able to buy in to the Medicare program. The Part A premium for these individuals is $192 per month.

7. John K. Iglehart, "The American Health Care System—Medicare," *The New England Journal of Medicine* (November 12, 1992): 1467–1472.

8. Katharine R. Levit, Gary L. Olin, and Suzanne W. Letsch, "Americans' Health Insurance Coverage, 1980–1991," *Health Care Financing Review* (Fall 1992): 31–57.

9. Iglehart, "The American Health Care System—Medicare."

10. Commonwealth Fund Commission on Elderly People Living Alone, *Medicare's Poor: Filling the Gaps in Medical Coverage for Low-Income Elderly Americans* (November 20, 1987). Additionally, of the 4.2 million eligible, 1.8 million are not receiving this assistance because they don't know it exists. Families USA Study, reported in *The Washington Post* (March 27, 1993): A6.

11. *Ibid.*

12. Kaiser Commission on the Future of Medicaid, *Medicaid at the Crossroads* (Baltimore: Kaiser Commission, November 1992).

13. Ibid.

14. In this case—*Alexander* v. *Choate*—the Medicaid restriction was challenged under Section 504 of the federal Rehabilitation Act of 1973 which prohibits discrimination against persons with disabilities by entities receiving federal funds. "Supreme Court Rules Hospital Stay Reduction Does Not Discriminate Against Handicapped," *Health Advocate* (Spring 1985): 10.

15. *McLaughlin* v. *Williams*, 801 F. Supp. 633 (S.D. Fla. 1992).

16. This requirement also covers discharges. A hospital cannot transfer or discharge anyone until their condition is medically stable. A consumer advocacy organization—Public Citizen Health Research Group—recently charged that the U.S. Department of Health and Human Services (HHS) has been lax in enforcing the law. The Department has never published final regulations for compliance, and of 268 hospitals found to have violated the law between 1986 and 1992, only 24 have been penalized. Reported in *The Washington Post* (May 20, 1993): A3.

17. B. Hahn and D. Lefkowitz, "Annual Expenses and Sources of Payment for Health Care Services," (AHCPR Pub. No. 93-0007). *National Medical Expenditure Survey Research Findings 14*, Agency for Health Care Policy and Research (Rockville, MD: Public Health Service, November 1992).

18. Joel Wisman, Constantine Gatsonis, and Arnold Epstein, "Rates of Avoidable Hospitalization by Insurance Status in Massachusetts and Maryland," *Journal of the American Medical Association* 268, No. 17 (1992): 2388–2394.

19. Emily Friedman, "Fifty Years of U.S. Health Care Policy."

20. Cynthia B. Sullivan and Thomas Rice, "The Health Insurance Picture in 1990," *Health Affairs* 10(1991): 104–115.

21. Janet O'Keeffe, "Health Care Financing: How Much Reform is Needed?" *Issues in Science and Technology* 8 (Spring 1992) 42–49.

22. This percentage represent persons with private insurance **only**; the percentage of all persons with private health insurance is higher because nearly 75 percent of Medicare recipients also have supplementary private coverage. Katherine R. Levit, Gary L. Olin, and Suzanne W. Letsch, "Americans' Health Insurance Coverage, 1980–1991," *Health Care Financing Review* 14(Fall 1992)31–57.

23. *Ibid.*

24. *Ibid.*

25. O'Keeffe, "Health Care Financing: How Much Reform is Needed?"

26. Slightly less than five percent of the population who are not workers or dependents of workers have employer provided coverage. Most of this coverage is for retired workers. Levit, Olin, and Letsch, "Americans' Health Insurance Coverage."

27. What is considered "experimental" may differ from insurer to insurer.

28. Estimates of the number of people under 65 years old who are under-uninsured range from 38 million (those who have insurance but have no limits on out-of-pocket expenditures), to 55 million (adding those who are at risk of being impoverished should they experience a major costly illness). U.S. Congress Office of Technology Assessment, *Medical Testing and Health Insurance*, OTA-H-384 (Washington, DC: U.S. Government Printing Office, August 1988): 162; Nancy DeLew, George Greenberg, and Kraig Kinchen, "A Layman's Guide to the U.S. Health Care System," *Health Care Financing Review* 14(Fall 1992)151–169.

29. Robert M. Saywell, Jr., Terrell W. Zollinger, David K. Chu, Charlotte A. MacBeth, and Mark E. Sechrist, "Hospital and Patient Characteristics of

Uncompensated Hospital Care: Policy Implications," *Journal of Health Politics, Policy and Law* 14, No. 2, (1989): 287–307.

30. Jack Anderson and Michael Binstein, "Insurance Company Bean Counters," *The Washington Post* (May 31, 1992), Outlook Op Ed.

31. For an extensive discussion of these types of insurance practices, see Donald W. Light, "The Practice and Ethics of Risk-Related Health Insurance: Caring for the Uninsured and Underinsured," *The Journal of the American Medical Association* (May 13, 1992): 2503–2509.

32. *Ibid.*

33. The U.S. Bipartisan Commission on Comprehensive Health Care, *A Call for Action* (Washington, DC: U.S. Government Printing Office, September 1990).

34. This incident occurred before the Americans with Disabilities Act (ADA) was enacted. Recently published guidance by the Equal Employment Opportunity Commission with regard to the ADA indicates that such exclusions will generally be considered discrimination under the ADA.

35. "Retiree Health Benefits: The Impact on Workers and Businesses." Hearing before the U.S. Senate Labor and Human Resources Subcommittee on Labor (March 2, 1993); Clint Willis, "How to Protect Your Retirement Money," *Money* (November 1991): 90–97, 100.

36. President's Commission for the Study of Ethical Problems in Medicine and Biomedical and Behavioral Research, *Securing Access to Health Care: The Ethical Implications of Differences in the Availability of Health Services*, Vol. I (Washington, DC, U.S. Government Printing Office, 1983). Quoted in Audrey Chapman, "The Right to Health Care: Reflections on a Series of Consultations," paper prepared for the AAAS Right to Health Care Project (1993).

37. Uwe E. Reinhardt, "Reorganizing the Financial Flows in American Health Care," *Health Affairs* (Special Supplement 1993): 172–193; Sally T. Burner, Daniel R. Waldo, and David R. McKusick, "National Health Expenditures Projections Through 2030," *Health Care Financing Review* 14(Fall 1992)1–29.

38. *Ibid.*, 19.

39. U.S. Department of the Treasury, *Financing Health and Long-Term Care. Report to the President and to Congress.* (Washington, DC: U.S. Government Printing Office, 1990).

40. Paul Torrens, *The American Health Care System: Issues and Problems*, 92.

41. There may also be a continuation of self-insurance by firms with a very large number of employees.

42. Economic Policy Institute Report, cited in *Health Care Reform Week* (Washington, DC: United Communications Group, May 17, 1993): 4.

43. Financing through a payroll tax would require an additional financing mechanism for early retirees who are not yet eligible for Medicare, and for other individuals under 65 years, who do not work but who have income from other sources.

44. Reported in Spencer Rich, "Payroll Tax-Based Health Plan Backed," *The Washington Post* (May 20, 1993): 20.

45. U.S. General Accounting Office. *Rochester's Community Approach Yields Better Access, Lower Costs.* Report to the Committee on Government Operations, House of Representatives. GAO/HRD-93-44. (Washington, DC: U.S. General Accounting Office, January 29, 1993).

46. There are also major concerns regarding the ability to accurately risk adjust. See Donald W. Light, "The Practice and Ethics of Risk-Related Health Insurance: Caring for the Uninsured and Underinsured," *The Journal of the American Medical Association* (May 13, 1992): 2503–2509.

47. Steven A. Schroeder and Lewis G. Sandy, "Specialty Distribution of U.S. Physicians—The Invisible Driver of Health Care Costs," *New England Journal of Medicine* 328, No.13 (1993): 961–963. See also, Kevin Grumbach and John Fry, "Managing Primary Care in the United States and in the United Kingdom," *New England Journal of Medicine* 328, No. 13 (1993): 940–945.

48. *Ibid.*

49. Paul Starr, *The Logic of Health Care Reform*, (Knoxville, Tenn.: Grand Rounds Press, 1992).

50. Melvin Konner, "We Are Not the Enemy: A Medical Opinion," *Newsweek* (April 5, 1993): 41.

51. John Immerwahr, Jean Johnson, and Adam Kernan-Schloss, *Faulty Diagnosis: Public Misconceptions About Health Care Reform* (New York: The Public Agenda Foundation, 1992).

52. Vicki Kemper and Viveka Novak, "The Great American Health Care Sellout," *The Washington Post* (October 13, 1991): C1.

53. Rep. Bernard Sander, "Guest Observer," *Roll Call* (June 3, 1993): 5.

54. Immerwahr et al., *Faulty Diagnosis.*

55. Public Broadcasting Service program on health care reform (date unknown).

56. Joseph S. Coyle, "Who Wins Under Clinton's Health Care Plan—and Who Loses," *Money* (May 1993): 98–105.

57. Larry Churchill, "Aligning Rights and Responsibilities," paper prepared for the AAAS Right to Health Care Project.

58. Presidents Commission for the Study of Ethical Problems in Medicine and Biomedical and Behavioral Research, *Securing Access to Health Care: the Ethical Implications of Differences in the Availability of Health Services.* Quoted in Audrey Chapman, "The Right to Health Care: Reflections on a Series of Consultations," paper prepared for the AAAS Right to Health Care Project.

59. "GOP Moderates to Clinton: Forget Mandated Employer Coverage," in *Health Care Reform Week* (Washington, D.C.: United Communications Group, May 10, 1993).

60. *Ibid.*

61. Immerwahr, et al., *Faulty Diagnosis: Public Misconceptions About Health Care Reform.*

62. In the U.K. National Health Service, capitation payments cover only those services provided by the general practitioners themselves. Other funds are used to provide specialist services, laboratory tests, and medications. In the U.S., physicians working under capitation contracts must almost always pay for these services out of the capitation fund. Kevin Grumbach and John

Fry, "Managing Primary Care in the United States and in the United Kingdom," 942.

63. Ideological opposition to government intervention in the "free" market is selective; for example, federal patent laws which protect private investment and tax subsidies for research and development are widely supported.

DAN W. BROCK

The President's Commission on the Right to Health Care

There is now a broad public awareness in the United States that we
are the only industrialized country besides South Africa that fails to
ensure access to health care to all its citizens. Some thirty seven million
Americans are without health insurance, and many millions more are
underinsured. Moreover,this failure is not the result of parsimonious
health care spending. Quite to the contrary, we spend a substantially
larger percentage of GDP—over fourteen percent in 1992—on health
care than does any other country. This failure to ensure universal
access to health care is increasingly widely regarded as morally unacceptable, an injustice to those denied access to care. Health care reform
to ensure universal access now appears more likely than it has in two
decades. As the public and political debate over health care reform
intensifies, how we conceptualize the moral claim of individuals to
health care can influence the direction and pace that reform will take.

Perhaps the most influential public study and report on access
to health care that focused on the ethical issues was *Securing Access
to Health Care* issued in 1983 by the President's Commission for the
Study of Ethical Problems in Medicine and Biomedical and Behavioral
Research.[1] An important feature of that report for the present project
exploring a human rights approach to health care is that the Commission explicitly chose to frame its analysis not in terms of moral or
human rights of individuals to health care, but instead in terms of a
societal obligation to insure adequate health care for all.[2] In this essay,
I shall first briefly summarize the Commission's ethical argument and
position regarding access to health care, offer some reasons that I
believe led to the choice of a social obligation, not rights, framework,
and then evaluate the Commission's own arguments for preferring
the language of social obligation. My conclusion will be that it was
both a philosophical and political mistake to use the language of obligation instead of rights—the Commission's own arguments strongly
support a moral or human right to health care, and rights language

has greater political force than the language of societal obligation. Despite my disagreement with this feature of the Commission's study, I believe that both the substance of its argument on access and its work in Chapter Two of its report in bringing together data on access have had a substantial, positive contribution to the public debate.

The Commission's Ethical Argument on Access to Health Care

What gives health care its special importance and makes access to it an ethical issue, a matter of equity or justice? The Commission cited four features. First, health care makes a central contribution to personal well-being "by preventing or relieving pain, suffering, and disability and by avoiding loss of life." (16) Second, health care can protect or restore "a person's opportunities, that is, the array of life plans that it is reasonable to pursue within the conditions obtaining in society." (16) Third, health care has the "ability to relieve worry and to enable patients to adjust to their situation by supplying reliable information about their health." (17) Finally, because all humans are subject to disease and die, health care "has special interpersonal significance: it expresses and nurtures bonds of empathy and compassion. . . and reflects some of [society's] most basic attitudes about what it is to be a member of the human community." (17)

The Commission took these respects in which health care is of special importance to show why health care ought to be fairly or equitably accessible to all, but they do not show what equitable access consists in. It considered three alternative interpretations of equitable access. Equity as equality would require that all persons have access to the same level of health care, that any health care available to some must be available to all. It rejected this interpretation of equity on the grounds that if the equal level was set high it would represent too great a drain on resources, while if it was set low individuals would have to be prohibited from purchasing more or higher quality services with their own resources. Either ethically justified inequalities in income and wealth, or differences in preferences for health care, can result in equitable inequalities in access to health care.

A second understanding of equitable access would be access solely according to benefit or need. This would mean "that everyone must receive all health care that is of any benefit to them." (19) Since health care is not the only good, it would be irrational to provide all beneficial health care without regard for its cost. "Equitable access to health care must take into account not only the benefits of care but also the costs in comparison with other goods and services to which those resources might be allocated." (19)

Instead, the Commission argued that equity should be understood as requiring access to an adequate level of health care, that is, "enough care to achieve sufficient welfare, opportunity, information, and evidence of interpersonal concern to facilitate a reasonably full and satisfying life." (20) This view avoids the difficulties the Commission found with the other two possible meanings of equity. Because an adequate level is not all beneficial care, it acknowledges the need for limits and for setting priorities, and because it is a limited moral requirement, it does not require prohibiting persons from purchasing health care that exceeds that level. The Commission argued as well that equity requires that an adequate level of health care be available to all without imposing excessive burdens on individuals, though again that is not to say that the burdens of securing an adequate level must be equal.

The moral obligation to ensure that everyone has access to an adequate level of health care, the Commission held, falls on society, understood in the broadest sense and as distinct from government. It is a societal and not merely an individual responsibility, most importantly because expensive, uneven, and unpredictable individual needs for care require "some social mechanism for sharing the costs." (23) Moreover, these differences in health care needs are not of a nature for which individuals can reasonably be held responsible. Many individuals will obtain an adequate level of care through health insurance acquired as an employee benefit or purchased in the marketplace, through charity, or through the efforts of state and local governments in subsidizing care for those unable otherwise to secure it. But these three means of securing access have failed to ensure an adequate level of care for all citizens, most importantly because of the high costs of health care and because services are not available in some geographical areas.

Because these other means of securing care have failed to ensure adequate care for all, the Commission argued that "the ultimate responsibility for ensuring that this obligation is met rests with the Federal government." (30) The Federal government "has a major responsibility for making sure that certain basic social goods, such as health care. . . are available to all." (31) The obligation is societally wide, not local, and only the Federal government has the necessary resources, can spread the burdens fairly of ensuring care to all, and can oversee a societal-wide program. The Commission went on to explore how much care is enough to be an "adequate level." It did not seek to specify precisely what care adequacy required, but instead to note the relevant criteria that should inform a public debate and determination of the specific content of adequacy. What is adequate is relative to an individual's health condition, and the overall determination of adequacy will take into account the overall benefits and burdens, interpreting each broadly, of securing different levels of care for all, including the non-health care goods and services that must be foregone to do so. It argued that there was no objectively correct relative importance to be given to these different costs and benefits. Finally, the Commission reviewed several common means for approximating adequacy, such as professional judgment, average current use, and lists of services, noting strengths and weaknesses of each.

This is a broad, though brief, summary of the Commission's central ethical argument about access to health care. It of course leaves out many details of importance. But of special concern here is the Commission's choice to frame its argument in terms of a societal obligation to ensure an adequate level of health care to all, instead of in terms of an individual right to an adequate level, the more familiar terms in which the debate had usually been carried on.[3] The Commission explicitly discussed and defended this choice and I shall address its argument shortly. But first I want to offer some observations by way of explanation of the causes of the Commission's choice, independent of its arguments in defense of the choice.

The Politics of a Report

I served as staff philosopher at the Commission from July 1981 through July 1982, with responsibility for the first draft of the "ethics chapter" of the access report, from the final version of which the summary above was drawn. In late spring another philosopher, Allen Buchanan, who had joined the staff at the beginning of 1982, assumed principal responsibility for this chapter since he would be continuing on staff after I left and through the completion of the access report. The following reasons thus represent in part conclusions I drew from my own experience, as well as from accounts of others, both published and informal, of the process.

The initial draft of the ethics chapter of the access report included an endorsement of a right to health care, while, as already noted, the final version of the report had shifted to endorsement of a societal obligation to secure an adequate level of health care to all, and explicitly rejected the rights approach. Apart from philosophical niceties about the relation of rights and obligations, some of which I will attend to later, why did it matter whether the Commission's position was framed in terms of a societal obligation or an individual right? The fundamental reason is that in the real world of politics and policy in the United States in the 1980s and 90s, the strongest moral claims, and in particular the strongest claims grounded in justice, were and are typically expressed in terms of rights, not obligations.

If people have a moral right to health care, that right grounds a moral claim they have to health care as their due.[4] That right also grounds an obligation on someone to secure that health care for them; in this sense, rights to something ground correlative obligations on someone else to secure, or not interfere with our enjoyment of, that something. If an individual's moral right is not secured, rights language directs our attention to the wrong, and typically as well the harm, done the individual whose right was violated. The right gives its possessor moral standing to demand what is his or hers by right, and if it is not forthcoming to complain that he or she was denied what morality required be secured for him or her. The failure to meet one's obligations, on the other hand, focuses attention on the agent who did not live up to his or her obligations, not the victim of that failure. Human rights, in particular, secure specific senses of equality, the respects in which the equal moral claims of all to particular treatment or goods must be respected.

While it is generally agreed that it is not possible for some people to have moral rights without some other people having correlative moral obligations, not all accounts of obligations are uncontroversially held to entail moral rights. A common example is thought to be the case of charity, to which the Commission made some appeal; it is often thought that we have an obligation to contribute to charity for the needy, but that no particular needy person has a moral right to charity from any specific other person. If so, then in the case of health care it need not follow from the societal obligation to secure an adequate level of health care to all, that individuals have a right to that health care, nor that they have a moral complaint against specific other persons if they cannot obtain adequate health care.

Moreover, while rights are typically taken to be the moral claims of individuals that warrant enforcement, by coercion or force if necessary, not all obligations are believed to warrant coercive enforcement. Finally, some may understand, though mistakenly in my view, that social obligations are only ideals that we should try to live up to, but that no wrong or injustice is done if we fail to realize fully the ideal.

This is not the place to assess in any detail the various philosophical claims about the nature of and relations between moral obligations and rights. My point now is only that in typical philosophical usage, as well as in political and public policy debate, the language of individual rights is employed to express stronger moral claims than the language of social obligations. This is why it mattered, and was understood to matter, whether the Commission endorsed a moral right of individuals to health care, or instead a societal obligation to secure access to health care for all. This is why commentators like Ronald Bayer and John Arras were correct to see the Commission's position as a retreat from the conclusions of previous commissions and commentators that had endorsed a right to health care. I believe the causes of this retreat were multiple, and so in that sense it was overdetermined. What were some of those causes?

First, one must recall the political climate in Washington in late 1981 and 1982 when the Commission was considering the shape its access report would take. This was early in the first Reagan administration when cutting taxes and social programs, while building up military expenditures and capacities, were at the top of the political agenda. In this climate, a proposal for a major new social program which would require major new expenditures would have confronted powerful opposing political currents. The weaker formulation of government responsibility for access to health care fit better the general political tenor of the times.

A second related factor was the replacement of a majority of Commissioners, all of whom had been appointed by a liberal Carter administration, by eight, out of a total of eleven, new Reagan appointees. Unlike some of the Commission's earlier reports, by the time the Commission was making final decisions on the form and content of the access report, the Reagan appointees were a clear majority. With some reports, this turnover in Commissioners had a relatively limited impact. In the report on forgoing life-sustaining treatment, for example, the combination of widespread demands, which cut across most political divisions, for some authoritative guidance on life-sustaining treatment decisions, together with recommendations which required no major new governmental initiatives or expenditures, resulted in recommendations which drew a consensus among Reagan and Carter appointees. But in the access report, responding to the large gaps in access to health care documented in the report would have entailed major new government expenditures and initiatives. This raised for some of the Commissioners the old bogeyman of "socialized medicine" to which they were strongly ideologically opposed.

Morris Abrams, the Chair of the Commission throughout its existence, believed strongly that the influence of the Commission's recommendations depended importantly on reaching consensus on them among all the commissioners. He thus continually pressed hard, some of us believed too hard at times resulting in excessive compromise and muddied instead of sharpened issues for public choice, to seek compromises that might resolve conflicts that developed over what the Commission's position should be. And the report, more than any of the other nine reports, generated such conflicts; it was the only report on which a Commissioner recorded a formal dissent, and there were threats from other Commissioners of dissents on the access report.

These conflicts were played out as well between a largely liberal staff responsible for drafting the report and the largely conservative Commissioners who gave directions to staff on the reports and who had to sign off on the final products. This conflict was deep and became acrimonious at times. Ronald Bayer quotes one staff member, dismayed by the "politicization" of the Commission process, as writing to Alexander Capron, the Commission's Executive Director: "I am sick and tired of wasting time drafting language to cater to the commissioners' ideological biases."[5] At one point several staff members working on the report considered the alternatives of mass resignation or issuing a separate staff report rather than accede to some of the Commissioners' wishes on the report. There was a continuous struggle between Commissioners and staff over the content and tone of this report, a struggle that was not replicated in any of the other reports. Most of the staff working on the report wanted more emphasis on the gaps in access to health care and probably supported some form of national health insurance. Most of the Commissioners, on the other hand, wanted a more positive picture of the existing health care system and less strong calls for any new government initiatives or programs. Ronald Bayer has provided substantial documentation of the sometimes subtle shifts in tone and wording made to satisfy the Commissioners.[6] The final product was a compromise between Commissioners and staff, but the Commissioners were in a strong bargaining position in forging that compromise. I should note, however, that this struggle between staff and commissioners was not principally over whether to frame the Commission's position in terms of rights, indeed some liberal staff opposed doing that (see the third and fourth reasons below), but rather over the overall tenor and political and moral position of the report. But given this larger struggle, a strong push by staff to frame the report in terms of rights to health care would not likely have been successful.

A third factor leading to the societal obligation formulation was a difference within the staff about framing the argument and position in terms of rights to health care. Specifically, Allen Buchanan, who replaced me with principal responsibility for the ethical argument on access, had significantly stronger reservations than I about the philosophical foundations of moral rights generally, and of their role in moral and political philosophy.[7] Buchanan had been a member of a philosophical advisory panel assembled by the Commission's first staff philosopher, Daniel Wikler, and had written a paper on the role of charity in providing health care for the uninsured which had generated significant interest in several of the Commissioners.[8] Substantial controversy remains in moral and political philosophy about the nature of rights, their relations to other moral concepts, how rights claims are to be grounded or justified, and how the more precise content of rights is to be specified. Moreover, it is positive rights, such as the right to health care, which require positive actions of others to satisfy the rights claim, as opposed to negative rights, which require only noninterference by others with the right holder's exercise of the right, that are most philosophically and politically controversial. In the case of positive rights, like a right to health care, how the precise content of the right should be determined is especially controversial.

Buchanan and I disagreed about the relative seriousness of these philosophical problems about rights, as well as about the degree to which these foundational problems were special to moral rights, or were more thorough going problems in ethics and political philosophy more generally. My own view was that there was more philosophical and public consensus on some right to health care, though substantially less consensus on how much health care there is a right to, with libertarianism and libertarians being the major exceptions. (The public consensus on some moral right to health care, however, was probably less broad and deep than it has become today as a result of public and policy debates over the last decade, together with a continued erosion in access to health care over that period.) There clearly is reasonable philosophical disagreement about the philosophical status of rights, but our differences probably led Buchanan to be more sympathetic to alternative formulations of responsibilities on access to health care in non-rights terms.

A fourth reason for the rejection of a rights approach was that from the earliest discussions of the project amongst staff the argument was made that it would be a political mistake to frame the Commission's position in terms of rights. More specifically, it was argued that when politicians and policy makers hear talk of rights to health care, they understand this to mean an unlimited legal entitlement to health care. In part, this results from a confusion between legal and moral rights, a point I shall return to in the next section. Since the Commission, including both the commissioners and staff, wanted to argue for a limited moral claim to health care, a claim to have access to an adequate level of health care, some staff believed that the rights formulation would be misleading about the nature of the Commission's position, and would thereby generate unnecessary opposition to the report. Regardless of explicit qualifications of any right as a limited right, it was concluded, many readers would hear an unlimited legal entitlement and therefore oppose the Commission's conclusions. There was and remains disagreement amongst staff about the likelihood and extent of this potential misunderstanding of the Commission's position if it had been framed in terms of rights. But the form of argument was not, I believe, illegitimate. It is appropriate for a public commission to consider how best to frame its position so as to enable it to move forward successfully in the political and policy process; how philosophers writing for an academic audience believe the argument is correctly framed is another matter and not a public commission's concern.

In sum then, there were multiple forces converging to produce a position framed not in terms of a moral right to health care, but rather as a societal obligation to ensure access to an adequate level of health care for all. (The latter formulation was perceived, whether correctly or not, to be weaker than the moral right to health care position). These multiple forces concern the empirical question of what were some of the main causes of the Commission rejecting the formulation of a moral right to health care. Whatever they may be, I want to turn now to evaluate the explicit reasons the Commission offered for rejecting the rights formulation.

A Moral Right to Health Care?

The Commission offered three reasons for rejecting a moral right to health care and I shall examine each in turn. The first reason was that "such a right is not legally or Constitutionally recognized at the present time. . . Neither the Supreme Court nor any appellate court has found a constitutional right to health or health care." (32, 33) On the face of it, this appears simply to be a confusion between moral and legal rights. While different commentators and theorists disagree about the nature and grounds of moral rights claims, as well as the criteria for determining which moral rights, if any, people in fact have, no one defends the position that a necessary condition of having a moral right is that such a right also be recognized as a legal right in some jurisdiction. That would make moral rights contingent on the vagaries of political and judicial processes in a way that no defender of moral rights believes them to be.

In political philosophy, at least some moral rights are considered to exist prior to governments and are not derived from any government action, but instead should guide and constrain legitimate government action. A particular moral right might not be acknowledged in law at all in a particular society at a particular time; for example, the moral right to equal respect and concern, and some more restricted right to freedom, were denied to slaves in the United States in the 19th Century. Other moral rights are only partially acknowledged in law; for example, as is true in the United States today according to those who believe that the moral right not to be killed does not permit capital punishment. On some theories of legal interpretation, most notably that of Ronald Dworkin, the proper interpretation of certain legal rights, such as the equal protection clause of the Fourteenth Amendment to the U.S. Constitution, involves appeal to an underlying moral right on which the legal right is based, in this example the right to equal respect and concern according to Dworkin.[9] But even supposing that some legal rights depend on underlying moral rights, that does not imply that a moral right presupposes an analogous legal right.

This first argument of the Commission then seems irrelevant to what is at issue, whether there is a moral right to health care. Moreover, if the question is whether there is a specifically human right to health care, the existence of a legal right is irrelevant as well. Most accounts of the nature and grounds of human rights take them to be one species of moral right, and all such accounts agree that the existence of human rights does not depend on prior legal recognition in any particular jurisdiction. Quite to the contrary, one central function of human rights, like moral rights generally, is to criticize the law at any particular time and place, and they could not play this role if their existence depended on prior legal recognition.

One possible explanation of the Commission's appeal to what appears an obviously irrelevant consideration is that Commission Chair Morris Abrams expressed the concern in hearings that if the Commission were explicitly to argue that there was a moral right to health care, this might be taken, even if mistakenly, by either courts or legislatures to be the same as, or the basis for finding, a legal right to health care.[10] Whether or not such a confusion was likely, it would have been a confusion that the Commission could have explicitly warned against, while arguing for a moral right to health care. To the extent that an argument for a moral right to health care might have been taken by legislatures as a reason, though not necessarily a sufficient reason, for enacting a legal right to health care, there would have been no confusion between moral and legal rights, but this possibility is no reason to believe there is not a moral right to health care.

The second reason the Commission offered for not formulating its position in terms of a right to health care was that such a right "is not a logical corollary of an ethical obligation of the type the Commission has enunciated." (32) There is a sense in which this claim is quite correct. As I have already noted, while moral philosophers are generally in agreement that moral rights do logically entail the existence of correlative obligations, for example a person's right not to be killed entails an obligation of others not to kill him or her, many believe that at least some ethical obligations do not entail a correlative right of the potential beneficiary of the fulfillment of the obligation. The Commission noted that there is more than one sense of the term "obligation" and that "[I]n the broad sense, to say that society has a moral obligation to do something is to say that it ought morally to do that thing and that failure to do it makes the society liable to serious moral criticism. This does not, however, mean that there is a corresponding right. For example, a person may have a moral obligation to help those in need, even though the needy cannot, strictly speaking, demand that person's aid as something they are due." (34) One basis on which this distinction between types of obligations is traditionally made is Immanuel Kant's distinction between perfect and imperfect duties.[11] Roughly, perfect duties morally require one to do the required action whenever the opportunity arises, whereas imperfect duties allow some exceptions based on one's own interests or inclinations. My imperfect obligation to aid the needy entails that I am morally required to aid the needy, but I have some discretion about which needy persons I aid. There are more needy people than I could provide significant aid to and if I were required to aid every needy person I could, this duty would consume all my efforts and life. This implies that I am not obligated to aid any specific needy person, nor could any specific needy person claim of me that I am morally required to aid him. I could have fulfilled my obligation by aiding some other needy person(s) and then neither he nor anyone else would have any unfulfilled moral claim to my aid, nor would anyone have any complaint that I had not fulfilled my obligation since, by hypothesis, I had. A perfect obligation to others, by contrast, requires the specific action on all occasions in which it could be performed, and so is owed to all specific persons regarding whom it could be done.

Could an argument analogous to the Commission's regarding the needy justify the Commission's claim that the societal obligation to ensure access to an adequate level of health care for all its members entails neither a right to health care of those members, nor that they could claim health care "as something they are due?" The nature of that obligation shows that it could not. The moral obligation the Commission defends is a societal obligation, presumably meaning it is assigned to society as whatever kind of collective organization or group a society is. And it is an obligation to ensure access to an adequate level of health care for all of its members. There is only one entity that has this obligation, the collective society, and each and every member of the society is required by that obligation to have access to an adequate level of health care. Thus, if some members of the society lack that access, there is no alternative individual or group besides the society who could be turned to instead as having a similar obligation. Moreover, since the obligation is not to provide access to some of its members, but to all of its members, if some members lack access, it cannot be the case that the society has fulfilled its obligation. There is none of the discretion or indeterminacy necessary for this to be an imperfect obligation, and so this cannot be the reason for claiming that the societal obligation entails no right to health care of its members. There might be other possible reasons for denying that the societal obligation entails a corresponding right, but the Commission does not offer any, and the one specific analogy it offers of an obligation entailing no right is not analogous and so fails to apply to the right to health care.

It is also worth noting that the Commission's assertion that society's members cannot claim access to health care from the society "as something they are due," is misleading as well. Sometimes moral claims to something we are "due" are claims of desert, claims that we deserve something as a result of something else that we have done; for example, you deserve some good thing like a prize because your performance is the best according to the rules of the competition, or you deserve a bad thing like punishment because you acted in a way prohibited by criminal law. But not all rights are grounded in a moral claim of desert for something we have done. One feature of human rights is precisely that they are not grounded in any such claim of desert for something an individual has done. They are not things people must earn by doing something, but rather moral statuses all people have simply in so far as they are human. Being human is sufficient to be due the particular treatment or benefit that a human right assigns us, in this case an adequate level of health care.

There is another sense in which individuals may make moral claim to a thing "as something they are due." We may use this formulation to indicate not that we deserve that thing because of what we have done, but to indicate that we are morally "due" or owed that thing from a particular individual(s), but not from others or just anybody, as a result of something they have done, for example promised to provide us with that thing or negligently harmed us and so now owe us that thing as compensation. To the extent that this is what the Commission intended by the language of what individuals are due, the reasons it offered for why this is an obligation specifically of society, and ultimately falling to the federal government, answers why access to health care is due individuals by society, or the federal government. In sum, the Commission has given us no good reason why the societal obligation to ensure an adequate level of health care is an obligation from which no right to health care follows. In the final section of this paper, I shall briefly suggest that such a right does follow from the Commission's argument for a societal obligation.

The third reason the Commission offered for not formulating its position in terms of a right to health care was that such a right

> is not necessary as a foundation for appropriate governmental actions to secure adequate health care for all. . . . [T]here are many forms of government involvement, such as enforcement of traffic rules or taxation to support national defense, to protect the environment or to promote biomedical research, that do not presuppose corresponding moral rights but that are nonetheless legitimate and almost universally recognized as such. In a democracy, at least, the people may assign to government the responsibility for seeing that important collective obligations are met, provided that doing so does not violate important moral rights. (33–4)

The Commission here is quite correct that many legitimate government activities, assigned to the government through democratic political procedures, do not, and need not, presuppose any moral right of the beneficiaries of these activities that the government undertake them. Moreover, it has offered, in my view, a persuasive moral argument why the society, acting through the government, morally ought to ensure that all its members have access to an adequate level of health care, and that argument makes no explicit appeal to a moral right to health care. To this extent, I have no quarrel with the third reason the Commission offered for its societal obligation formulation. (Its appeal to legal decisions protecting program beneficiaries from discrimination in existing public programs, including health care programs, could also be understood as supplementing a societal obligation argument, in effect arguing that such programs, once established, may commit the government to broader, perhaps societally wide efforts, though I will not pursue such a line of argument here.)

So long as the government morally must ensure adequate health care for all, why should it matter at all if there is also an individual moral right to health care of all members of society? If the societal obligation were fully equivalent in meaning to the individual right then to assert one would be equivalent to asserting the other; but they are not equivalent as the Commission itself insists and as I have suggested above, though precisely what the differences in meaning and implications are is philosophically controversial. I suggested above as well that the apparent differences between the Commission's use of "societal moral obligation" and the usual understanding of "individual moral right" make the latter the stronger moral claim, the claim that better recognizes the moral status of the victim of a failure to fulfill the obligation or respect the right.

It is a separate point, but important here as well, that the moral claim of all members of society to a right to health care tends to have greater rhetorical force and practical impact in political and policy contexts than does the claim of a societal obligation to ensure adequate health care for all. This might not be the case in all societies. In more communitarian societies, inhospitable to individualistic claims of individual moral rights and in which political debate is typically carried on in terms of societal responsibilities, societal obligation claims could have greater rhetorical force and practical impact in political and policy contexts. But in our own society, at this time in history, claims of moral rights nearly always have greater force in political argument, and greater potential for influencing practice and policy, as both the opponents and proponents of a right to health care, at the Commission and elsewhere, recognize and acknowledge. There is an important question then for how the Commission's argument about justice in health care should be formulated. Is their argument sufficient to establish a right to health care, even granting the Commission's claim that a moral case for the government ensuring adequate health care for all could also be established by its societal obligation argument? I shall briefly address this issue below. Even if the Commission's argument is inadequate to establish a right to health care, there may be other arguments which are capable of doing so, though what they might be is beyond the scope of my concern in this paper.[12] The last point the Commission offers in favor of its societal obligation approach is that an argument carried on merely in terms of assertions and refutations of a right to health care will be incapable of guiding policy. "[T]he nature of the right must be made clear and competing accounts of it compared and evaluated. Moreover, if claims of rights are to guide policy they must be supported by sound ethical reasoning and the connections between various rights must be systematically developed, especially where rights are potentially in conflict with one another." (34–5) These claims raise difficult and controversial issues about the role of moral philosophy and moral reasoning in public policy and in political deliberation, and about justification which cannot be pursued here. But the lack of persuasiveness of the Commission's claim that these considerations favor its societal obligation approach, can be most readily seen by simply substituting "societal obligation," as the Commission used it in its own broader argument, for "rights" in each of difficulties the Commission claims above for the argument framed in terms of rights. Whatever difficulties exist in specifying precise content, relative moral weight, and underlying ethical justification, for a right to health care, exist equally for a societal obligation to ensure access to health care for all, if either is to guide policy. There is no reason here for preferring the societal obligation approach.

A Right or A Social Obligation?

While the Commission did not conclude from its argument for a societal obligation to ensure access to adequate health care for all that there is also a right to health care, such a conclusion might, nonetheless, and I believe does, follow from its argument. There is space here to indicate only very briefly why that is so. As noted earlier, it is common in accounts of rights to distinguish negative rights, generally rights to noninterference by others, such as a right not to be killed, from positive rights, generally rights that require positive actions by others, such as a right to shelter or personal security. There is a consensus among nearly all moral and political theorists that moral or human rights go beyond negative rights and include some positive rights as well; the principal exceptions to this consensus are libertarians, who usually understand basic rights to include only negative rights.[13]

The common thread in different theories of moral or human rights is that those rights are to ensure the basic conditions necessary for a decent human life. It is because ensuring these conditions can require positive actions on the part of others, not just that others not interfere with us, that these theories typically include positive as well as negative rights. Defending a right to health care then will require showing that access to adequate health care is one of these fundamental conditions necessary for a decent human life. That is exactly the sort of argument the Commission provided in its account of the features of health care that give it special importance—its far-reaching effects on individual's well-being, opportunity, preservation of life, ability to plan, and security that we are the object of concern of others. Thus, personal security, shelter, and nutrition are also included in typical accounts of basic moral or human rights because they too have analogous, though different, special importance. They are what John Rawls called primary goods, necessary conditions for pursuing virtually any particular plan of life we may have.[14] Health care, at least basic health care, too has this fundamental role as a primary social good; without it, serious disease and illness impair our ability to pursue our goals and plans, whatever they may be. In the Commission's own words characterizing adequate health care, it is "enough care to achieve sufficient welfare, opportunity, information, and evidence of interpersonal concern to facilitate a reasonably full and satisfying life." (20)

Now a skeptic about rights to health care still might ask why there is a moral or human right to a good that has this special importance, whether it be health care or food, shelter, and personal security. Different moral and political theories will answer this skeptic in different ways, but what may be most important for political practice and public policy is that there is what John Rawls has called an "overlapping consensus" among these different theories that there is such a right.[15] Moreover, the proponent of a right to health care can correctly note that an exactly analogous skeptical question can be raised regarding the Commission's approach, why is there a societal obligation to ensure that all have access to a good with this special importance? The rights proponent is at no special disadvantage in answering this skeptic. As already noted, this still leaves both the rights and societal obligation accounts with the task of specifying the more precise content of an adequate level of health care, of distinguishing the different relative importance of different health care, of specifying the importance of this health care relative to other social goods, and of specifying the institutions and social programs that would ensure access to an adequate level of care for all. My point is that the rights approach is at no special disadvantage, in comparison with the societal obligation approach, in any of these tasks.

I want to conclude with a brief speculation about whether, in hindsight, the argument appears to have been correct that the Commission's asserting a right to health care would be less effective in practical policy terms than asserting a societal obligation to ensure access to adequate health care. My own view is that this claim was mistaken. I believe the Commission's ethical argument about access to health care has had some, but rather limited, influence on policy debates about health care reform over the last decade. It was not necessary to abandon the right to health care in favor of the societal obligation approach to make clear that there must be limits to what health care people should have access to. The Commission could have explicitly emphasized that a right to health care was a limited right, and the dominant importance that cost containment has come to have in our debates about health care reform would have ensured recognition that this must be a limited right in any case. Just because our strongest moral claims are typically expressed as rights claims, I believe the Commission could have contributed more effectively to the emerging consensus that access to health care must be ensured for all by defending a moral right of all to access to an adequate level of health care. In hindsight, it may well be that the Commission's most important contribution to building that consensus over the last decade was to bring together the data and evidence that has fostered greater public awareness of the magnitude of our failure to ensure access for all to an adequate level of health care.

NOTES

1.   President's Commission for the Study of Ethical Problems in Medicine and Biomedical and Behavioral Research, *Securing Access to Health Care* (Washington, DC: U.S. Governments Printing Office, 1983). All parenthetical pages references in the text to the Commission are to this report.

2.   Two of the best critical evaluations of the President's Commission's study of access to health care, to which I am much indebted here, are Ronald Bayer, "Ethics, Politics, and Access to Health Care: A Critical Analysis of the President's Commission for the Study of Ethical Problems in Medicine and Biomedical and Behavioral Research," *Cardozo Law Review* 6 (1984) 303–20, concentrating on the political issue and John D. Arras, "Retreat from the Right to Health Care: The President's Commission and Access to Health Care," *Cardozo Law Review* 6 (1984) 321–45, concentrating on the philosophical and ethical issues. My critical evaluation in Section III of this paper of the Commission's reasons for preferring a societal obligation instead of a rights approach is very similar to Arras' critique.

3.   For example, as the Commission noted: "In 1952, the President's Commission on Health Care Needs of the Nation concluded that 'access to the means for the attainment and preservation of health is a basic human right'."

4.   A good source of some of the philosophical literature on rights is Jeremy Waldron, ed., *Theories of Rights* (Oxford: Oxford University Press, 1984). On human rights see *Social Philosophy & Policy* 1, 2 (Spring 1984), the entire issue of which is devoted to human rights.

5.   Bayer, *op. cit.* 314.

6.   Bayer, *op. cit.*

7.   Allen E. Buchanan, "What's So Special About Rights?" *Social Philosophy & Policy* 2, 1 (Autumn 1984) 61–83.

8.   Other members of that panel were Allen Buchanan, Norman Daniels, David Gauthier, Alan Gibbard, Sidney Morganbesser, and myself (before I joined the Commission staff).

9.   Ronald Dworkin, *A Matter of Principle* (Cambridge: Harvard University Press, 1985).

10.   Abrams questioned extensively one witness, a law professor who had been invited to testify on a different issue, about whether the courts had ever held that there was a constitutional right to health care.

11.   Immanuel Kant, *Groundwork of the Metaphysics of Morals*, translated and analysed by H. J. Paton (New York: Harper & Row, 1964).

12.   See Norman Daniels, *Just Health Care* (Cambridge: Cambridge University Press, 1984).

13.   Robert Nozick, *Anarchy, State, and Utopia* (New York: Basic Books, 1974).

14.   John Rawls, *A Theory of Justice* (Cambridge: Harvard University Press, 1971).

15.   John Rawls, "The Idea of an Overlapping Consensus," *Oxford Journal for Legal Studies* 1 (1987) 1–25, and "Justice as Fairness: Political not Metaphysical," *Philosophy & Public Affairs* 14, 3 (1985) 223–51.

PART TWO

Health Care as a Human Right

VIRGINIA A. LEARY

Defining the Right to Health Care

Two contradictory and seemingly irreconcilable approaches to the concept of a "right to health care" presently co-exist in the United States. In the debate over health care reform, we hear, on the one hand, demands for a "right to health care" and, on the other hand, statements that demands for a "right to health care" are simply rhetorical, lacking in substantive content, are diversionary and fail to address the practical problems in the delivery of health care. Some commentators reject the concept of a "right to health care" on the grounds that it implies a "socialistic" approach which is incompatible with the prevailing American free market economy.

I argue in this paper that a rights based approach to health care should be adopted as the fundamental premise of a reformed health care system in the United States, rather than a market-based approach or a cost-benefit approach or an "ethical obligations" approach. The adoption of the premise of a right to health care would not resolve all the problems concerning health care in the United States, but such a premise would set the parameters within which practical decisions are made by providing goals, orientation and permissible limitations.

In his discussion of Medicare, Theodore Marmor has pointed out that "the United States legislated substantial extensions of the government's role in financing health care during the mid 1960s, but did so with only the vaguest clarity about its underlying rationale. . . Without understanding what right Medicare was to insure, the American public has been uncertain throughout over whether the program was a success or failure."[1] Canada focused on basic principles before deciding on the details of its present health care system. The report of the Canadian Royal Commission on Health Services, which led to the adoption of the present health care system in Canada, opened with a Section on "Basic Concepts." These basic concepts have provided guidance in the practical working out of that system which, despite stresses, has, to general agreement, provided equal access to medical care for all Canadians.[2]

Unless we think through our basic premises for a reformed health care system in the United States, we will adopt piecemeal reforms without clarity as to our ultimate aims. Ronald Dworkin has recently pointed out that very little attention had been given (to the date of his writing, December 1993) to the "profound issue" which arises in proposals for reform of the American health care system, namely, the issue of justice or fairness.[3] Issues of cost-containment and economics had dominated the discussion. The concept of a right to health care places issues of fairness, social justice and equity at center-stage in the reform of the health care system. Implications of such a right are further developed in later sections of this paper.

Differing Approaches to the Right to Health Care

Calls for "a right to health care" have come largely from public groups concerned with health care reform, philosophers, religious groups, ethicists and political figures. The 1991 campaign of Harris Wofford of Pennsylvania for election to the United States Senate focused political attention on the public demand for a reform of the United States health care system. Commentators attributed his successful campaign in large part to his emphasis on deficiencies in the American health care system. His campaign statement, "If criminals have a right to a lawyer, working Americans have a *right* to a doctor"[4] was widely quoted. Wofford is not the only political figure using the language of "rights" with regard to health care. John J. LaFalce, Congressman from the 32nd Congressional District in Erie County, New York, and Chairman of the House Small Business Committee, recently sent constituents "A Special Report" on Health Care in America headed by this phrase in bold type, "Health Care Should Be a Right not a Privilege."[5]

American Catholic Bishops issued a pastoral letter in 1981 affirming that every person has a basic right to adequate health care regardless of economic, social or legal status.[6] The Gray Panthers have been stirring up interest in health care reform for years with the slogan "Health Care is a Right". In a recent book on *The Right to Health Care*, philosophers Tom L. Beauchamp, Alan E. Buchanan and Norman Daniels wrote that they found value in the concept of the "right to health care" while expressing the need for detailed implications of such a right.[7] In the same volume, Robert M. Veatch puts forth a concept of health care based on an egalitarian theory of justice which closely approximates the concept of a "right to health care."[8]

Doubts as to the usefulness of the concept of a "right to health care" have been expressed primarily by health care professionals and economists as well as by some philosophers. Although some health care professionals support a "right to health care," those who are less sympathetic to the concept tend to focus on practical solutions to health care delivery and—when referring to fundamental principles— prefer the terms "equity" and "justice" rather than "rights."

Some perceive a "socialist" economic orientation in the term "right to health care" and reject the concept on ideological grounds. Thomas J. Bole views the "free-wheeling rhetoric of rights to health care" as "largely baseless" and suggests that the concept may appear to authorize "the coercive redistribution of individuals' resources."[9] He considers the concept of a right to health care as conceivably limiting the property rights of those whose resources will be used to promote care. The free-market approach to health care is also regarded favorably by H. Tristram Engelhardt, Jr., David Friedman and Hans-Martin Sass.[10]

During sessions of the 1992 consultation on the right to health care organized by the American Association for the Advancement of Science, Janet O'Keeffe questioned whether the language of rights would be effective or even useful in the effort to bring about major health care reforms and pointed out that, while the language of rights is popular, rights issues are rarely mentioned at the policy level where financing decisions are made.[11] Dr. H. Jack Geiger, who has long worked to bring health care to the less fortunate, contended, at the same consultation, that the establishment of a right to health care is of no functional consequence in the United States and that discussion concerning it diverts attention from the most important issues in health care reform.[12]

In 1983, the President's Commission for the Study of Ethical Problems in Medicine and Biomedical and Behavioral Research published their report entitled *Securing Access to Health Care*, explicitly rejecting the concept of a right to health care as an ethical basis for reforms of the health care system. In 1952, the President's Commission on the Health Needs of the Nation, stated that "access to the means for the attainment and preservation of health is a basic human right," but the 1983 Commission stated in its report that "it believes its conclusions are better expressed in terms of 'ethical obligations'" rather than rights.[13] The members of the 1983 Commission concluded that society has a moral obligation to achieve equity in health care, but stated that they had "chosen not to develop the case for achieving equitable access through the assertion of a right to health care."[14]

The Commission's rejection of the right to health care appears to have been based, in part, on the fact that such a right is not protected by the United States Constitution. Its discussion of the right to health care has been characterized as "very obscure."[15] Baruch A. Brody has pointed out that the distinction which the Commission makes between "a right to health care," which they reject, and "the social obligation to provide health care" which they favor is not supported by their argumentation. He remarks that the Commission's explanation that society has an obligation to provide health care but an individual would not have a right to that care seems "particularly inappropriate":

> If, as the Commission believes, society has an obligation to pro-
> vide some level of health care to all of the indigent, then it would
> seem that, as a correlative to that obligation, the group of the
> indigent have a right, which they hold against society as a whole,
> that that health care be provided. In short, it seems, contrary to
> the opinion of the Commission, that if the Commission is right
> about the ethical obligation to provide health care, then it is
> wrong about the existence of the correlative right to the health
> care in question.[16]

Brody suggests that, either the Commission reasoned badly on this whole topic, or that it found it "politically expedient" to make its case without resorting to the language of a right to health care. He favors the latter hypothesis.[17] During the 1980s, the concept of economic and social rights was not favored by the prevailing social philosophy of the Reagan Administration. In its approach to international human rights, the Administration rejected the concept of such rights, which include the right to health care, to education, to housing, and so on.

Largely missing from discussions concerning a "right to health care"—and surprisingly so —are representatives of the legal profession. Few lawyers or law professors have participated in the debate over the "right to health care."[18] The failure of the legal profession to address the subject of health care may be attributed to the fact that, unlike such rights as those relating to freedom of religion, freedom of speech and of the press and the right to fair trial, the right to health care is not among the rights protected by the Bill of Rights, the first ten amendments to the United States Constitution. There is indeed, as the 1983 President's Commission pointed out, no constitutionally recognized right to health care in the United States,[19] and only a limited statutory right for certain categories of persons.[20] Legal practitioners apply the law "on the books" and it is thus not surprising that they have not resorted to the concept of "a right to health care" which is, thus far, not a legal right in the United States. The failure of law professors to address the conceptual questions involved is less explicable, particularly in view of the numerous philosophical writings on the subject.

It has frequently been pointed out that the rights approach of the United States Constitution is based on an individualistic, liberal tradition in which social rights such as the right to health care have no place.[21] The framers of the American Declaration of Independence and the Bill of Rights of the Constitution used rights language—as we do today—to support demands for ending practices they deemed violative of human dignity. The language of rights has been used throughout American history in the battle against racism and sexism. If the language of rights is now being extended to include economic and social rights, it is because of a conviction that widespread poverty, homelessness, and a lack of health care are violative of basic human dignity, and rights language seems particularly powerful in the fight against them.

Social rights are not yet legal rights in the United States; they may someday become so as they have in many other countries. At the January 1992 annual meeting of the American Association of Law Schools—a meeting attended by hundreds of law professors—the plenary session was devoted to the subject, "Do we Need a New Economic Bill of Rights in the United States." The subject of economic and social rights—including the right to health care—is on the American agenda today. As moral rights—not yet legal rights— they are already invoked by many as a criterion for judging our treatment of social issues.

International Perspectives

The authors of a 1989 article in *The New England Journal of Medicine* observed that "Americans have no right to health care. In this respect we stand almost alone among the industrialized nations of the world."[22] It is striking that discussions of health care reform in the United States devote little or no attention to the concept of the right to health or health care in international instruments or in the constitutions or legislation of other countries.[23]

The controversy over the existence of a "right to health care" is largely absent in international organizations and in countries other than the United States. It is commonly assumed that such a right exists; it is enshrined in international conventions and national constitutions. The term "right to health," however, is more commonly used in other countries and in international legal instruments than the "right to health care." The latter is considered one aspect of the more inclusive concept of a "right to health." The terminology "right to health" is widely used in international human rights literature. In 1978, the prestigious Academy of International Law at The Hague organized a workshop on "The Right to Health as a Human Right"[24] and a recent scholarly publication of the Pan-American Health Organization (PAHO) is entitled, "The Right to Health in the Americas."[25] The "right to health" in this context is taken to include more than a right to health care; it relates to issues of health status as well as health care. The phrase "right to health," however, has been criticized since it is considered as implying that the government or some individual or group can guarantee good health, a manifest physical impossibility since no organization or person can do so. Yet the term as used in international instruments, legal writing and national constitutions and laws does not imply the impossible guarantee of good health; rather, it is a shorthand expression used instead of longer, more explicit and comprehensive statements relating to health care and health status. By encompassing health status it emphasizes that the health of individuals depends on factors such as adequate nutrition, clean water, adequate living conditions as well as on the provision of medical care.[26]

The authors of the PAHO publication, referred to previously, favored the terminology "the right to health protection" as a more explicit and precise terminology than the "right to health." They, nevertheless, opted for the term "Right to Health" as the title of their volume since it has become the more common international human rights terminology.[27]

The Constitution of the World Health Organization (WHO) contains a longer statement than the brief phrases "right to health" or "right to health protection." It states that "[t]he enjoyment of the highest attainable standard of health is one of the fundamental rights of every human being without distinction of race, religion, political belief, economic and social conditions." The WHO reiterated the assertion that health is a fundamental human right in the important Declaration of Alma-Ata, adopted at an international conference in 1978. Paragraph I of the Declaration reads,

> The Conference strongly reaffirms that health, which is a state of complete physical, mental and social wellbeing, and not merely the absence of disease or infirmity, is a fundamental human right. . . .[28]

Although the right to health care does not appear in the American Constitution or statutory law, the United States has committed itself to the concept as a member of the WHO. The Declaration of Alma-Ata adopts primary health care as an objective of WHO and its member States and provides that primary health care should be made "universally accessible to individuals and families in the community through their full participation and at a cost that the community and country can afford to maintain. . . " (Paragraph VI)

The International Covenant on Economic, Social and Cultural Rights (ICESCR) uses language similar to that of the WHO Constitution in committing ratifying States to "recognize the right of everyone to the highest attainable standard of physical and mental health" (Article 12). It provides that the steps to be taken by States Parties should include ". . . (c) the creation of conditions which would assure to all medical service and medical attention in the event of sickness." The Convention on the Right of the Child contains similar language. The phrase "right to health" in international instruments should thus be considered as encompassing the right to health care.[29]

Neither the International Covenant on Economic, Social and Cultural Rights nor the Convention on the Rights of the Child have been ratified by the United States, although both have been ratified by more than 100 countries, including the United Kingdom, France, Canada and Italy—all countries whose health systems, despite problems, provide minimum adequate health care to their citizens. At the World Conference on Human Rights in Vienna in June 1993, the new United States administration signaled a changed approach to the concept of economic and social rights by expressing strong support for the Covenant and the administration's intention to seek Senate advice and consent to ratification of the Covenant.[30] The ratification of the Covenant by the United States will constitute a binding legal commitment to the right to health, as well as other economic and social rights.

The United States voted for, and has consistently expressed support for, the Universal Declaration of Human Rights, adopted by the United Nations General Assembly in 1948, which provides in Article Twenty Five that "Everyone has the right to a standard of living adequate for the health and well-being of himself and of his family, including food, clothing, housing and medical care and necessary social services. . . ." While not a legally binding treaty, the Universal Declaration has great moral force and many of its provisions are now considered to be customary international law.

Many countries have adopted a right to health or health protection or health care as a basic premise of their health system. The Canadian Royal Commission which first proposed the adoption of the present universal health care system in Canada cited the language of the WHO Constitution as establishing one of the fundamental principles of a Canadian universal health care system. The PAHO publication on the Right to Health in the Americas contains information on the many countries in the Western Hemisphere which refer to the right to health in their constitutions.

Inadequate Alternatives

Invocations of a right to health care may, of course, be only political slogans or rhetorical statements with little content. Even as such, they give voice to the conviction that a different approach to heath care is required in the United States. But the expression of a right to health care should mean more than a mere slogan. In this section of the paper, I suggest some of the implications of a health based system as compared with two other prevalent approaches to health care (1) the market approach and (2) the cost-benefit approach. For reasons of limitation of space, these approaches, as well as the rights approach, are necessarily sketched briefly here, without extensive elaboration.

The market-perspective or market-orientation approach to health care regards health care primarily as a commodity to be marketed as any other good and not as a public good to be distributed equitably to all. In an essay entitled "Should Medicine be a Commodity?" David Friedman supports this approach,

In the course of this essay, I have attempted to make plausible a thesis many readers will find absurd—that health care should be provided entirely on the private market, just as shoes and potato chips are now provided. . . the market is, generally speaking, the best set of institutions we know of for producing and distributing things. The more important a good is, the stronger the argument for having it produced by the market. . . My conclusion is that there is no good reason to expect governmental involvement in the medical market, either the extensive involvement that now exists or the still more extensive involvement that many advocate, to produce desirable results."[31]

We have recently been reminded of the prevalence of this approach to health care in the United States. Arnold S. Relman graphically outlined the "new market-oriented health system marked by the rapid expansion of investor-owned medical facilities, free-standing centers for ambulatory surgery, sophisticated high-technology radiologic services, diagnostic laboratory services and investor-owned health maintenance organizations." He concluded that "[w]hat we see now is a market-oriented health care system spinning out of control. . . ."

The focus of Relman's lecture was on the unfortunate consequences of this market-orientation on persons in the health care professions who have traditionally regarded themselves as professionals in a service occupation and not as vendors in a business. In his view, health professionals should not only be competent and compassionate practitioners, "but also avoid ties with the health care market. . . ." He remarked, "If the present organization and incentives of our health care system make it difficult or impossible for us to practice in this way (and I believe they do), then we must join with others in examining ways of reforming the system."

Relman also cited other deficiencies of the market-oriented approach to health care, in addition to the high cost and the effect on medical practitioners. He pointed out that "[a]t least 15 percent of Americans have no health insurance and probably at least an equal number are inadequately or only intermittently insured. After all, a system that functions as a competitive marketplace has no more interest in subsidizing the uninsured poor than in restricting the revenues generated by services to those who are insured."[32]

The cost-benefit approach is the most common approach to social issues in the United States today.[33] Economic considerations—monetary calculations of costs and benefits—play a major role in this approach, although an attempt is made to take account of non-tangible benefits by giving them a quantitative value. This approach entails a presumption that an act should generally not be undertaken unless its benefits outweigh its costs. It may be considered an economic aspect of utilitarian social theory that suggests that the greatest good of the greatest number should be the guiding moral principle in making social choices.[34] The good of society in general prevails in this approach over the individual and his or her rights.

The current emphasis on cost containment in medical care and the concept of rationing of medical care tend to lend support to a cost-benefit analysis. The result is often a de-emphasis on the rights of individuals or a minority group in the name of the greater good of society in general. It has been often noted that cost-benefit analyses and rationing systems result in arbitrary discrimination against certain groups; the costs may be borne by one group and the greater benefits enjoyed by another group. The Oregon State system of rationing has been rightly criticized for discrimination against the poor.[35]

The utilitarian and cost-benefit approach to social issues, however, often includes an ethical orientation and has much to recommend it. We do not need to be reminded that controlling costs is an important issue in health care reform. Even if a rights-based approach is adopted, issues of costs must be weighed in many decisions. But as a fundamental or even major premise for the reform of our health system, it is deficient in its failure to emphasize and protect the dignity of individuals and minorities. Some social policies should be adopted because they are morally right and cannot be solely judged on the basis of cost-benefit analysis, particularly those conducive to greater respect for the individual person. The recent emphasis on increasing opportunities for the disabled and making public accommodations more suitable for them is an example of a morally right act which entails general costs for the community. Protecting workers from carcinogenic substances in the workplace entails extra costs for enterprises. Issues of costs are, obviously, not totally unimportant considerations in the adoption of these measures, but they should not be the primary focus. Societal measures to assist the disabled are increasingly based on a concept of the rights of the disabled, as measures for the safety and health of workers are increasingly based on conceptions of a right to health protection, rather than on utilitarian or cost-benefit analysis.

The emphasis on cost-containment and on rationing in health care is based on the perception of very limited resources for the allocation of health care. But the problem is, to an extent, one of priorities. Over-utilization of certain non-essential medical examinations, unnecessary surgical interventions and excessive expenditure on administration are most frequently cited as refuting the perception that only very limited resources are available for equitable apportionment of health care.

Health Care as a Right

How does a rights-based approach differ from the two methods previously outlined? Above all, treating health care as a human right means regarding the dignity of the individual and social justice as primary concerns. The rights-based approach also considers health care as a public good because of its importance for the life and dignity of the individual and not simply as a commodity to be allocated solely by market forces. This view also stresses the importance of non-discrimination in the allocation of health care and confers on the individual an entitlement to the right in question which should be protected through legislation or administrative measures. The concept of entitlement, in short, is derived from the concept of a right. Finally, recognizing a right to health care focuses special attention on the needs of vulnerable groups: the poor, minorities, and children.

The emphasis on the individual, rather than on the general good, and the emphasis on non-discrimination distinguish the rights approach from the cost-benefit approach. Regarding health care as a public good and not simply a market commodity, as well as the emphasis on non-discrimination, distinguish the rights approach from the market approach, which has demonstrably failed to provide equality of access to health care. Since one of the essentials of a rights-based approach is equitable access, the market approach is the contrary of a rights-based approach.

In many respects, the ethical obligation approach of the 1983 President's Commission resembles the rights-based approach to health care, but the former places a duty on the government, rather than conferring a right on the individual. The concept of "entitlement" is thus lacking. The difference is crucial in terms of enforcement of the ethical obligation. An example from the American constitutional system for protection of the rights contained in the Bill of Rights illustrates the importance of an entitlement. The American constitutional system establishes the right of the citizen to demand or claim the protections guaranteed by the Constitution. This can be done through legal action, administrative proceedings or other means of personal assertion of the right, as discussed below. There is a long history in the United States of providing various means for citizens to exercise their rights through individual assertion. Civil and political liberties and freedoms have been enhanced because of individual entitlement.

One of the most effective means of carrying out the "ethical societal obligations," referred to in the report of the President's Commission, would be to provide the opportunity for individuals to assert their rights. Americans are litigious and, as frequently noted, assertions of rights in the United States are often made in a contentious context in court cases. It is important to understand, however, that rights may be claimed in other ways and in situations of less conflict. In many countries, ombudsmen, in response to citizens complaints, raise issues of economic and social rights with regard to administration decisions. A policy of individual entitlement may, as well, create a greater opportunity for citizens or citizen groups to participate in the adoption of legislation based on a commitment to a right to health care. An individual entitlement may refer to the opportunity to bring a court case, but it is not limited to such means. Entitlements are contrasted with "privileges, personal ideals, group ideals and acts of charity" and they do not depend on the good will or cooperation of others.[36]

In the words of the Final Act of the Helsinki Conference on Security and Cooperation in Europe, individuals are entitled "to know and act on their rights." The individual must be provided with means to question the manner in which societal obligations are being carried out in the domain of health care.

Dr. Thomas Bodenheimer, a health professional supporting the concept of a right to health care, has written that a consensus formulation of that right means

> that society has a duty to allocate an adequate share of its total resources to health-related needs, and that each person is entitled to a fair share of such services as determined by medical need rather than by income, political power or social status. A simpler formulation would be: all people should have equal access to a reasonable level of health services regardless of income.[37]

Dr. Bodenheimer points out that the principle of health care as a right has two major implications for financing of health care: "(a) financial barriers to health care should not be greater for people who need more care than for those who need less care, and (b) financial barriers to health care should not be greater for people of lower income than for people of higher income."[38]

Charles J. Dougherty, professor of philosophy at Creighton University and author of a recent book on American health care, finds a basis for a right to health care in an egalitarian argument. He stresses that a fundamental aspect of the rights approach to health issues is "respect for the equal dignity of persons . . . [which] entails a commitment to equal access to the means necessary to cope with these burdens" of disease and death.[39]

Equality or non-discrimination is a fundamental principle of international human rights law.[40] If a particular good is considered as a right it must be granted to persons without discrimination on the basis of extraneous qualities. The Preamble to the Universal Declaration of Human Rights asserts that "recognition of the inherent dignity and of the equal and inalienable rights of all members of the human family is the foundation of freedom, justice and peace in the world." Article 2 provides that "Everyone is entitled to all the rights and freedoms set forth in this Declaration, without distinction of any kind such as race, colour, sex, language, religion, political or other opinion, national or social origin, property, birth or other status."

Rights are almost never absolute. They may be subject to certain limitations (for reasons of morality or health protection, for example); some may occasionally be derogated in times of emergency. But the concept of a "right" means that special attention must be given to the protection of what is considered a right and there must be strict, usually judicial, control over limitations and derogations. In the words of Ronald Dworkin, rights are "trumps" which generally, but not unfailingly, will prevail over other societal considerations. They create a presumption of special protection. A right to health care , as other rights, would not be absolute, but it would signify special attentions to any limitations on the right.

In practical terms, what do these generalities about health care mean? I have pointed out in the preceding section that practical measures concerning the disabled and concerning the safety and health of workers have been affected by approaching them in terms of rights. The final document adopted by the governments of the world at the

1993 Vienna World Conference on Human Rights stated that "Any direct discrimination or other negative discriminatory treatment of a disabled person is therefore a violation of his or her rights. The World Conference calls on governments, where necessary, to adopt or adjust legislation to assure access to these and other rights for disabled persons."[41] Attention to the needs of the disabled in terms of rights has and will have practical results in terms of legislation and assistance to their health needs.

The rights emphasis on non-discrimination would also have a practical effect on the adoption of particular programs of health care reform. Rationing systems and systems for cost-containment should be scrutinized with care for discriminatory aspects—particularly against vulnerable groups such as the poor, children, and minorities. A rights approach would argue for extension of whatever minimum health care is made generally available to American citizens to be made available also to other persons in the United States—including undocumented aliens.

The emphasis on entitlement in a rights-based approach means that creative means must be found to provide an opportunity for individuals to question and contest health care decisions. The use of ombudsmen to question administrative decisions has been referred to previously. The United States legal system provides many other types of means of raising issues concerning rights already recognized in the United States—similar means could be employed for protection of rights to health care.

A Critique of Reform Proposals

The persistent and pervasive criticisms of the present American health care system will lead to reforms. I have argued in this paper that a rights-based approach to health care should be adopted and that it will have practical implications for the choice of those reforms. Tom Campbell, a Scottish philosopher, has pointed out that rights discourse serves as a potent source of radical critiques of actual social arrangements and also as a powerful basis for working out and presenting alternative institutional practices.

In what manner then can the concept of the right to health assist us as a radical critique of our present and future health care system? I suggest that it may do so by using as a criterion for judging proposed reforms the five principles outlined in the previous section as implicit in a rights-based approach to health care, with special emphasis on non-discrimination, social justice, entitlement and rejection of a total market-based approach.

It may be that a number of proposed reforms meet these criteria. I suggest that general acceptance of the present health care system in the United States with only minor specific adjustments will not meet them. The present health care system does not provide equal access, is market-oriented and is discriminatory on the basis of financial status. It does not provide individual entitlement to health care. Tampering slightly with the system will not be sufficient. Over-emphasis on cost-containment may focus attention away from the important aspects of equity and entitlement.

A final caveat. The concept of health care does not solve all the problems implicit in any health care system. What it does provide is fundamental premises and criteria. And fundamental premises are important, but practical problems remain even with the choice of a rights-based system. Even if all are to be granted equal access to minimum care, we must decide what constitutes that minimum care. Ronald Dworkin has attempted to develop a methodology for working out the content of a minimum package of health care benefits which should be universally provided, using a "justice" approach. He finds the Clinton Plan "more promising for justice than any realistic alternatives yet proposed."[42] His justice criterion for judging reform plans is consistent with the rights-based approach developed in this paper.

The critics of the concept of the "right to health care" are correct in pointing out that some very important issues are not resolved by adopting a concept of the right to health care. How does one, for example, guarantee that all geographic areas will be provided with the necessary medical manpower and what methods of financing should be adopted. However, they err in minimizing the importance of the basic premise which will inform the working out of details of the health care system.

Can such a health care system exist? We have an example nearby. The Canadian government has adopted a rights-based approach for its health care system. We know that problems exist in the Canadian health system, as they will in any humanly devised system, but an overwhelming majority of Canadians believe that they have an excellent health care system, in contrast to the perception of Americans of their health care system. There are problems of financing, of waits for elective surgery (exaggerated in the American media), and perhaps of dissatisfaction among some health care professionals. But as an individual who has lived in Canada and been a participant in its health care system, I can attest to its virtues. On the basis of the criteria of equality and non-discrimination and adequate provision of minimum health care, the Canadian system ranks very high. American society is not Canadian society, and we may implement a rights-based approach to health care in a different manner. But we have on our doorstep a good rights-based health care system. We should learn more about it.

Americans are pragmatic. We prefer to look at specific proposals and ignore theory, but fundamental principles will underlie whatever health care system we adopt. It will be based on a market-approach or a utilitarian approach or a rights approach. A rights approach most satisfactorily recognizes the intrinsic dignity of the human person and should be the basic premise of our health care reforms. While we are a pragmatic people, we are also citizens of a nation that has traditionally placed importance on human rights. The time has come to extend the concept of rights to encompass health care.

NOTES

1. Theodore R. Marmor, "The Right to Health Care: Reflections on its History and Politics," in Thomas J. Bole and William B. Bondeson, *Rights to Health Care* (Dordrecht: Kluwer Academic Publishers, 1991), pp. 27, 38.

2. For an excellent discussion of the Canadian health care system, see John K. Iglehart, "Canada's Health Care System," *The New England Journal of Medicine*, Part I: July 17, 1986, vol. 315, No. 3, pp. 202–208; Part II: Sept. 18, 1986, Vol. 315, No. 12, pp. 778–784; Part III: Dec. 18, 1986, Vol. 315, No. 25, pp. 1623–1628.

3. Ronald Dworkin, "Is Clinton's Plan Fair", *The New York Review of Books*, January 13, 1994, p. 20.

4. See, *inter alia, The Economist*, November 16, 1991, 27. Underscoring mine.

5. Congressman John J. LaFalce, "A Special Report, The Issue: Health Care in America," September 1991.

6. U.S. Catholic Conference, "Health and Health Care", 1981, cited in Jose Lozano, M.C., "Health Care in the United States and Social Teachings of the Catholic Church," Physicians for a National Health Program newsletter, October 1991, 2–3.

7. Tom L. Beauchamp, "The Right to Health Care in a Capitalistic Democracy" Alan E. Buchanan, "Rights, Obligations and the Special Importance of

Health Care" Norman Daniels, "Equal Opportunity and Health Care Rights for the Elderly'', in Bole and Bondeson.

8.   Robert M. Veatch, "Justice and the Right to Health Care: An Egalitarian Account" in Bole and Bondeson.

9.   Thomas J. Bole, III, "The Rhetoric of Rights and Justice in Health Care" in Bole and Bondeson.

10.   H. Tristram Engelhardt, Jr., "Virtue for Hire: Some Reflections on Free Choice and the Profit Motive in the Delivery of Health Care"; David Friedman, "Should Medicine be a Commodity? An Economist's Perspective"; Hans-Martin Sass, "My Right to Care for My Health—and What About the Needy and Elderly'', in Bole and Bondeson.

11.   American Association for the Advancement of Science (AAAS), Consultation on the Right to Health Care, Summary and Assessment, Session III, Washington D.C., Dec. 4, 1992.

12.   AAAS, Consultation on The Right to Health Care, Assessment and Summary, Session I, Washington, D.C., September 18, 1992.

13.   President's Commission for the Study of Ethical Problems in Medicine and Biomedical and Behavioral Research, *Securing Access to Health Care*, (Washington, D.C.: Government Printing Office,1983), vol. 1, p. 4.

14.   *Ibid.*, 33.

15.   Baruch A. Brody, "Policy Debate and the Right to Health Care" in Bole and Bondeson, p. 116.

16.   *Ibid.*, p. 117.

17.   Brody states that he does not take a position for or against the right to health care, but argues that it should not be viewed as the central question in moral examination of issues of health policy. Brody, p. 114.

18.   Professor Charles Fried of Harvard Law School is one of the few law professors to have written on the subject of the right to health care. A number of law professors have published widely on health care issues, but not on the concept of the right to health care.

19.   See William J. Curran, "The Constitutional Right to Health Care", *New England Journal of Medicine*, 320 (March 23, 1989) 789.

20.   "..[T]he federal and state and state governments have established certain categorical and needs-based programs, Medicare and Medicaid, in particular, and those qualifying for these programs may be said to have legal rights to the benefits they convey. There are also laws and regulations that forbid the denial of health care on discriminatory grounds and that mandate that certain levels of care be given to certain categories of needy individuals—handicapped newborns, for example. And a growing trend in the American law of torts may amount to a virtual guarantee of needed emergency care at a hospital emergency room under some circumstances" (footnotes omitted). Charles J. Dougherty, *American Health Care, Realities, Rights and Reforms*, (New York: Oxford University Press, 1988), p. 30.

21.   See Ian Shapiro, *The Evolution of Rights in Liberal Theory* (New York: Cambridge University Press, 1986); Ronald Dworkin, *Taking Rights Seriously*, (Cambridge: Harvard University Press, 1978).

22. D. M. Berwick and H. H. Hiatt, "Who Pays", *The New England Journal of Medicine*, volume 321 (1989), 541–542.

23. See, for example, Bole and Bondeson. There is only a passing reference to the Universal Declaration of Human Rights in one of the chapters and no mention of the International Covenant on Economic, Social and Cultural Rights. Although the Canadian health care system is referred to in a number of the chapters, no reference is made to the fundamental premise of a right to health care, enshrined in the WHO Constitution, on which the system is based. See Royal Commission on Health Services, Canada, 1964, Volume 1, 6.

24. Rene-Jean Dupuy, ed., *The Right to Health as a Human Right*, Workshop, Hague Academy of International Law, 1979.

25. Hernan L. Fuenzalida-Puelma and Susan Scholle Connor, eds., *The Right to Health in the Americas: A Comparative Constitutional Study*, Scientific Publication No. 509, (Washington, D.C.: Pan-American Health Organization, 1989).

26. For a more detailed discussion of the terminology "right to health" see Virginia A. Leary, "Implications of the 'Right to Health' " in Kathleen Mahoney and Paul Mahoney, eds., *Human Rights in the Twenty-First Century: A Global Challenge*, (Boston; Dordrecht: Nijhoff, 1993), pp. 481–494. See also Brody, p. 124, emphasizing that health care is not the only important element that contributes to a longer and healthier life.

27. Fuenzalida-Puelma and Connor, p. 599.

28. Declaration of Alma-Ata, adopted at the International Conference on Primary Health Care, September 12, 1978, WHO.

29. But see, Tom L. Beauchamp and Ruth R. Faden, "The Right to Health and the Right to Health Care", *The Journal of Medicine and Philosophy*, 4 (1979) 118–131, suggesting that the concept of the right to health does not imply a right to health care.

30. "Democracy and Human Rights: Where America Stands", Remarks by U.S. Secretary of State Warren Christopher at the World Conference on Human Rights, Vienna, June 14, 1993.

31. David Friedman, "Should Medicine Be a Commodity? An Economist's Perspective", in Bole and Bondeson, pp. 301–303.

32. Arnold S. Relman, "Shattuck Lecture—The Health Care Industry: Where is it Taking Us?" *The New England Journal of Medicine* 325 (September 19, 1991) 854–858.

33. For an ethical critique of cost-benefit analysis in relation to environmental, safety and health regulation, see Steven Kelman, "Cost-Benefit Analysis: An Ethical Critique", *Regulation*, 5 (January/February 1981), 33; and responses to his analysis by James V. DeLong, Robert M. Solo, Gerard Butters, John Calfee, Pauline Ippolito and Robert A. Nisbet, *Regulation*, 5 (March/April 1981).

34. Kelman, 34: "Utilitarianism is an important and powerful moral doctrine. But it is probably a minority position among contemporary moral philosophers. It is amazing that economists can proceed in unanimous endorsement of cost-benefit analysis as if unaware that their conceptual framework is highly controversial in the discipline from which it arose—moral philosophy."

35. See David J. Rothman, "Rationing Life", *The New York Review of Books*, March 5, 1992, 32 at 36: "But the Oregon venture makes apparent how treacherous are the politics of rationing. The plan affects only the Medicaid population—only the poor therefore bear the burden of the cutbacks and they, in reality, subsidize the extension of medical coverage to other poor people. . .Thus, the one target is low-income women and their children."

36. Beauchamp and Faden, 119.

37. Thomas Bodenheimer, "Should We Abolish the Private Health Insurance Industry?" *International Journal of Health Services*, 20 (1990) 200.

38. *Ibid.*, p. 201.

39. Dougherty, 31.

40. Anne F. Bayefsky, "The Principle of Equality or Non-Discrimination in International Law" *Human Rights Law Journal* 2 (1990) 1–34.

41. Vienna Declaration and Programme of Action, UN World Conference on Human Rights, 25 June 1993, para. E(1).

42. Dworkin, p. 25.

Robert M. Veatch

Egalitarian Justice and the Right to Health Care

My task is to sketch out what an egalitarian account of justice looks like as it applies to health care, what conceptual and ethical problems it raises, and what its implications might be for a right to health care for the United States.[1] An egalitarian account is one that focuses on an interpretation of the moral principle of justice emphasizing some kind of equality, usually equality of individual well-being. This analysis shall suggest that an egalitarian account is one in which people are given opportunities for equality of well-being. This raises deceptively complex questions such as whether there must also be opportunities for equality of *medical* well-being, whether a second tier of "luxury" health care services could be purchased with discretionary funds, whether there is an objective standard for determining if people are equally well-off, and whether people should be permitted to trade away their entitlement to health care in order to buy goods in other areas that they value more highly. This analysis shall suggest that the emerging debate over global budgets provides a fruitful context for exploring these issues and that an egalitarian allocation of a global budget will look quite different from one devoted to maximizing the medical good done based on outcomes measures and cost-benefit analysis.

The Concept of Justice

In the debate over justice and the right to health care in contemporary health care ethics two terms are controversial, rights and justice. The first is the use of the term *right*. Sometimes the starting point is to spell out certain characteristic obligations that tend to make actions right. These are often called *principles*. Justice is one such principle. The frame of reference is the one who is obligated to act in a certain way toward another. Rights-claims then derive from the

106

obligations. Obligations are seen as morally prior and rights derivative. The other possible starting point is to focus on the bearer of the rights, who can be seen as the source of a derivative obligation. Whether we focus on rights or obligations as prior is debated in ethical theory, but, for our purposes, the matter need not be settled here. Hence, whether one speaks of the obligation to provide health care or the right to health care, will not be critical for these purposes. Similar matters are at stake.[2]

The term justice is used in two quite different ways. The problem goes back as far as Aristotle. He distinguished between *justice in the broad sense* and *justice in the narrow sense*.[3] In the broad sense justice is more or less a synonym for "the right course of action." But justice is also used in a much narrower sense to refer to fairness in distribution.

Contemporary ethical theory that relies on ethical principles recognizes that there are a number of principles—including respect for autonomy and production of good (beneficence) and perhaps others such as fidelity to promises, veracity or truth telling, and avoidance of killing. In such lists often the principle of justice appears. The right course is the resultant of the combined influence of these principles (based on some theory of ranking or priority of principles).[4] Hence what is right (just in the broad sense taking into account all competing principles) may not be the same as what is the morally most just distribution (just in the narrow sense focusing only on the pattern of distribution).

Thus there are two quite separate questions to be addressed: First, concerning only the principle of justice as fair distribution, what rights exist and, second, concerning all principles (justice and the others as well) what rights exist?

The Meanings of Justice

Justice (in the broad sense) is recognized as supporting different patterns of distribution. Some of these really reflect the distributional implications of other principles such as autonomy or utility. Others view justice as an independent principle that provides an independent basis for distributing resources. One's right to health care will depend on which focus is chosen.

If justice refers to a pattern of distribution of resources that is supported by other ethical principles, justice must be used only in the broad sense meaning the morally right arrangement. For example, those who give highest or sole priority to the principle of autonomy (or liberty) will consider the "just" arrangement to be whatever results from appropriation of unowned resources or from trades or free-exchanges of goods fairly possessed.[5] The result will be that the morally right arrangement will be whatever results from free-market deals provided no unfair appropriation has taken place. For those who give priority to liberty, to say that an arrangement is just is to say nothing more than that it is morally right based on the supposed dominance of the principle of liberty or autonomy.

Likewise, those who hold that maximizing aggregate utility is the highest or sole ethical principle will consider the "just" arrangement to be the one that most efficiently maximizes the aggregate net good. Mill specifically acknowledged that the "just" arrangement of social resources is simply the one that maximizes the total good.[6] For utilitarians to say that an arrangement is just is to say nothing more than that it is morally right based on the supposed dominance of the principle of utility.

Neither of these views really gives justice—in the narrow sense—any role as an independent ethical principle. An egalitarian account is one of a group of approaches that takes an independent ethical principle of justice seriously. This independent principle must specify a pattern of distribution that is morally right *even if it conflicts with autonomy or with the maximizing of the aggregate good.* It is amazing how often the current debate over the allocation of health care resources presumes that the allocation that respects autonomy or maximizes aggregate good will automatically be the morally right allocation. This overlooks the very real possibility that, at least according to those who affirm an independent principle of justice, the most just allocation may not be the one that maximally respects autonomy or maximally promotes the aggregate social good.

There are several possible independent bases for arranging benefits and harms in a society other than in order to respect autonomy or produce maximum aggregate good. Aristotle names allocations based on free birth, wealth or noble birth, and excellence.[7] The dominant basis for an independent principle of justice in contemporary ethics is none of these. Rather it is based on some notion of equality. When existing patterns are very unequal, such as with health status, egalitarian justice would distribute on the basis of need, that is, in a pattern necessary to move toward equality.[8] It would target for those who are worst off, striving to make them more equal, insofar as possible, to other people. The notion of being poorly off (or worst off) is central to egalitarian allocation theory. Being poorly off generally is taken to refer to individuals who score lowest in the amount of well-being they possess, either medical well-being or, more plausibly, total well-being.

Some examples of how distribution based on egalitarian justice will differ from one based on maximizing aggregate good may help here. The current enthusiasm for outcomes measures is probably based on utilitarian benefit-maximizing intuitions. Insofar as outcomes research is used to allocate medical resources and assign priorities, the working assumption is that if we can figure out which health care interventions will do the most good on balance, we will know which ones should get priority. Similarly, the use of cost-benefit analysis to assign priorities strives to maximize the net social benefit per unit of investment.[9] Supporters of this use of outcomes research and cost-benefit analysis do not consider the possibility that some particularly poorly off patients may have high priority claims of egalitarian justice even though the interventions that may help them are less efficient in maximizing the total net good done with scarce resources.

In the Oregon experiment many people express the poorly thought out intuition that simple "basic" services such as immunizations deserve moral priority over high tech interventions such as bone marrow transplants because the former are more efficient in producing aggregate health benefit. The original formula used by the Oregon Health Services Commission calculated cost and divided by net benefit for each diagnosis-treatment pair—an approach grounded squarely on utilitarian assumptions. The revised formula, which dropped cost from the formula, still measured aggregate net benefit. It then ranked the diagnosis-treatment pairs based on this aggregate benefit. Only later were treatments grouped subjectively by the commissioners into categories and "eye-balled" to introduce any element of justice into the rankings. By contrast egalitarian justice would strive to give priority based on how poorly off patients were in each diagnostic group prior to treatment. The Commission had data estimating how poorly off patients in each diagnosis-treatment pair were prior to treatment but chose not to make any formal use of this information. For example, it could have used the same computer to calculate the standard deviation from average well-being for patients and arranged priorities so as to minimize the variation. Or it could have simply ranked diagnoses on the basis of pretreatment quality of well-being giving highest priority to those lowest on the scale.

Consider another example of how egalitarian justice can conflict with efficiently maximizing the good done. In allocating scarce organs such as kidneys for transplant, one possible goal would be to maximize the amount of benefit obtained from each organ. Assuming, for the moment, that benefit is limited to health benefit (such as years of life expected per organ transplanted) the goal would be to give the organ to the person needing it who could be expected to get the most years of life from it. This would make use of such factors as tissue typing—giving the organ to the person with the closest tissue match because that is known to predict likelihood of graft survival.

However, this benefit-maximizing strategy poses a serious ethical problem from the point of view of the egalitarian. It is known that all races do not match equally well to the pool of donors. In particular blacks and hispanics do not match up as well. This means that an allocation that strives to get as many years of aggregate survival as possible per graft will, de facto, be a whites-first policy. Egalitarian justice rejects the suggestion that it is just or right to allocate organs on the basis of expected graft survival just because it would efficiently maximize the net good.

There is an even more controversial implication of trying to maximize the number of years of survival per graft. Since elderly people do not do as well with organs and will probably die relatively soon of other causes even if the graft takes, an allocation that maximizes years of survival would give priority to young persons. (It is also true that, on average, men do better than women and middle class patients do better than lower class so that the utility maximizing allocation would be the one that give organs to young, white, middle class males.) Egalitarian justice rejects the suggestion that it is just to allocate organs in this way even if it is maximally efficient in adding years of life. In general, egalitarian justice rejects the goal of maximizing the aggregate social benefit as the criterion of either justice or rightness in allocations of health care.

Egalitarian justice as an independent principle comes in two forms. The first, grounded in the work of John Rawls, subordinates maximal production of aggregate benefit to arrangements that, among other things, benefit those who are least well off. This Rawlsian approach is often referred to as egalitarian.[10] The interesting case is the one in which the best way to improve the lot of the worst off persons is to actually increase inequality. Consider, for example, a mass disaster in which a physician skilled in emergency medicine was known to be among the victims. Assume that she was less injured than the others and if she were given first priority in the rescue effort she would be available to help rescue others. They would be helped more than if the physician were not given special priority. Assuming, however, that the physician was better off to begin with and would get even greater benefit by being rescued first, the steps necessary to benefit the worse off would actually increase the inequality. If the Rawlsian difference principle can be extrapolated to create rules for priority in rescue (a controversial move that Rawls sometimes has been known to question), then the supposedly egalitarian difference principle would, in this case, actually have just the opposite effect. It would increase rather than decease inequality by arranging resources so as to benefit the least well off.

A more radical or true egalitarianism in health resource allocation claims that the just allocation is the one that makes persons more equal even if it does not maximize the benefit to the worst off. Its principle is that X *is right (prima facie) insofar as it contributes to opportunities for equality of well-being.*

Several features of this egalitarian principle of justice need to be noted. It holds, at least for now, only prima facie. That is to say, this tells us what is a just allocation, not necessarily what will be morally right taking into account principles that may compete with justice. Second, in order for this egalitarian principle of allocation to be used there must be some objective standard for interpersonal comparisons of how well off people are. It, in effect, presumes some objective standard of well-being. We shall see in a moment how to avoid some of the controversy that implies. Radical egalitarianism differs from Rawlsian justice in identifying variation in well-being as morally relevant, not simply how well off the worst off are.

Rawls has actually incorporated the criterion of maximizing benefit as well as equality in his difference principle. His so-called second principle of justice actually strives for equality except when everyone benefits from inequalities. That may be a plausible way to integrate the principle of justice with the principle of utility, but it is not just striving for equality. It is egalitarian justice subordinated to utility when (and only when) it serves the utility of the worst off to abandon equality. True egalitarians prefer to leave the integration of egalitarian justice with utility to a later step when conflicts among principles must be reconciled. They insist that justice strives simply for opportunities for equality of well-being insofar as possible.

Compare this with the concept of autonomy. There are times when autonomy may have to be sacrificed to promote other principles. We do not pack those compromises into the very definition of autonomy. Rather we hold to a pure definition of autonomy while acknowledging that sometimes autonomy may give way. Likewise, an egalitarian holds to the notion that a just allocation is one that targets for the worst off in a way that will give them opportunities for greater equality of well-being. Whether the just allocation is also the morally right allocation remains to be decided at a later stage in the analysis.

Trades and Tiers: Implications for Health Care

Thus far this analysis has suggested that an egalitarian principle of justice supports the view that people have a prima facie right to resources needed to give them opportunities for equality of well-being. That leaves open the question of how this principle of justice intersects with other ethical principles to determine what is right. It also leaves open the question of the implication for allocating health care.

Applying the egalitarian principle of justice to health care is more complex than may appear. Surely, the goal is not to give everyone equal amounts of health care. But should the goal be to give everyone equal health status? This analysis has already suggested that all that is at stake for an egalitarian is the opportunity for equality, so should the goal be opportunities for equal health status?

Some people are fortunate enough that they have very good health without the benefit of any significant health care services. If everyone is to have equal health status than we either have to get everyone up to their level or bring the very healthy down to a lower level. The former is impractical; it would take resources beyond what is available. The latter makes no sense. What is usually sought is some decent minimal level of health, beyond which there is no entitlement right to resources needed to improve further. The decent minimum may have to be set arbitrarily, but, once set, the goal would be to give everyone whatever health care it takes to bring them, to the extent possible, up to that decent minimum. A true egalitarian would start with the medically worst off—those who score lowest on a pre-treatment quality of medical well-being scale—and treat until they are brought to the next level, at which time this new, larger group of worst off is then targeted. As a practical matter, we can probably set a list of services that are covered under the notion of decent minimum and then provide all such services. This is essentially what Oregon is doing, although, as has been suggested, there is strong evidence that they are not ranking their list on the basis of who is worst off. Their primary criterion is efficient production of medical benefit.[11]

That still leaves two problems: (1) what should happen if someone wants to trade a piece of their entitlement to get some other nonhealth good and (2) what should be done with those who want to use private discretionary resources to buy a second or higher tier of health care? First, let's consider the ethics of trading some below-the-decent-minimum health care for other desired goods.

If the goal of egalitarian justice is opportunities for equality of well-being, this does not necessarily imply that there must be equality in each sphere of well-being. Some might have unusual amounts of well-being in housing, other in the arts, still others in special gourmet food, others in health. As long as opportunities for total well-being are about the same the egalitarian should be satisfied. This means that, in principle, egalitarian justice need not strive for equality of well-being in the health sphere. If, for example, people received vouchers for health care or health care insurance and chose to trade them for other goods they value outside of health care or sell them, their total well-being probably would not decrease and, to the extent that they trade and spend wisely, it is likely to increase, at least in the short run. Is there any moral reason that trades of health care for nonhealth care goods should be proscribed? Two arguments against trades have to be taken into account.

First, as a practical matter health care is quite different from other goods that people need to promote their well-being. In rough terms people's needs for food, clothing, shelter, and recreation are about the same. If everyone received the same dollar income, there is no reason why an egalitarian should insist that people spend the same amount in each of these areas. Bracketing some modest variations in marginal utility functions, each person's total well-being would be about the same, even if expenditures in various areas differ significantly as long as the total is the same.

Health care is quite a different matter. The amount needed to achieve equality of medical well-being is radically different from one person to another. In theory one might be able to assess initial well-being among individuals including one's physical and mental assets as well as familial and social assets. Those with physical and mental deficits might be compensated to level the playing field before everyone receives an equal share of remaining resources. Education is the only other sphere where needs differ as greatly among persons. In both cases we might have to distribute resources needed to compensate for very unequal starting points before distributing remaining resources equally. After such compensation, if people did not choose to spend exactly the same amounts on health care and health insurance the egalitarian should not care.

However, as a practical matter permitting trades could lead to impossible problems even if one accepted the idea that justice required only opportunities for equality of total well-being. There would be initial problems of how to quantify how poorly off people are. That is the least of our problems, however. Efforts at establishing quality-adjusted life year (QALY)[12] and quality of well-being index (QWBI)[13] scales reveal considerable skill in making such interpersonal comparisons. The real problem would be in trying to track entitlements. Some people would have received compensation for a medical need that they chose to spend on some other good preferring to suffer the medical deficit. They would have had an opportunity for equality of health, but have chosen not to take it. They would have compensatory improvement in some other sphere of well-being, but would continue to manifest the medical deficit. Another person presenting the same medical problem who has never been provided an opportunity to have the problem addressed would be in a different moral situation. Two people with medically identical problems, thus, could stand in radically different positions from the standpoint of egalitarian justice. The only way to tell the difference if trades can be made or health care entitlements sold would be to develop an elaborate computerized tracking system by which persons could be followed throughout their lifetimes.

The problem is even worse. Some people who are treated for a medical condition discover that the treatment fails. If they do, then they are surely—according to egalitarians—entitled to another shot using some alternative treatment. The one who has traded the original opportunity away, however, would never know whether he was in the group for which the first treatment would have failed thereby being entitled to the second try. The only practical way out of this chaos is, say the egalitarians, to recognize entitlements to health care services themselves, banning trades for other goods even if they would be preferred and even if no significant inequalities in overall well-being would result from the trades.

There is a second, more theoretical argument against trades of health services for other goods. Let us assume that an egalitarian would favor allocations that grant a right to opportunities for overall well-being equal to that of others (up to the decent minimum) and that, in a perfectly just world, there would be no problems introduced if people with different tastes got together to make their trades.

It is still not clear what an egalitarian would do in a less than perfectly just world such as the one in which we live. There is good reason to suppose that other goods (or generalized media such as money that can be used to purchase other goods) will not be distributed in a completely just manner. That leads to the problem of what allocation of health care is just when the underlying social allocation of other goods is inequitable. The problem is particularly acute when there is a chance that politically the health care allocation can be made more just than the allocation of other goods.

In such a world, if those who have too small an allocation of other goods wish to trade their health care vouchers for other things and can increase their well-being by doing so, would it be just—and would it be right—for them to do so?

The answer will depend on how one ought to behave in a less than perfectly just world. One approach is to hold out for those parts of a social policy as they would exist in a just society even though such arrangements might not be in people's interests in a less than perfect world. This is what the social historian Ernst Troeltsch has referred to as the "absolute or ideal" position.[14] In allocating health care this would lead to a policy of allocating that health care to which one would be justly entitled in a just world even though the world is not presently just. The other approach would be to readjust the allocation policy to take into account that when the worst off do not have their fair share of other goods, they would be better off if they traded some of their just entitlement to health care for other goods they need more. This is what Troeltsch has referred to as the "relative" position. It is not obvious which approach is better. In any case, it is not necessarily irrational to insist on citizens getting their full just entitlement to health care, thus banning trades if the political process permits such allocations for health care but not other goods.

The second question raised by egalitarianism is what should happen with those who wish to use private, discretionary funds to buy additional health care above the decent minimum? In a truly egalitarian world the problem might not exist because there might be no discretionary funds. All such funds might be taxed away to be redistributed to those with the greatest need. On the other hand one can imagine an egalitarian world in which some resources distributed according to egalitarian principles could be used on a discretionary basis. In an egalitarian world, should people be permitted to use such discretionary resources to buy some additional health care?

They would not need to use such resources to buy health care needed to get to a decent minimum; that would already be provided. But they might want to get beyond that point. If people are permitted to buy frivolous luxuries with discretionary funds, why should they not be allowed to buy luxurious levels of health care as well? Of course, if the decent minimum level is set too low, it might be argued that some of the services above the line are not appropriately called luxuries at all, but if the line is properly drawn, then, by definition, one would not have an entitlement to those medical services above the line. They might reasonably referred to as luxuries in the sense of not being goods to which one is entitled.

In the real world, of course, a second tier will be available. We are not in danger of becoming such an egalitarian society that people will not be able to buy face lifts, private hospital rooms, and designer drugs such as TPA. These drugs promise slight extra margins of benefit, but at costs so high that they would not be considered part of the decent minimum. But would people be permitted in a hypothetical egalitarian world to make such second-tier purchases?

Radical egalitarians are often wrongly accused of striving for a world in which everyone is exactly the same. This has been shown to be a false accusation. All that the egalitarian wants is opportunities for equality of well-being, not sameness. If people can be equal while having different mixes of goods, there is no reason why a world of equal well-being would be a world of sameness.

Nevertheless there are potential problems for an egalitarian if the relatively well off are permitted to buy a second (or third) tier of care. As long as what is being bought is conceptualized as a luxury, there is no problem in principle with permitting such purchases with discretionary funds assuming some such exist. But the problem will arise if those funds are used by the relatively well-off to tie up scarce, irreplaceable resources needed for the medically worst off. If the wealthy buy off the best surgeons, the best researchers, and the best of scarce drugs or organs for transplant, then a policy tolerating these second-tier purchases would jeopardize the care needed by the worst off. Moreover, if the wealthy buy their way out of the standard system, those with the talent and power to correct flaws in it may have lost the incentive to bring about necessary changes in it. Egalitarian justice would not automatically oppose a second tier of health care, but it would be skeptical and seek assurance that permitting a second tier would not jeopardize the prior right of those who are not getting the decent minimum.

Justice, the Right to Health Care, and Global Budgets

The problem of justice and a right to health care may arise not at the level of deciding what lists of services should be covered in order to give everyone an opportunity for a decent minimum health status; it may arise at the microallocation level in the emerging concept of "global budgeting." Many health care systems now handle the problem of rationing by providing an administrative unit with a global, predetermined budget.

This budget will purposely be somewhat below what a clinician would like to have in order to provide every conceivable benefit to every patient in the system. The reason is that some health care services provide very marginal benefits per unit of investment or provide benefits for people who are already quite healthy. In a world of scarcity a government or an insurer should provide only enough funds so that the significant needs are met leaving some marginal ones unmet.

Examples of this global budgeting are numerous. The DRG system used by Medicare provides a fixed reimbursement per patient in a diagnostic group for a given hospital. The medical service—say, cardiology—ends up with a fixed budget which it then has to spread among its patients. Likewise, HMOs accumulate premiums from subscribers leaving them with a fixed pile of money to spread among their patients. The Canadian system relies on global preset budgets; The Clinton administration's health plan may rely on something similar.

The problem is that it is morally necessary that the total should be less than the total amount that the clinicians would like to have to do everything they would like to do for every patient. Some set of rules—implicit or explicit—must be available for each service to allocate its fixed, limited pool among its patients. The allocation will be a function of the implicit ethic of those administering the service's budget. Different ethics—utilitarian and egalitarian, for instance—will allocate the pool differently. Moreover, there is good reason to assume that those who administer such medical service budgets have unique, atypical ethics that lead them to allocate in peculiar ways. What are the ways different ethics might allocate?

The utilitarian administrator of a medical service would take his global pool of resources and spread them among patients in whatever way would produce the greatest aggregate net benefit. The formula would be:

$$\text{maximize } \Sigma \ (QWBI_a - QWBI_b)$$

where $QWBI_a$ is the individual quality of well-being index score after treatment and $QWBI_b$ is the individual quality of well-being index score before treatment. This would simply maximize the sum of the changes in individual quality of well-being.

While that would maximize the total net good done with the service's available resources and thus satisfy utilitarians, it would not distribute health resources equally to each patient. It would not distribute care on the basis of need. It is the nature of illness that those who are sickest and thus can be said to have the greatest need are often also inefficient to treat. Although decreasing marginal utility applies in many areas of life, it often does not in health care. Those who already are relatively well off may get more benefit per unit of health resources than those who are worst off.

How would egalitarians spread the resources available in a global budget of a health care service? They would begin by asking which patients are worst off and do what they can to raise their well-being.

One approach would be simply to target those with the lowest $QWBI_b$. Other approaches also have egalitarian plausibility. For example, one might imagine for each patient the most that health care could do for them assuming resources were unlimited. One would ask "What would be their maximum quality of well-being obtainable

($QWBI_{max}$)?" Then one could try to hold constant for all patients the ratio of the good actually done to the maximum that could be done:

$$\frac{(QWBI_a - QWBI_b)}{(QWBI_{max})} = k$$

This formula would treat each patient equally in the sense of giving each one the same percentage of his or her maximum possible health benefit. It would, of course, raise the well-being of some who are already quite well off, thus not being truly egalitarian.

Another formula that would be more egalitarian without giving absolute priority to the worst off would be:

$$\frac{(QWBI_a - QWBI_b)}{(QWBI_{max})} = 1/k \, (QWBI_b)$$

In this arrangement the ratio of the amount of benefit provided to the maximum possible benefit would be inversely proportional to the pretreatment quality of well-being. Those who start the worst off get the greatest proportion of their possible benefit.

The most just arrangement may not finally be the morally right arrangement when other moral principles such as beneficence are taken into account. Recognizing this, the formulas above nonetheless offer potential for telling us what it is to which each person has an entitlement right, taking into account the moral objective of producing good as well as distributing it justly.

There is one final problem in trying to determine health care to which one might have a right from the point of view of egalitarianism. The methods that rely on assessment of health care benefits using quality of well-being scales and similar devices all assume some objective standard of what counts as a health benefit. In fact we know that what some count as a significant benefit others consider useless or even an outright burden. There may be no accessible standard objective list of what is a health benefit. If so, then any generalized calculation of QWBI for a particular diagnosis and treatment is, at best, an average view. Individuals may differ significantly on how beneficial they think the treatment would be. This has radical implications.

Any single list of services covered in an insurance plan, such as the Oregon list or any Blue Cross or HMO list, will be evaluated differently by different people. From the egalitarian perspective this is disturbing. We set out to treat people equally in the sense of trying to give people opportunities to rise to at least a decent minimum health status, but, since different people will evaluate the services differently, providing any one list of covered services will necessarily leave people feeling subjectively unequal in their health status.

With some simplifying assumptions, there may a solution available, however. Perhaps we can assume that equality of resources will more or less produce opportunities for equality of outcome. A case can be made that, adjusting for inequalities in the natural lottery, all that egalitarian justice requires is equal resources[15] and that with equal resources opportunities for well-being will be about equal.

If that is true, then giving people equal dollars in purchasing power for a health insurance policy should give them approximately equal opportunities for health status provided there is open enrollment and community rating, and a wide range of lists of coverages is available. Each person could choose his or her own preferred list of services provided that the total cost for the average person was the same regardless of the list chosen. An entitlement for, say, $3000 in insurance probably would do the job. Some people who have a strong preference for low tech lifestyle counseling could opt for a plan rich in such services but proportionally lower in high tech, end-stage treatment for cancer or kidney disease while others with opposite preferences could choose plans with opposite biases. Some plans would exclude abortion (for those who considered the service of no value or immoral). Their coverage would have those funds available for some other desired service normally left out of insurance coverage. We would all have different plans, but, assuming equal resources tend to buy equal overall satisfaction provided there is open enrollment without differences in premium, we should end up about equal.

The lists would all have to meet certain minimum standards. They would have to cover all those services required to fulfill obligations to others, treatment for infectious disease, for example. Emergency room service would have to be included not because everyone desires it, but because society cannot be left stranded trying to guess at whether someone in an accident has selected a plan with such coverage. Justice would require that certain services, treatment for certain conditions of the elderly, for example, could not be excluded, in order to avoid adverse selection problems. These, however, are all problems already faced in any open enrollment environment.

This egalitarian approach to health insurance is neutral regarding whether the insurance is offered by private markets or by a single government payor. The only condition would be that whoever offers it—private companies or government—would have to offer multiple lists all meeting certain minimal conditions and all costing the same on an open enrollment, community-rated basis. As long as each list satisfied certain criteria of justice—making sure that certain conditions everyone would consider to offer the poorest quality of life were covered—this multiple list, equal price, open enrollment, community-rated insurance system may be the only way we can provide all people with opportunities for equality of well-being, at least up to a decent minimum. That is what an egalitarian account of a right to health care might look like.

Conclusion

If this analysis is correct, an egalitarian account of a right to health care is one that permits opportunities for equality of well-being. This is not necessarily incompatible with allocations of health care in which some people are permitted to trade away their entitlements to health care and others are permitted to use discretionary funds to buy a second, luxury tier of health care. Nevertheless, even if in theory such unequal health outcomes are compatible with an egalitarian principle of overall justice, there are strong practical reasons why trades of one's entitlements should be proscribed and there are also some practical reasons as well as theoretical reasons why permitting people to buy a second tier of health care with discretionary funds should be questioned.

If global budgets for health care plans are emerging as the wave of the future, it will be necessary to understand how different ethical principles will allocate these budgets differently. An egalitarian account supports an arrangement whereby individuals are entitled to a fixed dollar amount of health insurance made available in such a way that people could choose from multiple equal-valued lists of services on a basis of open enrollment and community-rating.

NOTES

1. This paper draws upon and extends the analysis of earlier work I have done on egalitarian theories of justice as they apply to health care. See Robert

M. Veatch, *The Foundations of Justice: Why the Retarded and the Rest of Us Have Claims to Equality*. (New York: Oxford University Press, 1986); Robert M. Veatch, "Just Social Institutions and the Right to Health Care," *Journal of Medicine and Philosophy* 4 (No. 2, June 1979): 170–173; Robert M. Veatch, "Justice and the Right to Health Care: An Egalitarian Account," *Rights to Health Care*. Thomas J. Bole III and William B. Bondeson. (Dordrecht: Kluwer Academic Publishers, 1991), pp. 83–102; Robert M. Veatch, *A Theory of Medical Ethics*. (New York: Basic Books, 1981).

2.   Ruth Macklin, "Moral Concerns and Appeals to Rights and Duties." *Hastings Center Report* 6 (5, 1976): 31–38.

3.   Aristotle. *Nicomachean Ethics*. Martin Ostwald, trans. (Indianapolis: The Bobbs-Merrill Company, Inc., 1962), Book V.

4.   On the major theories of balancing or reconciling conflict among ethical principles see Veatch, *A Theory of Medical Ethics*, chapter 12. One approach is to try to collapse all principles into one underlying fundamental principle. Utilitarianism has tried to do this. Another approach has been to "balance" the competing principles. Another is to attempt to rank principles in priority (or lexical) order. This effort was long thought to have been a failure until John Rawls made a powerful case for such a ranking in John Rawls, *A Theory of Justice*. (Cambridge, Massachusetts: Harvard University Press, 1971), pp. 40–45.

   I have attempted to extend the notion of lexical ranking of the principles by first grouping those principles that strive to maximize aggregate consequences (beneficence and nonmaleficence) combining them geometrically and then combining by balancing those that do not strive for maximizing aggregate consequences. At that point I have claimed that the result of balancing nonconsequence maximizing principles can be lexically ranked above the consequence maximizing ones.

5.   Robert Nozick, *Anarchy, State, and Utopia* (New York: Basic Books, Inc., 1974); Tristram H. Engelhardt, *The Foundations of Bioethics*. (New York: Oxford University Press, 1986).

6.   John Stuart Mill, "Utilitarianism." in *Ethical Theories: A Book of Readings*. A.I. Melden, ed. (Englewood Cliffs, New Jersey: Prentice-Hall, Inc., 1967), pp. 391–434, chapter 5.

7.   Aristotle. *Nicomachean Ethics*, V,3.

8.   Christopher Ake, "Justice as Equality." *Philosophy and Public Affairs* 5 (No. 1, Fall 1975): 69–89; Hugo A. Bedau, "Radical Egalitarianism." in *Justice and Equality*, pp. 168–180. Edited by Hugo A. Bedau. (Englewood Cliffs, NJ: Prentice Hall, 1971).

9.   The Hastings Center, Institute of Society, Ethics and the Life Sciences, "Values, Ethics, and CBA in Health Care," in Office of Technology Assessment, Congress of the United States, *The Implications of Cost-Effectiveness Analysis of Medical Technology* (Washington: Office of Technology Assessment, 1980), pp. 168–185.

10.   Allen Buchanan, "Justice: A Philosophical Review." *Justice and Health Care*. Edited by Earl Shelp. (Dordrecht, Holland: D. Reidel Publishing Company, 1981), pp. 3–21.

11. Robert M. Veatch, "Should Basic Care Get Priority? Doubts About Rationing the Oregon Way." *Kennedy Institute of Ethics Journal* 1 (September 1991, No. 3): pp. 187–206.

12. Abraham Mehrez and Amiram Gafni. "Quality-adjusted Life Years, Utility theory, and Healthy-years Equivalents", *Medical Decision Making* 9 (1989) 142–49; Richard Zeckhauser and Donald Shepard. "Where Now for Saving Lives?" *Law and Contemporary Problems* 40 (1976): 5–45; Jan Acton, "Measuring the Monetary Value of Lifesaving Programs." *Law & Contemporary Problems* 40 (1976): 46–72.

13. R. M. Kaplan and J. W. Bush. "Health-Related Quality of Life Measurement for Evaluation Research and Policy Analysis." *Health Psychology* 11 (1982): 61–80.

14. Ernst Troeltsch, "Das stoische-christliche Naturrecht und die moderne profane Naturrecht." In *Gesammelte Schriften*, IV (Tubingen: Verlag J. C. B. Mohr (Paul Siebeck), 1925), pp. 166–191.

15. Ronald Dworkin, "What is Equality? Part 2: Equality of Resources," *Philosophy and Public Affairs* 10 (Fall 1981): 283–345.

JACK DONNELLY

International Human Rights and Health Care Reform

The right to health care is firmly entrenched in the major international human rights documents. For example, Article 25(1) of the Universal Declaration of Human Rights declares "Everyone has the right to a standard of living adequate for the health and well-being of himself and of his family, including food, clothing, housing and medical care. . .". Likewise, Article 12 of the International Covenant on Economic, Social and Cultural Rights recognizes the right to "the enjoyment of the highest attainable standard of physical and mental health. . . . [including] the creation of conditions which would assure to all medical service and medical attention in the event of sickness."[1] These two documents, along with the International Covenant on Civil and Political Rights, are the principal international documents in the field of human rights.

These obligations have been accepted by most countries. For example, over 90 states, including most of the countries of Europe (most of which also accept more detailed regional health care obligations through the European Social Charter), are parties to the Covenant. The United States, by contrast, is not a party to the Covenant or to any other international legal instrument that recognizes a right to health care.

International law, however, should not be seen as a solution, or even very much help, in reforming the United States health care system. With very few exceptions, obligations in international law are voluntary. This is most evident in the case of treaties, executive agreements, and similar instruments, which are the principal source of contemporary public international law. States are free to chose to become a party to a treaty or not. A state that chooses not to recognize a right to health care violates no international legal obligation. And even if it did, there is the notorious problem of enforcing public international law. For example, the international "enforcement" provided by the Covenant extends no further than the requirement to submit periodic reports to a Committee on Economic, Social and Cultural Rights.

International law can point to retrograde American policies. This may be of some domestic political importance. For example, it may be useful to counter arguments that the competitive position of American industry would be harmed by recognizing and implementing a right to health care. In general, though, international law reflects, rather than shapes, the understandings and practices of states, even in states whose practices are as deviant as those of the United States in the area of health care. One might even argue that if Americans come to see health care as a right—and a basic human right at that—it is likely that international legal obligations either will be voluntarily accepted or will not make much difference to political practice in the United States.

If health care does come to be seen as a human right rather than a contingent benefit, however, the chances for radical health care reform are likely to be improved. For better or worse, ours is a rights-oriented society. We believe not only that in most circumstances rights are the highest form of political claim, but also that most important political issues are issues of rights. Whatever the virtues or defects of this assumption, and the implicit moral and political theories that it reflects, it is a political fact. Therefore, establishing a plausible case for a right to health care is likely to increase the power of demands for health care reform.

My argument will proceed at three levels. At minimum I want to show that a right to health care is not qualitatively different from human rights well recognized in the U.S. This will involve addressing some standard arguments against recognizing economic, social, and cultural rights. A related, but somewhat more ambitious argument, will emphasize substantive similarities between a right to health care and certain well recognized human rights. This involves an indirect positive argument for the right to health care. I will also argue more directly for recognizing a human right to health care.

Although this last argument is obviously theoretically the most important, it is also, obviously, the most problematic. Therefore, the bulk of my attention will be focused on the other two levels of argument, which in any case are politically at least as important. Much of the resistance to a right to health care in the United States, in so far as it involves objections of principle, seems to rest on mistaken conceptions about the nature and character of economic, social, and cultural rights. Addressing such conceptions, I believe, may actually make a more important contribution to the ongoing political debate on health care in the United States than any direct argument for a human right to health care.

A Human Right to Health Care

Human rights, as the term suggests, are the rights one has simply because one is a human being. Exactly how "being a human being" gives rise to rights, though, is theoretically obscure and problematic. The formulation of the International Human Rights Covenants— "these rights derive from the inherent dignity of the human person"— is no less problematic.

In my own work,[2] I have argued that human rights represent one type of conception of human dignity, based on equal and inalienable rights held by all individuals against society and the state. They are a moral ideal, coupled with a social practice—individual rights/ entitlements held against the state and society—to realize that ideal. They reflect a particular political conception of what it means to be a *human* being.

A list of human rights specifies our current minimum understandings of the political conditions necessary for a life *worthy* of a human being. Human rights rest on an account of a life of dignity to which human beings are "by nature" suited, and the kind of person worthy of and entitled to such a life. And if the rights specified by the underlying theory of human nature are implemented and enforced, they should help to bring into being the envisioned type of person.

Such an understanding aims to reconcile the moral universality of human rights with their obvious historical particularity. The very concept of human rights entails that they are universal rights. All human beings have the same human rights. (They either are or are not human). But what those rights are—any particular list of human rights—is historically and geographically contingent. Within these limits of time and place, however, human rights are universal, minimum requirements for living a life of dignity. I call this the relative universality of human rights.

Henry Shue has developed the useful idea of "standard threats."[3] A list of human rights reflects dominant contemporary social understandings of the most important standard threats to human dignity. This clearly implies that lists of rights will change over time, in response to changing social conditions (new or newly recognized threats to dignity) and changing social understandings of what it means to lead a life worthy of a human being.

The evolution of lists of human rights might be viewed as expressions of an improving understanding or discovery of an unvarying core of human nature. More plausibly, lists of human rights may be seen as social constructions. The very idea of human nature, as it serves as a source of human rights, is a fundamentally moral, socially constructed, notion. Psycho-biological facts about human beings set outer limits, but "human nature," in the relevant sense, is largely a social product. It concerns what it means to be a *human* being, which is more something that we create through our social life than something we discover or uncover.

How can we characterize our contemporary list of internationally recognized human rights? Elsewhere I have argued[4] that the list of rights recognized in the Universal Declaration of Human Rights and the International Human Rights Covenants reflect a particular conception of human dignity based on the requirement that the state treat each person with equal concern and respect. For example, personal rights to nationality and to recognition before the law, along with rights to life and to protection against slavery, torture and other inhuman or degrading practices (Universal Declaration, Articles 3, 4, 5, 15) can be seen as legal and political prerequisites to recognition and thus respect. Rights to equal protection of the laws and protection against racial, sexual and other forms of discrimination are essential to *equal* respect. (Universal Declaration, Articles 1, 2, 7) Equal respect for all persons will be at most a hollow formality without personal autonomy, the freedom to choose and to act on one's own ideas of the good life. Therefore, freedoms of speech, conscience, religion, and association, along with the right to privacy, are recognized. (Articles 12, 18–20) Rights to food, health care, and social insurance (Article 25) are required to make equal concern and respect a practical reality rather than a mere formal possibility.

The idea of equal concern and respect certainly is philosophically controversial. It does, however, have a certain inherent plausibility. It is closely related to the basic conceptual fact that human rights are equal and inalienable. It also offers a plausible interpretation of the common claim that human rights derive from the inherent dignity of the human person. Nonetheless, the idea is historically contingent—

most societies at most times simply have not believed that each and every person, simply because she is a human being, is entitled to equal concern and respect from the state[5] —let alone the particular specification of what such concern and respect involves.

Consider the case of the right to health care. If one conceives of death and disease as the result of sin or inferiority, as divinely caused (whether by evil forces or as punishment for evil), or as a result of forces beyond human comprehension or control, a human right to health care would be at best an incoherent notion. Likewise, in a Hobbesian state of nature, where simple survival is problematic and society rudimentary if it exists at all, it would be at best a cruel hoax to recognize a right to health care.[6]

In our world, however, there are readily available means to prevent, treat, and cure many diseases and injuries. We do not see disease as an unfathomable, or unconquerable, force, let alone as divine retribution for our sins. Health and longevity have come to be seen as the norm rather than a blessing of unusually good fortune. We think of disease as something to be treated. Untreatable diseases are viewed as a research challenge, perhaps even an affront to both the sufferer and society. And in developed Western liberal democracies, overpowering social needs or interests (e.g., extreme scarcity or lack of social order) do not politically preclude delivering considerable quantities of medical care to those who require it. Denial of access to health care thus amounts to imposing needless suffering, a terrible affront to minimum dignity. Health care therefore is (ought to be recognized as) a human right.

Some people would refer to the state of health care in the United States as a denial of basic human needs. This suggests an alternative route to justifying a right to health care. Personally, I do not find needs-based theories of human rights helpful. No scientifically established list of human needs provides justification for anything like an adequate list of human rights, and any other sort of list sacrifices the objectivity that is one of the great attractions of using needs as a basis for rights. If one does work from a needs theory, though, health care becomes one of the most basic of human rights (especially if operating with Maslow or other hierarchical needs theory). A "human need" is perhaps best defined as something that is requisite to the health or flourishing of human beings. Therefore, a right to health care would obviously be one of the most fundamental human rights.

A variety of other theoretical cases might be advanced. But I want to move beyond general or abstract theoretical arguments for the right to heath care to examine analogies with well-established human rights.

Analogies to Recognized Human Rights

Rights to life and to security of the person, which are firmly recognized in the United States as human rights, are very closely analogous to a right to health care.

The right to life is usually conceptualized in the U.S. as a right not to be killed. Our typical focus is on state violence, the right to life providing protection against arbitrary deprivation of life by the state. But the right to life also implies state protection against private violence. If the state willfully and systematically fails to protect people against violent assaults, it clearly violates the right to life. This is most obvious in the case of politically tolerated death squads. But deaths resulting from the systematic failure of the police to provide levels of protection similar to that received by the rest of society or an elite group are also violations of the right to life (not to be killed).[7]

Denial of certain forms of health care can clearly and directly lead to death. When the care could be provided at modest cost, the rights violation is very closely analogous to failure to police. Death results from denial of a generally available social service to a particular segment of society. When that care could be provided at no net cost—as many people argue is the case in the United States today—we face a particularly objectionable violation.

Likewise, the right to security of the person provides not merely protection *against* the state but protection *by* the state. In the United States, this is often expressed as the obligation of the state to protect "law and order." A state that systematically fails to protect large segments of society against violent private assaults (assuming the existence of more or less readily available societal resources to provide such protection) violates the right to security of the person no less surely, although somewhat less directly, than if it directly terrorizes the population or if it tolerates systematically abusive police practices.

Denial of access to health care often produces results very similiar to violent assault. The victim suffers preventable injury or debilitation as a result of the failure of the state to provide a generally available social service to some segment of society. And numerous American families face far greater threats to their security from lack of health insurance, or worry about the loss of insurance, than from the risk of being mugged while walking in their neighborhood. Given the high level of American spending on health care, such suffering and insecurity represents a particularly objectionable violation of basic human dignity.

These violations are additionally problematic because they involve blatant discrimination. In the United States, health care is not randomly distributed, but rationed on the basis of employment and income. The American welfare system formally guarantees access to the poorest in society. Therefore, some of the most severe problems of access may not lie at the very bottom of society. Certain segments of the working poor and those temporarily unemployed but not ordinarily considered "poor" are probably at least as severely affected. Nonetheless, the denial is systematic, well-known, and thus a form of invidious discrimination.

Analogies with the rights to life and security are especially telling because these rights are often thought of as functional prerequisites to the enjoyment of other rights and thus unusually important human rights. Although I am leery of such arguments—they often are taken to suggest that politically dangerous priority should be given to these rather minimal rights—it is true that without protection of these rights, the value of other rights usually is radically reduced. Therefore, these analogies suggest that the case for a human right to health care is particularly strong.

The Status of Economic and Social Rights

No analogy, however, is perfect. Many Western, and especially American, conservatives, have argued that economic, social, and cultural rights are qualitatively different from civil and political rights. In its strongest form, this involves the claim that economic, social, and cultural rights, including the right to health care, "belong to a different logical category," are not really *human* rights.[8] I will argue, however, that such arguments are almost entirely without merit.

Critics of economic, social, and cultural rights often argue that they are substantively less important than civil and political rights. The classic example used in such arguments is the right to paid holidays, which is recognized in Article 24 of the Universal Declaration of Human Rights. This right certainly is far less important than, say, the right to life. But the full enumerated right—the right to "rest, leisure, and reasonable limitation of working hours and periodic holidays with pay"—is very important. Consider, for example, the horrors of sixty hour work weeks, fifty two weeks a year in nineteenth century factories, or twentieth century "sweat shops" in the garment industry in the United States.

One can easily point to more minor civil and political rights. For example, Article 10 of the International Covenant on Civil and Political Rights proclaims the right of juveniles to separate prison facilities. In every country of the world, far fewer people have suffered from penal confinement as juveniles in the company of adult criminals than from the denial of reasonable rest and leisure.

In any case, the right to paid holidays is hardly the typical economic and social right. Consider, for example, the internationally recognized human rights to food, work, and social insurance —and, of course, health care. While there are differences in importance between different internationally recognized human rights, they simply do not correspond to the distinction between economic, social, and cultural rights and civil and political rights.

A second strand of criticism of economic, social, and cultural rights rests on arguments of practicality. For example, Maurice Cranston argues that "there is nothing especially difficult about transforming political and civil rights into positive rights," but that in most countries it is "utterly impossible" to realize most economic and social rights.[9] Both sides of this claim are indefensible.

In countries such as China, Cuba, Zaire, Somalia, Serbia, and North Korea today it would be almost obscene to say that it is relatively easy to transform civil and political rights into positive rights. Likewise, in the recent past people in South Africa, the Soviet Union, Guatemala, Argentina, and literally dozens of other countries have in fact found it extremely difficult to transform internationally recognized civil and political rights into effective rights in national law. Conversely, many of the impediments to implementing economic and social rights are political. For example, there is already enough food in the world to feed every person. Universal implementation of the right to food would "only" require redistributing existing supplies.

Arguments of practicality rest on the moral maxim "ought implies can." If it is impossible to do x, one does not have an obligation to do x. But "can" or "impossible" here refers to something very much like physical impossibility, not mere political ease or difficulty.[10]

For most internationally recognized economic, social, and cultural rights, the resources are available in almost all countries to make substantial progress toward implementing most civil and political and economic, social, and cultural rights alike. The argument that the obligation is relieved because of impossibility is therefore largely irrelevant.

It is certainly true that health care (and other social services) at the level provided in much of Western Europe cannot be universally implemented. But there is no reason why the right to health care need be conceptualized in such terms. Internationally recognized human rights are specified in rather general terms. When it comes to the details of implementation, there is a considerable range of legitimate variation. And this is as true of civil and political rights as economic, social, and cultural rights. Certainly no one would claim that in every country the right to a fair trial entails free legal assistance, numerous levels of appeals, and all the other niceties that characterize the contemporary American system of criminal law. Even most poor countries can make substantial progress in health care with modest additional expenditure. And in any case, the impediments to implementing a right to health care in the United States are almost entirely political. They do not even approach the sort of impossibility entailed by ought implies can.

The United States does not underspend in the area of health care. Some 14 percent of the gross national product, over $800 billion, goes to health care annually. The nation spends 170 percent more on health care per person than Great Britain, 120 percent more than Japan, 90 percent more than West Germany, and 40 percent more than Canada. Rather than underspend, we allocate an inordinately large share of medical resources to some groups and a remarkably small share to other groups.

There are, of course, political reasons for this pattern of allocation. One may even argue that it reflects the individualistic ethic that is at the core of much of American political culture. But these "practical" political problems are irrelevant to the status of health care as a human right.[11] The United States *can*, if it chooses, provide universal access to health care, significantly improving the quality of life of tens of millions of Americans at little additional financial cost. Arguments of impracticality simply hold no weight.

A third line of criticism of economic, social, and cultural rights rests on the claim that there is a qualitative difference between "negative" civil and political rights and "positive" economic and social rights. Negative rights, it is argued, require only the forbearance of others to be realized. Violating a negative right thus involves actively causing harm, a sin of commission. Positive rights require that others provide active support. Violating a positive right thus involves only failing to provide assistance, an alleged lesser sin of omission.

All human rights actually require both positive action and restraint by the state if they are to be effectively implemented. Some, though, are admittedly relatively positive, and others are relatively negative.[12] But even the distinction between relatively positive and relatively negative rights does not correspond to that between civil and political and economic and social rights.

What is it that the state is to abstain from doing to realize the right to periodic and genuine elections under a system of universal and equal suffrage? Clearly the right to vote is a largely positive right. So is the right to trial by a jury of one's peers. It can be claimed or demanded of the state, often at considerable expense. Trial by jury, or the right to effective legal remedy for violations of fundamental rights, simply is not a mere liberty that rests on state abstention.

Consider also the (civil) right to protection against racial discrimination. If it is to be more than an empty formality, the state must not merely abstain from discriminating but actually provide *protection against* discrimination. This often requires extensive, difficult, and costly intervention (e.g., affirmative action programs and even reverse discrimination). Other "freedoms from" also may require substantial positive endeavors if they are to be effectively realized. "Simply" abstaining—or, more accurately, *assuring* that certain things are not done —often requires considerable work over an extended period. In fact, if it really were easy to abstain, the right in question probably would not be very important (at least in that context).

Conversely, most economic, social, and cultural rights contain a substantial "negative" component. For example, the right to marry and found a family largely requires the state to abstain from interfering. It is no more "positive" than the right to freedom of religion. The rights to participate in the cultural life of the community and to share in the benefits of science and technology are about as negative (or as positive) as the civil right to nondiscrimination. The right to rest and leisure requires "only" restraint (on the part of employers). The right to food could in many circumstances be much better implemented if governments would simply stop encouraging the production of cash crops for export. Arguments for the efficiency of markets imply that governmental restraint may contribute significantly to realizing economic and social rights.

But regardless of how the negative-positive distinction is made with regard to internationally recognized human rights, we still must address the contention that (relatively) negative human rights have some sort of theoretical priority. This amounts to an argument that what is done to people is less important than how it is done.

Let us grant that the use of different means to the same end can influence our moral evaluation. Let us grant, for example, that it is in some sense worse to kill people than to let them die, to actively and directly injure them than to allow them to be injured. Nonetheless, it is still of great moral significance to let people die (or suffer)—at least when one is aware of their impending death (or injury), possesses the resources needed to prevent death, and is not severely constrained from acting. The offense is especially great if the resulting deaths (or injuries) are systematic.

This is precisely the case with access to health care. Despite our immense wealth and considerable spending on health care, the performance of the United States as measured by such standard statistical measures as life expectancy and infant mortality is dismal. The United States ranks (from best to worst) 19th in infant mortality, and 9th in life expectancy. A large part of the explanation for such figures is inadequate access to health care by the poor, especially the nonwhite poor. For example, a nonwhite infant in the United States is twice as likely to die as a white infant.

We know full well the consequences of not treating access to health care as a basic human right. The experience of other developed liberal democracies shows that there are alternatives. We have the resources available (probably already even being spent) to alter the situation dramatically. Yet we have more or less freely *chosen* not to act. This willful refusal to prevent well documented and relatively easily preventable suffering may be in some way qualitatively different from directly and actively causing similar suffering. The difference, however, is of relatively minor significance in any overall evaluation.

We should not be misled by misplaced analogies with personal moral or legal relations. Let us grant that no individual is obliged to go out of her way to prevent the death or injury of another person. This is no reason to hold that the state is similarly free of obligations. Quite the contrary, the state is obliged to provide a considerable array of protections for the life and personal security of all persons who fall under its jurisdiction. For example, as we saw above, a state that fails to provide basic law and order usually is responsible for the violations of rights that they "merely" allow, through inaction, to occur.

The state, of course, is not obliged to protect every person against all possible threats to life or security. Denial of guaranteed access to health care, however, is neither an obscure nor an uncharted threat. Certainly we must admit that there is a point at which the diminishing returns of further investments in protective services can no longer be justified, especially when we take into account the competing demands the state faces for the use of its scarce resources. The dismal comparative health care performance of the United States, however, indicates that we are no where near the point of diminishing returns. In fact, comparison with other developed countries suggests that with a reorganization of the system, we would likely see positive and increasing marginal returns.

In other words, even granting qualitative differences between killing and allowing to be killed, maiming and allowing to be maimed, the differences are swamped by the similarities in the case of state action with respect to access to health care. So long as we are willing to grant a state obligation to engage in vigorous and often expensive efforts to prevent and punish private theft and violence, the case for a parallel right to health care remains strong.

A rather different type of argument against economic, social, and cultural rights focuses on the substance of the underlying values that civil and political and economic, social, and cultural rights seek to realize. It is often argued that civil and political rights are specially concerned with the value of liberty. Economic, social, and cultural rights, according to this argument, are directed toward realizing the value of equality.[13] Such arguments are typically made to argue for equal emphasis to the two categories. It is easy enough, however, for American conservatives, especially those with any sort of libertarian bent, to turn this distinction into a critique of economic, social, and cultural rights *because* they favor equality over liberty.

Most if not all internationally recognized human rights in fact foster both liberty and equality. Let us grant, though, that some are directed principally towards fostering liberty and others towards equality. Once more, however, we find that this categorical distinction fails to correspond to that between civil and political and economic, social, and cultural rights.

For example, the (civil and political) rights to equal protection of the laws and protection against discrimination are *primarily* concerned with equality. The rights to due process and trial by a jury of one's peers aim to assure equal justice for all. Even classical civil liberties such as the freedoms of conscience, religion, speech, press, assembly, and association are largely concerned with equality. They do protect a sphere of personal autonomy, allowing individuals to form and pursue their own understandings of the good life. But in actual political practice, they principally protect the autonomy of minorities and those out of power; that is, the equal rights of all to make and act on important life choices.

Conversely, most economic, social, and cultural rights have a significant "liberty" dimension. The right to health care aims to liberate people from the indignities and constraints of avoidable or curable diseases. Many other economic, social, and cultural rights can also be seen as efforts to free individuals from material needs or common social or economic risks and dangers. For example, Article 11 of the International Covenant on Economic, Social and Cultural Rights speaks of "the fundamental right of everyone to be free from hunger." Some economic, social, and cultural rights are even primarily liberties. Consider, for example, the right to the free choice of marriage partners, the liberty of parents to choose schools for their children, the right to gain a living by work one freely chooses or accepts, and the rights of individuals to form trade unions and of trade unions to function freely.

A World Without Rights

A very different way to approach the question of the status of economic, social, and cultural rights is to ask what a life with only civil and political rights would look like. Without certain minimum economic and social guarantees, a life of dignity is clearly impossible, at least in modern market economies. Even strong conservatives in the Reagan Administration stressed the importance of a "safety net" of economic and social rights for "the deserving poor." Many even recognized it as a matter of right, not charity or compassion.

It is certainly possible to imagine societies with alternative conceptions of health care. Britain before World War II, for example, was a society in which dominant social understandings of human rights and dignity did not include universal access to high quality health care. This, however, is no longer the case anywhere in the so-called developed world, with the partial exception of parts of the United States. The reason, I would suggest, is that we have come to understand the direct and indirect threats to human dignity posed by the denial of access to medical care, and the striking similarities with other recognized rights (standard threats). Health care thus presents a classic case of the process I discussed above of transformations of lists of human rights in response to evolving social understandings of the conditions for and threats to human dignity.

None of this should suggest that we cannot or should not classify different types of human rights. But any differences between economic and social rights and civil and political rights are no less important than differences within each broad class of rights. Furthermore, there are striking similarities across these two classes of human rights. For example, the right to work is a right to economic participation very similar to the right to political participation. Likewise, the (civil and political) right to life and the (economic and social) right to food can be seen as two different means to protect the same value.

There may even be good reasons, in some contexts, to classify human rights as civil and political rights and economic, social, and cultural rights.[14] It is clear, though, that there are no fundamental analytical distinctions between civil and political and economic, social, and cultural rights. Therefore, the analogies between the right to health care and rights to life and security of the person carry their full force. On substantive theoretical grounds, the case for a human right to health care is a strong one.

NOTES

1. The Universal Declaration, a resolution adopted by the United Nations General Assembly on December 10, 1948 is the most widely cited statement of international human rights norms. Although not legally binding, it is widely accepted as authoritative by most states. The two International Human Rights Covenants, which were opened for signature and ratification in 1966 and entered into force in 1976 largely give greater detail to the norms of the Universal Declaration. They also create legally binding obligations on the

more than 90 states that are parties (although they provide no mechanisms for coercive international enforcement of these obligations).

2. See Jack Donnelly, *Universal Human Rights in Theory and Practice* (Ithaca: Cornell University Press, 1989), Part I.

3. Henry Shue, *Basic Rights: Subsistence, Affluence, and U.S. Foreign Policy* (Princeton: Princeton University Press, 1980).

4. Donnelly, *University Human Rights*, Chapter 4.

5. For an extended argument to this conclusion, see Donnelly, *Universal Human Rights*, chapters 3 and 4.

6. One might still want to recognize guaranteed health care as some sort of ideal that although obviously unattainable in this lifetime was still of great substantive importance to a life of dignity. I would suggest, though, that it would be a serious error to talk of it as a human right, at least as we ordinarily use that term. A human right is something that each person can claim to be entitled to receive from her society. In a truly Hobbesian world, were one ever to exist, anything beyond a right to life could not be plausibly claimed, and in a pure state of nature even that right could not be effectively claimed.

7. Similarly, I would argue that allowing people to die of starvation when food is or could be made available is also a violation of the right to life. A standard objection to such examples relies on the distinction between killing and allowing to die. This counter-argument is addressed below.

8. Maurice Cranston, *What Are Human Rights?* (New York: Basic Books, 1964), 50.

9. Maurice Cranston, *What Are Human Rights?* (London: The Bodley Head, 1973), 66–67.

10. If we were to apply the standard of political difficulty, civil and political rights would sometimes end up being denigrated. For example, in China or Cuba today it is much easier to make progress on implementing rights to health care or education than rights to freedom of the press.

11. Even if we were to consider political impediments relevant to the theoretical status of a right, this line of argument would fail. The United States could implement universal health care with far fewer immediate and long-term political problems than, say, the Chinese would face in effectively implementing a human right to freedom of the press.

12. The right to health care clearly lies on the positive side of the spectrum, although it is possible to create systems that implement the right to health care primarily through private insurance systems, with the state regulating the market and acting as an insurer of last resort.

13. Many then go on to argue for a third "generation" of human rights (e.g., to development, peace, and a clean environment) that emphasizes the value of solidarity. See, e.g., Stephen P. Marks, "Emerging Human Rights: A New Generation for the 1980s?" *Rutgers Law Review* 33 (Winter 1981): 435–452 and Karel Vasak, "Les différentes catégories des droits de l'homme," in A. Lapayre, F. de Tinguy, and K. Vasak (eds.), *Les dimensions universelles des droits de l'homme* (Brussels: Bruylant, 1990).

14.   The underlying idea that politics and economics are fundamentally separate spheres of social life, however, is so patently absurd that I suspect that little more underlies this conventional classification than complementary misguided ideologies.

LARRY R. CHURCHILL

Aligning Rights and Responsibilities

Is there a moral right to health care? Most Americans think so. They rank health above wealth and achievement as "the greatest single source of happiness."[2] And ninety one percent say they believe that "everybody should have the right to get the best possible health care— as good as the treatment a millionaire gets."[3] This is not surprising. Every industrialized democracy except the United States and the Republic of South Africa recognizes a right to health care. In all other countries, universal access to basic health services is assured as a matter of public policy, even though in practice many countries fail to achieve that objective.

Though not always called a *right*, health care is seen in these other countries as a basic good no one should be without. In the United States there is no general, legal right to health services. Still, most U.S. citizens see health care as central to their concept of a good, or even a minimally tolerable, life.[4] Being denied health care services is hazardous to a person's well-being. But of equal importance, denial of health services is an assault on one's self-respect. In short, while most Americans believe health care should be a right, this moral conviction is not reflected in the law, or in any organized government program to provide general health services to the population.

If health care is to become a *tangible* right in the United States, a way must be found to define the scope of that right. A system of health care which entitled all citizens to all possible services would be financially infeasible. We currently spend fourteen percent of our Gross Domestic Product (GDP) on health care, yet twenty five percent of the population is unserved or underserved. If we were to provide health coverage to everyone and leave other aspects of the system unchanged, health expenditures would immediately rise to twenty percent of the GDP. No one believes this is economically possible, let alone practical. There is growing consensus that financial and administrative reforms are needed, such as reducing the paperwork, eliminating duplicative diagnostic testing, and reducing both patient and physician incentives for excessive care. Yet even if all the financial and administrative efficiencies we might devise worked perfectly, there would still be a need to limit the services to which persons would be entitled under a right to health care.

In a previous work I sought to articulate a working principle for a right to health care, that is, a principle which affirms access to care as fundamental, yet also recognizes that there are limits to the level and kind of services to which any person can be entitled.[5] Need, I argued, is the essential criterion for access and cannot be superseded by financial, social worth, or other considerations. But not all needs can be met, and in the United States our seemingly insatiable appetite for health services means that the desire for higher levels of well-being and reassurance quickly turn into needs. So a full rendering of a right to care must contain provisions for parsimony in defining access and need. A right to health care based on need means, then, a right to equitable access based on need alone to all effective care society can reasonably afford.

The term "equity" is used to signal proportionality, as opposed to sheer numerical equality. Because needs vary among people—often dramatically—a policy of strictly equal access would not be equitable.

Equity "based on need alone" is intended to signal the morally arbitrary nature of race, gender, income and other differences as criteria for access to care. Any given person's needs are equivalent to anyone else's. No one holds a prior place in the health care queue because of social worth or wealth. Whatever hierarchy of needs is devised to distribute services cannot be calculated to privilege persons because of their social or financial power.

The term "effective care" calls into play a profound limiting device. It is intended to curtail useless treatments and duplicative testing, and also to substantially curb high-tech interventions of marginal utility. Making this criterion work would require a much greater degree of professional consensus than we now enjoy about what services are truly important, not to mention a way of reducing so-called "defensive medicine" through tort reform. Yet such consensus and reform are a necessary part of any change in health care than hopes to contain costs, not just the one I propose.

Finally, the phrase "what society can reasonably afford" is designed to signal that some pressing needs in health care will inevitably not be met. No modern society anywhere has devised a way to meet all the health needs of its population. Needs, even when sheered of aspirations for higher levels of well-being and reassurance, will always outrun the ability to meet them. Unless we are willing to cripple or eliminate other social programs, health care must be limited in a prudent balancing of health services with education, housing, social services, highways and dozens of others. This necessary restriction on the extent of services provided does not, however, mitigate the idea of a right to some level of services. As Beauchamp and Faden have put it, a right to health care is inalienable (it cannot be taken away) but not absolute. It can be overridden by other social priorities and is always contingent on the amount of resources society is prepared to allot to the provision of health services.[6]

In sum, the creating of limits to the right of access—limits which can be affirmed as fair—is pivotal. Without some realistic and morally cogent notion of limits, all talk of a right to health care is utopian. A variety of ways to limit services can be imagined—by a person's age, by the effectiveness of services, by their cost, and so on. Whatever ways are chosen must be ethically, as well as economically, coherent. That is, a *right* to health care must be correlated with some sort of *responsibility*. For example, Richard Lamm, the former governor of Colorado, has suggested that age could be used as a limiting criterion for a right to health care. If that were the case, the elderly would have a duty not to use expensive resources near life's end.[7] While many disagree with Lamm's proposal, he is correct in suggesting that *duties* or *responsibilities* are a critical part of any workable health care system.

In brief, affirming a right to health care is important but of limited practical help. The essential next move is to discern what a workable right would be, which means specifying the limitations on that right, and what those limits require of people morally. In what follows I will examine two ways of aligning rights and responsibilities, and will argue for a Response Model over a Good Behavior Model. These are only two of many possible ways to consider the issue, but examining these two ways will help clarify what values we should consider in thinking about allocating health resources.

The Good Behavior Model

Rights, we typically think, have corresponding responsibilities. For example, the right to freedom of expression entails a corresponding duty not to defame or slander others. Refraining from defamation and slander not only marks the boundary of free speech but is a moral responsibility which makes free speech socially viable as a right. In a similiar fashion, it is the exercise of responsibility that makes a right to health care socially viable. Not surprisingly, some parts of our society increasingly perceive responsibility in health care as a responsibility for good health practices. Here the logic of responsibility holds that accountability for our health is justified by what we know about the effects of individual lifestyle choices on health status.[8] I call this way of thinking the Good Behavior Model, because it implies that *the right to health services is forfeited, or at least weakened, by indulging in behavior damaging to one's health.*

The attraction in this way of thinking is obvious. Individuals clearly do have some control over their own health status and their need for medical services. The extent of this control marks the extent of individual responsibility. Many illnesses and injuries are seen as problems that persons inflict upon themselves through bad health behaviors. Smoking, excessive alcohol consumption, overeating, and high-cholesterol-and-low-fiber diets are only the chief examples. Driving without seat belts, riding a motorcycle without a helmet, and unprotected sexual activity are additional examples of lifestyle practices that are associated with disease and disability.

The problems which result—lung cancer, emphysema, cirrhosis of the liver, coronary artery disease, gastrointestinal cancers, motor vehicle injuries and fatalities, and a variety of sexually transmitted afflictions—are perceived as caused by choices to live in an unhealthy way. Such diseases add both to societal ill health and to health care expenditures.

In the Good Behavior Model, smokers, for example, would have a lesser right to treatment for lung cancer than non-smokers enjoy. They might lose their claim to these resources altogether. Alcoholics would relinquish any claim to liver transplants, helmetless motorcycle riders would have diminished access to emergency medical services, drug abusers to coronary care units, and so on.

This sort of thinking received a substantial boost in 1991 from the then Secretary of Health and Human Services, Dr. Louis W. Sullivan. In his "Foreword" to *Healthy People 2000*—the United States Public Health Service document which was intended to set "the Nation's disease prevention and health promotion agenda for this decade"—Dr. Sullivan endorsed the Good Behavior Model in its causal form, and thereby aided those who would endorse it as a criterion for access to care, or as a criterion for payment for care received. Sullivan's basic point was that "personal responsibility, responsible and enlightened behavior by each and every individual, truly is the key to good health."[9] He followed this claim with a litany of the health hazards of smoking, alcohol and drug abuse, and the importance of fitness and good nutrition. Asserting that "we can control our health destinies in significant ways," Sullivan finally commended what he called a "culture of character," namely, a way of thinking and acting that would reflect responsible health practices. Building this "culture of character" he contended, was "an absolute necessity."

There is no question that Sullivan is correct, but to a far more limited extent than his rhetoric suggested. Yet the problem is not so much his inflated statements about personal control over our health destinies. Rather the pitfall in his thinking is signaled by his moralizing language. Health problems, he says, result from deficient "character," from lack of responsibility for one's health habits. To be sure, he does not argue for good character as a criterion for access to care, but all that he says lends credence to this conclusion. To single out individuals as responsible is, of course, to deflect attention away from governmental inaction and professional neglect of the poor. The language of individual moral fault-finding becomes an idiom to cover ineptness in social policy. But the central point is that Sullivan invites us to embrace a logic which begins in "good behavior" and which threatens to end in denial of care for the impoverished sick because of their profligate behavior. It is a short step from the premise of a "culture of character," implying that the ill have created their own health problems, to the conclusion that therefore they do not merit treatment. A "culture of character" is easily correlated with inaction toward (and advice for) the "undeserving sick."

A central problem with the Good Behavior Model is its exaggerated notion of control. While the Good Behavior model has its roots in the American reverence for self-reliance and individual responsibility, control over one's health status and the extent of one's need for medical services is far from complete. Some behavioral factors in ill health may be only partially voluntary—for example, addiction to cigarettes, alcohol, or controlled substances. Other behavioral risks are embedded in cultural dietary traditions, or in poor nutrition or living and working environments associated with socio-economic status. An individual's responsibility cannot exceed his or her ability to choose. Hence, assignment of responsibility for health status and the need for medical care must take account of the multiple factors involved in disease causation, whether behaviors contributing to ill health are voluntary or non-voluntary, and whether they are individually chosen or socially sponsored choices.

Efforts to base access to health care (or payment for health services) on individual responsibility for one's health care are very slippery. Such efforts frequently exaggerate our knowledge of causes or ignore multiple factors in the causes of diseases. They also run the risk of blaming the victim. Dan Beauchamp argues, "Victim-blaming misdefines structural and collective problems of the entire society as individual problems, seeing these problems as caused by the behavioral failures or deficiencies of the victims."[10]

In sum, responsibility for one's health status should be the focus of substantial educational and public health efforts. Active promotion of healthy lifestyles and sound health habits is altogether laudatory. Yet to step beyond this educational mission and invoke characterologic language and behavioral flaws is dangerous. It leads to basing allocation or financing decisions on Good Behavior thinking and results in a system that is punitive toward the sick. Responsibility for individual health-related behaviors is only one dimension of a just overall health policy. If taken by itself, and as way of curtailing rights to services, it will lead us in the wrong direction.

The Response Model

In the face of limited health care resources, the key individual responsibility is for realistic expectations and wise use of these resources. This is the health-related responsibility of citizenship. It is the obligation to think of health care services not only as an individual and private benefit but as a social and public good as well.

This connection of a right to health care with responsibility for judicious use can be called the Response Model of linking rights and responsibilities. *Rights to health care are granted by a society, and in response the individual takes responsibility to use only his or her fair share.* Responsibilities are individual expressions of response toward maintenance of the social or common good. Rights cannot be sustained without responsibilities, just as individuals cannot be sustained without social support.

The Response Model requires a new way of thinking. It requires assent to the idea that a health care system must be shaped and defined by the health needs of the population rather than the personal needs and preferences of professionals or powerful consumers. In many countries, this means tolerance for waiting periods for non-emergency surgery, and curtailment of treatment for some conditions which satisfy personal needs but have little or no bearing on the health of the population. This includes, for example, treatments for baldness, cosmetic procedures, and very expensive treatments of marginal utility near the end of life.

Consider Canada. There, the supply of hospitals, surgeons, and intensive care units is limited, so there are fewer solid organ transplants. Or consider the United Kingdom. There are waiting periods for elective surgeries such as hip replacements, and a limited supply of money and facilities for CT scanners. There is less aggressive chemotherapy and radiation treatment for advanced cancer. Yet all citizens of both Canada and the United Kingdom are provided access to a primary care physician and their general health status is as good or better than ours in the United States. Ultimately, deciding which health services to provide and which to forgo is a public policy question. The point is that in *any* system, some services will have to be limited if there is to be equity of access and proportionate funding left for schools, roads, defense, and the like.

A viable and fair health care system is something in which all citizens have a stake. We all share a common human vulnerability to disease, disability, and death. We are all poor predictors of the time or extent of our need for health services. We all support through tax dollars the creation and maintenance of the various institutions of health care, including hospitals, nursing homes, and the education of health professionals. And we all have a stake in a healthy populace above and beyond the stake we have in our personal health. This shared vulnerability and investment in creating the means of medical and social assistance point to a responsibility for judicious use of the resources for health that we possess. The responsibility individuals have is not only for healthy lifestyles but also for their general expectations and specific demands on a system that is understood to be finite.

This responsibility of individuals must be grounded in their awareness that health resources will *always* be scarce relative to needs. No modern society has yet devised a way to meet all the health needs of its citizens. Individuals can help by adopting prudent health habits, but even more so by accepting more equitably priced health insurance (that is, not disproportionately expensive for the poor, the unemployed, or the sick), and by forming more realistic expectations for what the system can provide.

Individuals will assume responsibility for using and supporting a health care system only when that system is seen as equitable and just. In short, this health-related civic responsibility for prudential use and equitable burden of cost will be impossible without a general right of access to adequate health care for all. The current patchwork system which allocates health services by price, by age, and by employment status, and leaves a quarter of the population underinsured or uninsured, cannot inspire a sense of responsibility, either individual or collective. The result is a consumer-oriented approach to health care, one that encourages us to satisfy all of our personal health needs without regard to what effect this has on the well-being of others.

Conclusion

Developing a viable and fair health care system does not mean simply providing coverage for the medically indigent, important as that is. Given the escalating costs of health care, more of the same for more people is a recipe for economic disaster. Reforms to the system in financing and organization are essential, but they are not sufficient. These organizational reforms must be accompanied by reforms in our thinking.

One reorientation needed is linking a right to health care services with responsible use of those services, and avoiding the erroneous and punitive Good Behavior Model. The notion that a right has to be earned by good behavior, as this forfeiture model portrays it, undermines it as a right and makes it ultimately a commodity granted to the behaviorally worthy. Such a health care system would be just as morally flawed as one that granted a right to health care on the basis of race or gender. The Good Behavior Model, in sum, focuses on the grounds for disqualification, whereas the Response Model focuses on the civic virtues to be exercised in receiving care.

The Response Model allows us to talk of health care as a social good, and not just as an individual good, because the response of judicious use and acceptance of limits is a response to a social policy of fairness. This opens the way for a non-commercial concept of health care as part of the social and public world which, as Hannah Arendt says, we all hold in common without anyone owning it.[11]

During the next decade, we will likely see profound changes in the organization and financing of health care. Some believe that national health insurance with centralized control and management, will prevail, while others—looking at the initiatives of Oregon and elsewhere—believe that each state will become its own organizational unit for health policy. In either case, realigning rights and responsibilities is essential.

NOTES

1. An earlier and shorter version of this essay appeared in *North Carolina Insight* (November, 1991). The research and writing was supported by the Charles E. Culpeper Foundation through a Scholarship in Medical Humanities.

2. Louis Harris, *Inside America* (Vintage Books, New York, 1987), 40.

3. Louis Harris and Associates for the Harvard Community Health Plan Foundation and the Loran Commission, *Making Difficult Health Care Decisions* (June 1987), 8.

4. Arthur Barsky, "The Paradox of Health," *New England Journal of Medicine* (1988) 318: 414–418.

5. Larry R. Churchill, *Rationing Health Care in America: Perceptions and Principles of Justice* (Notre Dame, Ind.: University of Notre Dame Press, 1987), 94ff.

6. Tom Beauchamp and Ruth Faden, "The Right to Health and the Right to Health Care," *Journal of Medicine and Philosophy*, 4 (June, 1979), 121–122.

7. Richard Lamm, "Critical Decisions in Medical Care: Birth to Death," *Southern Medical Journal* (1989) 82: 822–824.

8. An earlier form of this discussion of rights linked to individual responsibility for health was published in *Innovative Partnerships for Affordable Health Care*, program and background papers for the National Governors' Association Meeting, Sept. 23–24, 1990, Washington, D.C., 48.

9. Public Health Service, *Healthy People 2000: National Health Promotion and Disease Prevention Objectives* (Washington, D.C.: U.S. Department of Health and Human Services, Pub. No. (PHS) 91-50213, 1991).

10. Dan Beauchamp, "Public Health as Social Justice," *Inquiry* 13(1976)4–6.

11. Hannah Arendt, "Public Rights and Private Interests," in Michael Mooney and Florian Stuber, eds., *Small Comfort for Hard Times: Humanists on Public Policy* (New York: Columbia University Press, 1977), 104.

AUDREY R. CHAPMAN

A Human Rights Approach to Health Care Reform

What does it mean to speak about a right to a basic and adequate standard of health care? The concrete requirements and implications of affirming a right to a basic and adequate standard of health care are as follows:

1. A right to health care based on the principle of universality requires that a basic and adequate standard of health care be guaranteed to all citizens and residents.

A. A secure entitlement requires legal recognition. While legal recognition by itself cannot guarantee secure and meaningful access to basic health care, legislative provision of a guaranteed standard of health care is a necessary prerequisite. The neglect of the recommendations contained in the 1983 Presidential Commission report on *Security Access to Health Care for All* suggest that underscoring society's ethical obligations may or may not be translated into a change in public policy. In contrast, a legal right imposes binding obligations on one or more levels of government.

B. A secure and meaningful right to health care requires elimination of all grounds for exclusion. The principle of universality acknowledges that all persons, without regard to their purchasing power, social status, or personal merit, are entitled to basic and adequate health care. Conversely, it does not accept the validity of the current practice of denying coverage to many of those with the greatest need of health care. A human rights approach, based on justice rather than efficiency, does not recognize any valid grounds for withholding health care from the poor, the unemployed, or individuals with preexisting conditions or hereditary proclivities to disabilities or illness.

C. The principle of universality mandates that all citizens and residents be covered. Although many countries distinguish between

149

citizens and non-citizens or citizens plus legal residents and others in according rights, excluding some residents, like nondocumented aliens, imposes a form of discrimination that is inconsistent with human rights criteria. By doing so, governments deny basic health care to some of the most disadvantaged individuals and groups. It is also counter-productive because it increases the likelihood that others will be exposed to communicable diseases. Moreover, in the United States, many of those who are precluded from receiving preventive and primary health care services will eventually be treated less effectively in hospital emergency rooms at far higher cost.

D. In an affluent society, it is appropriate that the standard package of benefits guaranteed to all citizens and residents be set at a generous and comprehensive level.   The right to health care is society specific, defined in relationship to the level and type of resources available. In an affluent industrialized society, like the United States, the standard package available to all citizens and resident should be set at a generous and comprehensive level. Such a standard of health care should include full preventive and primary services and most types of acute care, reproductive, long-term care, and mental health services. A basic entitlement package needs to provide for special needs of the disabled and disadvantaged groups as well as the general needs of the population.

2. A rights approach would emphasize the equality of all persons and their inherent right to health care as the framework for health care reform.

A. Human rights are predicated on a recognition that all members of society have equal moral claims and have to be treated as such.   The principle of equality underscores the importance of providing uniform standing and status to all Americans within the health sector. A human rights approach would not necessitate that all health care resources be distributed according to a strict quantitative equality or that society attempt to provide equality in medical outcomes, neither of which would in any case be feasible. Instead, the universality of the right to health care requires a specific entitlement be guaranteed to all members of our society without discrimination.

B. Health care requires a national system based on a standard set by the federal government that does not vary according to the resources of specific states or regions. An entitlement established by the federal government has to be uniform in all parts of the country. Current variations in funding levels and benefits by states should not be incorporated in a new and more equitable national health care system. To achieve this uniformity, the federal government will have to levy a broad-based tax that will redistribute resources within the health care system.

C. *To promote equality, there should also be a single-tier health care system rather than a dual-tier system in which the poor are given a different standard of health care than the middle class.* Multiple option or tiered systems tend to result in class stratification. More affluent people, who can afford to do so, pay extra for plans offering better coverage and freedom to choose the best doctors, while the poor are left with cheaper, lower quality health care. Because it is highly unlikely that Americans will accept a system that lacks options for extra services, it is important to provide safeguards and incentives within health care reform to assure as much equity as possible. In health care systems which provide comprehensive basic packages of benefits, permitting citizens to purchase extra care on the side, such as Great Britain, Sweden, or Canada, most users and providers stay within the mainstream system.

3. *By employing rights language, the provision of health care would be understood as a fundamentally important social good to be considered differently from other goods and services.*

A. *In applying a rights designation, a society assigns priority to a particular human or social attribute and accepts responsibility for its promotion and protection.* Rights discourse accords moral criteria related to achieving true universal access and redressing historical inequities in the health care system greater importance than cost containment as the motive force for health care reform. A right approach would also have implications for health care reform. To assert that a particular goal is a right does not imply that its claim is absolute, but it does confer a considerable advantage in the competition for scarce resources and governmental attention. Or to put another way, "rights are strong considerations that *generally* prevail in competition with other concerns."[1]

B. A logical corollary of health care being understood as a fundamentally important social good is that the health care system itself should be evaluated by a social or community standard.   A primary goal of the health care system is promoting the general health and well-being of the population as a whole. Designating health care as a right therefore changes the status of health care from a commodity regulated primarily by market forces for the financial benefit of health care providers to a social good to be distributed according to principles of justice.

To be judged by a social or community standard means that the basic structure of the health care system would be evaluated according to its ability to promote the general health of the population as a whole. The current health care system does not fare well when assessed by this standard. Proposals for health care reform also need to be rigorously evaluated to their ability to contribute to the promotion of the general health of the population. This public interest standard constitutes a very different approach than politics as usual in which special interests with money and political influence typically prevail at the expense of the common good.

C. A health care reform initiative designed to assure a meaningful and secure health care entitlement requires a new paradigm that places a greater emphasis on health protection, prevention of disease, and community-based and oriented primary health care services.   The dual goals of universal coverage and cost containment cannot be achieved within a health care system that focuses on expensive curative medicine delivered by specialist physicians. Moreover, to promote the general health of the population as a whole, public policies need to place a priority on improving health conditions. Comprehensive health protection would include measures to improve air quality, significantly reduce exposure to toxic substances, assure greater workplace safety, discourage substance abuse, eliminate the availability of guns and weapons, and cleanup water supplies. Major investments in preventive health services, such as inoculations, early detection screening for disease, and regular checkups, would be another component of the strategy.

4. A human rights approach focuses particularly on the needs of the most disadvantaged and vulnerable communities.

An egalitarian account of justice applied to health care, such as Robert Veatch offers in his article in this volume, requires a pattern of distribution that confers priority on the disadvantaged and those with the greatest needs. The principle is that an allocation is right *prima facie* in so far as it contributes to opportunities for equality of well-being.[2]

    A. A human rights approach therefore implies both nondiscrimination and affirmative action to rectify historical inequities in access to health care. Measures of affirmative action taken with a view to eliminating a legacy of discrimination do not contravene the principle of equal rights.[3] Improving the health access of those who have historically lacked equal opportunities for health care and bringing them up to mainstream standards benefits the entire society. To be consistent with a human rights approach, health care reform should be designed to eliminate instances of discrimination and to promote the positive enjoyment of equal rights.

    B. Because a human right is a universal entitlement, its implementation is measured particularly by the degree to which it benefits those who hitherto have been the most disadvantaged and vulnerable and brings them up to mainstream standards. A health care reform seeking equal access and opportunities for disadvantaged and vulnerable groups would be quite different from changes which focus on protecting the insurance coverage and benefits of individuals and groups (like the middle class) which have hitherto been among the "haves." Because the current health care system disproportionately benefits some groups, (notably whites, the affluent, and the insured) and systematically disadvantages others, (primarily the poor, the uninsured, and various racial and ethnic minorities) reforms which focus particularly on improving the health status of "have nots" would generate more fundamental structural changes. It would go beyond plugging loopholes to recrafting a health care system capable of being as responsive to the needs of the disadvantaged as the present system is to the health needs of the middle class.

    5. By establishing a clear individual entitlement to health care, a rights approach would empower individuals and groups to assert their claims.

    Claims to health care would be a matter of right, and not regarded as a privilege, a matter of charity, or an optional service.[4] As Annette Baier points out, "The language of rights directs attention to individual persons, and to them not as duty-bearers or contributors to the human task, but as beneficiaries or claimants to a share of what is produced by the performance of that task." She goes on to observe that "the language of right pushes us, more insistently than does the language of duties, responsibilities, obligations, legislation and respect for law, to see the participants in the moral practice as single clamorous living human beings, not as families, clans, tribes, groups, classes, churches, congregations, nations or people."[5] A rights approach offers a normative vocabulary that facilitates both the framing of claims and the identification of the right holder. This means that the addressees of the rights or duty-bearers, in this case the federal and state governments, have a duty to provide the entitlement, not to society in general, but to each member. This standing has very important implications for efforts to seek redress in cases where the entitlement is not provided or the right violated.

A. A human rights approach empowers or facilitates individuals and groups to make claims and receive entitlements. That a human rights approach empowers individuals and groups to make claims is an important consideration in a situation where there are historical inequities in access to health care. Lack of insurance coverage is but one of the ways that the current health care system does not meet the needs of minorities, the urban poor, and persons with disabilities. Hospitals and other providers choose sites, offer services, and engage in a host of other practices to draw patients who are less likely to get sick and to discourage uneconomic patients.[6] Providers often treat minorities with rudeness and inattentiveness. Because the health care system is so complex and requires organizational skills, those who are poorly educated or lack fluency in English are frequently ill-equipped to see that their needs are met. Moreover, studies indicate that groups which have experienced long-standing oppression and hold little hope for improved conditions tend to have worse health status than those who are poor but more hopeful in their outlook.[7]

B. Enabling individuals and groups to claim these rights requires ongoing education and the establishment of institutions and procedures that facilitate claiming these entitlements. Informing and educating rights holders as to the nature of their rights and how to secure them is a major responsibility of the governments providing funding and services. Improving the accessibility of health services through such measures as using vans, providing services in schools, expanding and relocating primary care sites to local neighborhoods is another component. Providing incentives for people to use certain services might be another approach.[8]

6. A meaningful and secure right requires that health care be affordable and publicly financed.

A. Recognition of a right to health care mandates that society remove financial barriers to basic and adequate health care. Access to the basic and adequate standard of health care guaranteed to all citizens and residents should not vary depending on financial resources. The quality and scope of basic health services provided would need to be the same for all persons regardless of their financial status.

B. A human rights approach also assumes a social or public responsibility for financing basic health care services. A right to health care mandates that benefits or entitlements be uniform or related to need but that financing reflect an ability to contribute. One of the two primary ways that society acknowledges public responsibility for financing is by accepting the principle of social insurance in which the healthy subsidize the sick. Community ratings which set equal premiums for all members of the group accomplishes this goal. The second is by collectivizing revenues for health care through a broad-based progressive tax. A public, single-payer system of national insurance would be the simplest way to achieve these objectives.

C. Additionally, the means by which the health care system is financed would need to be equitable and fair. Taxes, premiums, and patient cost-sharing rates should be set at levels that do not impose burdens that are linked to income and ability to pay. Because even modest premiums may be unaffordable for those with low incomes, the system will also need meaningful public subsidies for these groups. If employers are required to provide health insurance, small businesses with low profit margins may need to receive some form of subsidy.[9]

D. A formulation of the right to health care which links the scope of the entitlement to the resource levels available in a particular society also implies that the total cost of health care is affordable on a societal

level. The objective is to seek a national consensus on a cost conscious standard of health care. This could best be accomplished
through a new paradigm for health care emphasizing preventive and
primary health care services and utilizing family practitioner physicians (general practitioners), nurse practitioners, and other professionals rather than relying on specialist physicians. Containing health care
costs also requires limiting fees and provider profits. The price of
helath care, understood as a human right, should not be left to the
market.

7. *A human rights approach underscores the importance of public
participation in shaping health care policy and of major health care
institutions being accountable to the broader public.*

A. *There needs to be meaningful public consultations about goals
and options related to health care reform.* The recognition of a new
universal legal entitlement requires a new political consensus. It is a
political action in the most profound sense through which a community redefines the nature of its ties and its obligations to its members.
Thus setting the agenda for health care reform cannot and should not
be the prerogative of medical professionals, health care providers, or
public policy elites. The legitimacy of both the process and the specific
definition of the right depends on the broadest possible involvement
of its citizens. Meaningful participation entails the careful design of
a process through which issues are identified and forums provided
that encourage citizen input into the debate. Moreover, these debates
should hear the voices of the heretofore voiceless: the homeless,
migrant workers, poor urban residents, the disabled, and those who
live in remote rural communities. Various mechanisms including hearings, community forums, and surveys could continually assure public
input into health care reform as well as data to help evaluate implementation.

B. *Health care consumers should be representative on all decision-making boards so that oversight and control are not the prerogative only of health care professionals.* To assure public participation,
all decision-making bodies should be required to have public representatives, at least some of whom have background protecting consumers'
interests. Community-based and oriented primary care networks
would offer a meaningful way to achieve public participation on an
ongoing basis. While the communities would in most cases be geo-

graphically defined, it might also be possible to have some "magnet" centers that would cater to groups with special linguistic or cultural needs. Like school boards in many localities, community-based and oriented primary care centers could better enlist residents' or subscribers' input and participation in management, priority setting, and identification of innovative delivery mechanisms.

 C. *A human rights approach entails the accountability and transparency of major institutions in the health sector.*   Institutions, particularly those which set policies and standards, need to be publicly accountable and data about their operations publicly accessible. Public participation and accountability should be the standard at all levels of the health sector—federal, state, and local/regional. Federal and state boards at the very least should publish annual state of the nation's health reports which outline the major decisions they have made and evaluates implementation of the health care reform. A variety of other mechanisms, including open hearings and surveys should be incorporated into the operation of the system.

 8. *A rights formulation translates into a series of obligations on the part of the federal and state governments.*

 Recognition of rights claims implies duties for both individuals and governments. In the case of a recognized legal right, the relevant governmental authorities assume a major responsibility. Language of the International Covenant on Economic, Social and Cultural Rights, for example, vests parties to the covenant with the responsibility to achieve the full realization of the rights enumerated in this instrument. Under the federal system in the United States, the obligations associated with recognizing a right to health care would be shared by federal and state governments.

 A. *The framework, priorities, and orientation of the health care system must be consistent with a human rights approach.*   An entitlement to a basic and adequate level of health care requires both legal recognition and structural reforms to rectify inadequacies and inequities in the current health care system. The responsibilities of government encompass formulating a framework or plan through which to promote progressive realization of health care as a human right, as well as undertaking specific policies and actions intended to achieve that goal. In addition, legal recognition means that the content of the right should be used as a standard of evaluation for all public policy formulation. Finally, governments have the duty to set a framework conducive to private individuals and groups contributing to implementation.

B. The achievement of universal coverage has the highest priority and therefore should be achieved in the shortest possible time. Preferably universality should be coterminous with the initiation of health care reforms. Another possibility would be to vest immediately all persons with rights, with benefits gradually phased in over time. Recognition of a right would provide individuals with legal standing if the government deferred granting entitlements beyond the designated period.

C. With regard to health care, the duty to respect the equality of all persons is associated with a responsibility not to discriminate. Where there is a legacy of discrimination or inequities related to a right, governments have a particular responsibility to rectify and redress this pattern. In the United States, this translates into the need for a vigorous affirmative action policy with regard to health care, one component of which would be to give priority to problems of minority, disadvantaged, and underserved individuals and communities. Another component would be to evaluate systematically whether proposed public policy changes would have a beneficial impact on the health status of these communities. Concerted efforts to address and compensate for the unequal distribution of health care facilities would be a third requirement.

D. The obligation of government has a positive component to remove obstacles to or barriers to access, a kind of affirmative action applied to the health care sector. Although health care reform proposals typically focus on expanding health insurance coverage, providing universal health insurance coverage will not assure access to appropriate health services. Among the problems that would have to be addressed are the uneven distribution of health care providers and facilities, particularly the lack of quality health care in urban centers and rural areas; the inappropriateness and cost of the prevailing acute care paradigm which neglects preventive services; and financial and nonfinancial barriers that inhibit the poor, ethnic and racial minorities, and the disadvantaged from having equal access to health care. Meaningful health care reform should both provide incentives for physicians to practice in underserved areas as well as to redistribute health care facilities more equitably.

E. With regard to health care, the duty to protect in a narrow sense relates to preventing other institutions and individuals from violating the health care rights of individuals and communities.   In a wider context, the duty to protect includes the establishment of policies conducive to health protection, such as effective regulation to preserve or restore clean air and water, reduce exposure to toxic substances, and assure workplace safety.

F. A duty to fulfill also obligates government to develop a plan with a timetable and specific goals through which it can move toward progressive realization of a full right to basic health care.   While it would be unrealistic to expect a government to implement immediately all components of a major restructuring of the health care system, it cannot indefinitely delay the process. Given its importance, universal coverage should be given first priority.

G. Monitoring the implementation of a right to health care and using these data to revise public policies is another important obligation of governments.   This requires the development of appropriate standards and indicators to assess the achievement of the right to basic health care, the use of a database that permits disaggregation into appropriate categories, and regular evaluation creating time series data. Some of this monitoring could be accomplished through national health care surveys. It would also require the design of special research tools and projects, particularly to monitor the status of the homeless, migrant workers, and some ethnic minorities.

9. A rights approach provides potential recourse for those who experience violations.

A human rights formulation accords right-holders a special protected status. Having a right gives its possessor moral standing to demand the entitlement which is due, and, if it is not forthcoming, to complain that she or he was denied what morality required. If an individual's moral right is not secured, rights language directs our attention to the wrong done. In contrast, the failure to meet one's

obligations focuses attention on the agent who did not live up to her/
his obligations, and not on the victim of that failure.[10]

*A. A simple appeals process not requiring legal counsel needs to
be incorporated into the health care system.* When a right becomes
a legal entitlement, an individual or group whose rights are being
violated can institute legal action to secure the right. In situations
where an entire category of persons are having their rights violated,
class action suits may be filed on behalf of the group. Because legal
suits are time-consuming and expensive, it would be preferable for
alternative mechanisms to be provided, such as ombudspersons with
the power to hear and act on complaints. An effective monitoring
system that could evaluate the extent to which the right to health
care was being implemented successfully as a basis for public policy
changes would also be very important.

*B. There also should be the possibility of legal recourse as a
last resort for individuals and groups.* Legal redress may provide a
significant potential means of securing the rights of an individual or
groups. The possibility of legal action also many offer incentives to
respect rights. To secure such a right, it will be necessary to provide
legal aid to those who lack required financial resources.

*10. The rights approach advocated in this study balances individ-
ual needs with the common good thereby making the viability and
effectiveness of the health care system a shared concern and responsibility.*

*A. The claiming of rights implies associated responsibilities for
individuals and groups.* Because individuals within a democratic
society have a dual status as right-holders and duty-holders, they
have an obligation collectively to promote and protect the health care
system. To hold a right is to have a reciprocal obligation to the society
that grants the right. This has several implications. First, it requires
that all members of society keep claims to a reasonable and affordable
level. Second, it means that individuals, as well as governments, have
duties as well as rights. One duty is personal responsibility for one's
own health. Another duty is to be sensitive to the health care needs
of others and a collective responsibility for meeting the needs of the
most vulnerable and disadvantaged members of society. Third, establishing the framework and basic structure of the health care system

becomes a social rather than a private prerogative. Health care institutions belong to the society collectively and are not the exclusive private property of the providers who control them.

One aspect of individual and collective responsibility is to have realistic and appropriate expectations regarding health care. The right to health care is not an unlimited and open-ended entitlement. A societal commitment to health protection and improvement does not necessitate a constantly increasing investment of the gross national product to health care at the expense of other goals. Nor does it imply that the goal is perfect or optimal health for each of its members. It most likely means that the standard for treatment of chronic illness be "care" rather than "cure." There also need to be corporate decisions about other sensitive and difficult issues, one of which is investment of resources in futile care. Currently vast resources are invested in active treatment of terminally ill patients, often prolonging death rather than extending life, and not infrequently ignoring the patient's own directive.

B. The primary goal, the highest priority of the health care system should be that of fostering the common good and collective health of society, not the particularized good of individuals. Health should be understood as a common benefit,[11] as well as an individual right. A primary goal of the health care system should be to promote the general health of the population as a whole. Any individual right to health care should be understood as a component of a broader effort to protect and improve the public's health. It has been suggested that a society has a sufficient level of health when its citizens are healthy enough to pursue common purposes and participate in the life of its private communities. An alternative way of conceptualizing a sufficient level of health would be that poor health of constituent groups is no longer an impediment to the functioning of social and political institutions.[12]

C. Health care reform initiatives should therefore provide incentives for promoting health lifestyles. Positive incentives are very different, however, from the "good behavior model" of limiting health care benefits. According to this approach, the right to health services is qualified or lost by indulging in behavior damaging to one's health. In the good behavior model, smokers would have a lesser right to treatment for lung cancer than non-smokers enjoy, and driving without a seat belt would be grounds for forfeiting payments for treatment for motor vehicle-related injuries. As Larry Churchill points out, the problem with the "good behavior" approach is that it is based on an exaggerated notion of control. Many behavioral factors related to unhealthy lifestyles are embedded in cultural dietary traditions and in living and working environments associated with socio-economic status, not in personal decision-making. Assignment of responsibility for health status is also far more complex than this model implies; there are usually multiple factors involved in disease causation. Moreover, the good behavior model deflects attention away from governmental inaction and professional neglect of the poor, both of which are far greater determinants of health outcomes.[13]

NOTES

1. James W. Nickel, *Making Sense of Human Rights: Philosophical Reflections of the Universal Declaration of Human Rights* (Berkeley: University of California Press, 1987), pp. 16–17.

2. See Robert M. Veatch's contribution to this volume.

3. This point has been made by interpreters of the International Covenant on Economic, Social and Cultural Rights. According to Philip Alston, Chair of the U.N. Committee on Economic, Social and Cultural Rights, "Measures of affirmative action taken with a view to eliminating discrimination do not contravene the Covenant." His comments are in "The International Covenant on Economic, Social and Cultural Rights," United Nations Centre on Human Rights, *Manual on Human Rights Reporting* (New York: United Nations, 1991), p. 47.

4. Virginia A. Leary, "Conceptualizing and Promoting the Right to Health Care," paper presented at the Symposium on the Right to Health Care, Annual Meeting of the American Association for the Advancement of Science, February 7, 1992.

5. See Annette Baier's forthcoming *Passions of the Mind* to appear with Harvard University Press.

6. See Daniel Wikler's contribution to this volume.

7. Herbert Nickens, M.D., "The Needs of Minorities," Roundtable: Perspectives on Defining a Minimum Adequate Standard of Health Care," AAAS Right to Health Care Consultation, November 13, 1992.

8. Many of these measures were suggested by Herbert Nickens, *Idem.*

9. On these points see Janet O'Keeffe's article in this volume.

10. See Dan Brock's article in this volume.

11.   Daniel Callahan, *What Kind of Life: A Challenging Exploration of the Goals of Medicine* (New York: Touchstone Books, 1990), p. 110.

12.   *Ibid.*, pp. 189–190.

13.   See Larry Churchill's discussion in his article in this volume.

PART THREE

Defining a Basic Standard of Health Care

Part Four

Defining a Minimum Standard of
Health Care

MARY ANN BAILY

Defining the Decent Minimum

Most people agree that health care is a good of unusual importance. For individuals, health care plays a vital role in preventing pain and suffering, preserving the ability to live a normal life, providing information, and relieving worry. For society, health care can avert social costs associated with disease and disability, and contribute to the achievement of social goals. Finally, health care's importance in individual lives makes access to health care of deep symbolic significance, reflecting the concern members of society feel for one another.

For these reasons, there is broad support for a public role in ensuring access to health care. In justifying this role, some focus on the individual's claim on society, framing the issue in terms of a right to health care. Others focus on society's duty to the individual, framing the issue as one of social responsibility. Still others emphasize the pragmatic benefits to society from a healthy population and an enhanced sense of community.

Whatever the justification for a public role in ensuring access, a central question is: Access to what? The benefits of health care vary in importance, from the preservation of life to the elimination of minor inconvenience, and some highly beneficial care is extremely costly. Society's resources are limited. To guarantee universal access to all care of any benefit would be prohibitively expensive, compromising the ability to spend resources on other important social goods which might even have more impact on health through, for example, better nutrition or safer transportation. It seems reasonable to conclude that society must guarantee access only to a limited level of care. This level is variously referred to as a "decent minimum," "basic care," or "an adequate level," with the content determined in reference to the reasons for considering health care to be "special."[1]

In the United States, all parties to the current debate on health care reform seem to accept this approach to ensuring access. Nevertheless, translating it into practical policy is proving difficult and controversial. Reaction to Oregon's plan for restructuring the provision of health care to the poor illustrates this. Many who accept the objective—to guarantee a "basic level of care" to everyone while setting fair limits on the care provided at public expense—nevertheless have serious reservations about the methods Oregon is using to pursue it.

This paper considers issues in the implementation of the decent minimum approach to access to health care. The paper does not pretend to be a rigorous examination of the intellectual foundations of the approach or a detailed description of specific health care reforms. Rather, it offers some reflections on the practical task of structuring a real health care system to define and deliver adequate health care to all Americans.

Characteristics of the Adequate Level

What *is* an adequate level? Generalizations about what it should look like flow naturally from the logic of the arguments justifying the approach to guaranteeing access. The various arguments differ in important respects. It is beyond the scope of this paper to evaluate their relative merits, and in any case, agreement on any one justification for the decent minimum is unlikely in a pluralistic society like the United States.[2] For this discussion, what is important is the fact that the different arguments have practical implications in common.

One such implication is that the adequate level of care varies with health condition. All the arguments for an adequate level approach imply that the importance of health care—the extent to which it is special—depends on an individual's health state. Therefore, any system to define and deliver a basic level of care must be able to vary the care according to individual need; a decent minimum cannot be simply an amount of money or a fixed amount of care.

The adequate level of care also varies with the availability of resources in the society. All the arguments imply that the benefits of health care must be weighed against costs in the light of competing uses for resources; poor societies cannot be expected to set as high a standard of adequacy as rich societies. In tempering the definition of adequacy to available resources, the priorities and values of society's members are important in guiding the trade-offs they would make among different kinds of health benefits, and between health benefits and other social goods.

Definition of adequate care for a particular health condition requires specification of the kind, the amount, *and* the quality of health care to be received. Given resource constraints, an adequate level of treatment may mean no treatment at all for some health conditions, and quality will not necessarily be the highest possible.

Therefore, the task of specifying an adequate level is one of describing a standard of care, not an insurance benefit package. This is a critical point. Discussions about the meaning of a right to health care or of equitable access to care have often focused on access to health insurance and the need to guarantee everyone "basic coverage." When asked to define "basic coverage," advocates tend to respond with a laundry list of service categories: hospital care, physician services, diagnostic tests. A list of services does not, however, define an adequate level of care any more than a list of foods defines an adequate diet. Setting fixed limits on quantities is not a solution, since it does not adjust coverage to health status. When pressed for specifics, therefore, advocates sometimes delineate specific condition-related care that should or should not be covered. For example, prenatal care, periodic screening mammograms, immunizations, well-child care, and kidney dialysis are included; cosmetic surgery, heart and liver transplants, and long-term ventilator support for the permanently unconscious are not.

A particularly detailed example of a condition-related approach is the Oregon plan. Its creators have developed a list of over 700 "condition-treatment pairs" and ranked them in order of importance. State budget constraints then determine how much of the list is covered in a given year, and thus the definition of the adequate level. Critics have noted, however, that there is still considerable heterogeneity among patients who fall within a particular condition-treatment group. This means that some patients in funded high-priority categories would receive far less treatment benefit in relation to cost than some patients in unfunded low-priority categories. The list also fails to address the specific content of the items covered. For example, for prenatal care, how many visits are provided? What level of practitioner delivers the care? What happens during each visit? Finally, diagnostic effort must be expended to determine the patient's category. There is no fixed limit on this expense, even as there is tight restraint on treatment of the conditions identified.

The problem is, the "decent minimum" should not be seen as a list of conditions and treatments to be developed once and for all and imposed on the health care system. Only when the adequate level is seen as an entire standard of care can appropriate trade-offs be made among health benefits and between health benefits and other kinds of benefits can be made. Given this, defining adequacy requires detailed information on both medical technology and preferences, with the definition open to constant revision, since medical technology, resource availability, and preferences vary over time. What is needed, in other words, is an ongoing *process* capable of defining a *standard of care* that *evolves over time* to incorporate changes in technology, preferences and resource availability.

Defining Adequacy

Such a process requires the cooperation of health care providers. Providers are the experts on the medical alternatives available to treat a health condition and the content of each alternative as it influences cost. They are also in the best position to assess the condition of an individual patient and determine which alternatives are relevant. The easiest way to ensure that the specification of the adequate level is flexible enough to respond to individual situations is to give providers the authority to fine-tune it at the patient level. Conversely, if an inflexible standard of care is defined and imposed without provider cooperation, only very intrusive supervision can prevent them from undermining it if they choose. Since physicians and other providers must play an active role both in the definition of the standard of care and in its administration at the bedside, and the standard of care cannot include everything of benefit, provider ethics must allow providers to limit beneficial care (i.e. to ration care).

The active cooperation of patients (or more broadly, all actual or potential users of health care) is also required. As citizens, they must contribute their views on the standard of care that is morally required for all. As patients, they must accept the fact that in exchange for guaranteed access to this standard, at times their access to care above the standard may be restricted, by ability to pay or by other means (i.e. by price or non-price rationing).

The process must be linked to the political process. In the United States, this is an obvious way to incorporate societal preferences. More important, if access to an adequate level is to be guaranteed to all, the coercive power of government is required to ensure that funds are available to subsidize those who cannot afford to pay for their own care, and to ensure that this financial burden is equitably distributed.

In sum, the process must define a cost-conscious standard of health care that reflects societal and individual views on priorities and satisfies the moral imperatives inherent in the concept of guaranteeing access to a decent minimum. Ideally, the process treads the narrow path between "cookbook medicine," with rigid rules and little choice for doctors or patients, and "cost-benefit analysis at the bedside," with doctors trying to take cost into account based on their own prejudices and patients insisting on maximal care, without guidance from society about social priorities and balancing individual preferences with social goals.

Implementation of an Adequate Level

Can a real health care system be structured to yield such a process? If the process must achieve perfect harmonization of disparate beliefs about the moral basis for the specialness of health care, the benefits and costs of different services, and the appropriate trade-off between health benefits and other benefits, the answer is certainly "no." If the goal is more realistic—a process that defines an approximation to an adequate level, achieving a compromise among different views that leaves most Americans reasonably satisfied—the answer is a cautious "perhaps." One way to search for such a process is to examine real or proposed health care systems guaranteeing universal access to some level of care and ask how the level is set.

A "two tier" system, with radically different standards of care for the poor and for the better off, is one possibility. Access to the standard of care for the poor can be means-tested, or it can simply be so minimal that only those who cannot afford another alternative will use it.

Some developing countries, for example, have a public system used only by the poor, in which the standard of care is low, and a more lavish system, usually private (although it may be subsidized indirectly with public funds) used by those of higher economic status. Such a system is most natural in countries with a highly polarized income distribution, many poor and a few rich, with a large gap between them. Under these conditions, a radical difference in the standard of living between the two groups is taken for granted and the difference in the standard of health care received follows as a matter of course.

The allocation of resources to the public health care system is the key determinant of the guaranteed standard of care in such a system. The total budget and the division of resources among different kinds of care are influenced by the preferences of those using the system, since the provision of health care helps maintain grassroots support for a political regime. Pragmatic economic considerations also enter in, leading, perhaps, to an emphasis on family planning and control of diseases that reduce labor productivity. The main determinant of the decent minimum, however, is likely to be the priority assigned to the well-being of the poor by the rich, who have a disproportionate share of political and economic power.

Most industrialized democracies have made a different choice; they provide a publicly sponsored, cost-conscious but comprehensive standard of care to all. If such a system were truly a single-tier system, with the same standard of care prevailing everywhere and no additional care available outside the system, it would exemplify a strict egalitarian approach to access, rather than a decent minimum approach. In reality, however, there is nearly always some additional care available to those able and willing to pay, although the extent and the terms on which such care is available vary significantly across countries.[3] Therefore, such decent minimum systems guarantee a level of care generous enough to satisfy the great majority of the population.

The complexity of the process used to set the standard of care is interesting. Americans tend to assume that the decent minimum must be determined by a "central czar," or at least a "central committee," far removed from the patient, and then imposed on the delivery system, as in the Oregon plan.[4] Yet this is actually rare in other systems.

Consider, for example, the British National Health Service, an example of "socialized medicine," in which the government not only finances but also provides health care. In a book published in 1984, Henry Aaron and William Schwartz described how the standard of care was determined at that time.[5] They found that even in this "socialized" health service, there was no single, central authority making all the decisions. Instead, a system of interlocking levels operated with different mechanisms at different levels. At the top was a global budget for the entire health service determined by the Treasury and approved by the Cabinet and House of Commons—in other words, through a political process in which health care competed with other goods. At the bottom were the general practitioners, paid on a capitated basis and serving as gatekeepers to the system. In between were regional and district planning authorities and the hospitals. The regions received fixed budgets which were then allocated by planning authorities that included physicians and non-physicians. The hospitals also received fixed budgets which were allocated by the medical staff, composed of salaried physicians working directly for the hospital.

This complex process has many of the characteristics essential to defining and delivering adequate care. First, it is a process, not a static allocation, in which the level of care provided evolves with changing technology and societal preferences. Second, there is a political mechanism for determining the overall availability of resources to the sector and weighing health benefits against other uses of resources. Third, both physicians and non-physicians participate in the allocation process at the middle levels, where trade-offs are made among various health benefits. And fourth, the use of physicians as gatekeepers for individual patients ensures that the care provided varies with health condition.

In contrast to Britain, Canada combines public financing of care with private provision.[6] Each province establishes and administers its own health care system, guided by federal principles requiring universal, portable[7] coverage of all medically necessary care with no cost sharing in a publicly run and publicly accountable system. The provinces pay for all covered medical care, subsidized by federal block grants covering about 40% of expenditures. The provincial authorities decide how much money will be spent on health care, what services to cover in addition to physician and hospital care, and how to finance the province's share of expenditures. They set physician fees and annual budgets for hospitals and approve or disapprove hospital acquisition of certain equipment and specialized services. Family practitioners (about one-half the total physician supply) serve as gatekeepers to the system; if a patient visits a specialist without a referral from a primary care physician, the specialist is paid only the non-specialist fee. Within this framework, however, the determination of the details of the standard of care is left to providers and patients, with limited oversight by utilization review committees monitoring physician practice patterns that deviate significantly from the average.

Managed Competition

An approach that has not been fully implemented anywhere but is currently receiving serious attention in the United States is "managed competition." Like many terms used in health policy, the term means different things to different people, a fact which undoubtedly contributes to its political appeal. To most people, it means a system in which there is an explicit acceptance of multiple tiers. There is a bottom tier that is guaranteed to all, but above it is an array of different standards of care, the result of market choices by individuals made in accord with their personal financial circumstances and preferences.

The approach has been articulated most clearly in the proposals for health care reform associated with Alain Enthoven. His various proposals differ in important respects; for concreteness, we consider the original proposal, Consumer Choice Health Plan (CCHP).[8] In this plan, consumers are given incentives through the income tax to join health plans. Each health plan is a kind of mini-health service, which sets a standard of care for its members based on the premiums paid on their behalf. Competition among health plans leads to a distribution of standards of care that reflects consumer preferences. A system of government regulation is designed to ensure that the health plans compete on quality and price, rather than in less socially desirable ways (for example, by devising ways to skew plan membership toward people in better than average health, or exploiting the difficulties of consumers in acquiring information about the differences among plans).

What makes this a method of setting an adequate level is the provision for the poor and for others who would have difficulty obtaining health insurance in a purely private market. These people are allocated purchasing power to enable them to join health plans. A complex set of regulations ensures that the poor and the high-risk will belong to health plans that also serve middle class Americans and that they will receive a certain basic list of services.

CCHP has been criticized for providing only a list of required basic services rather than specifying amounts in relation to health condition as well. The list of services clearly does not specify adequacy, but in CCHP, the health plans determine the details of the standard of care their members receive, and they are subject to a set of incentives and regulations conditioning their behavior that are supposed to produce a standard of care that is at least adequate. The "decent minimum" of care is not set explicitly; rather, it is the least generous level provided in a plan, which, given the rules, must have been freely chosen by a substantial number of middle class people, who presumably have the financial means to have made other choices if they so desired.

As with the British and Canadian systems, the CCHP embodies a process of defining adequacy in which the standard of care guaranteed to all can evolve over time. Physicians serve as gatekeepers, adjusting the care provided to individual patient need but operating within organizations that have financial incentives to weigh the benefits of care against the costs. Rather than a political or bureaucratic process, the preferences of consumers expressed in the market in their choice of health plan, backed by their freedom to change plans if dissatisfied, are expected to determine trade-offs among health benefits and between health and other goods. The government's role is limited to maintaining the conditions necessary to allow consumers' preferences to influence the outcome and assuring that everyone has the resources to join a plan.

Later versions of the managed competition approach impose somewhat more structure on the market process for defining the decent minimum of care. In a consensus document on the broad outlines of "managed competition" as of 1991, prepared by the "Jackson Hole Group,"[9] a central concept is that of the "Uniform Effective Health Benefits" package, the basic insurance package that must be guaranteed to all. Although the concept is still a list of insured services, the language in which it is described brings it closer to that of a standard of care. Moreover, an administrative structure defines the basic package and ensures its availability. It includes three private non-profit entities, a Health Standards Board, an Outcomes Management Board, and a Health Insurance Standards Board; the first two are sponsored by insurer, employer, consumer and health provider groups, and the third by insurer, employer and consumer groups. These Boards provide information to a National Health Board, an independent federal agency which defines the basic package as well as the regulatory framework for channeling market competition along socially desirable lines.

The discussion above of how the different systems determine the decent minimum is simplified. The object is merely to demonstrate that the process of setting the guaranteed level of care is dynamic and layers of decision making are involved. In each system, there is a complex combination of political, administrative, and market decision-making, with the balance of these quite different from one system to another. None relies primarily on an Oregon-style process of setting a committee to work drawing up a list of condition-treatment pairs to be covered.

Judging Adequacy

These systems set a level of care, but is it adequate? How good an approximation to adequacy are these systems likely to achieve, especially as adapted to an American setting? Viewed from this perspective, all of the systems are clearly imperfect.

There has been long-standing suspicion of "two-tier" medicine in the United States when it is defined as a system in which a political process dominated by "the haves" sets a minimal standard of care for "the have-nots." There are several pieces to this suspicion. There is concern that such a system would not meet the moral obligations of society toward its most vulnerable members. Americans are comfortable with class differences in goods such as housing, clothing, and transportation, but many do not accept differences in the standard of health care, unless the differences can be characterized as "amenities" or "luxuries" (such as cosmetic surgery and orthodontia, private hospital rooms, attractive service environments, convenient locations, and short waiting times for services). The special importance of health care leads them to believe that health care should be more equally distributed than it would be given the distribution of income and normal market forces.

There is also an element of self-interest. Americans recognize that private markets allow them only limited ability to protect themselves and those they love from unexpected changes in their medical and financial circumstances. They are aware that they or those close to them might find themselves using the bottom tier. Since they can more easily contemplate accepting a diminished living standard than a minimal standard of health care, there is a social insurance motive to guaranteeing a level of care that is not too minimal.

Nevertheless, although these views are widely held and should support a generous definition of adequacy, many people fear that in an imperfect political system, the guaranteed standard will be set too low. Experience with other public services used only by the poor shows that even when there is a public commitment to a generous standard of service, and such a standard is set initially, it tends to erode as interest groups with more political power assert their claims on public funds. Thus, a major objection to the Oregon plan was the perception some people had that it was a process in which the "haves" were setting the standard of care for the "have nots," with the inevitable result a morally unacceptable level of care.

The other examples have in common the fact that they peg the standard of care to the average citizen's, or the middle class's, preferences. At first sight, one might argue that this goes too far in the other direction, setting a standard that is too high. Much of the appeal of the decent minimum approach in the United States is the freedom it seems to offer to abandon the goal of mainstream medical care for the poor, an ideal that has seemed too expensive to achieve and that has therefore been an obstacle to the achievement of universal access to care. The key point is, however, that these systems set a *cost-conscious* standard of care for the middle class. Each has built-in pressure to consider cost as well as benefit in setting the standard of care. By contrast, all observers agree that a major problem with the American health care system is the ingenious way in which its structure dilutes the incentive of decision-makers to weigh the benefit of care against the cost. In fact, the average American is not even aware of the full cost of the access to care he has.

In sum, there is considerable appeal in an approach that (1) identifies the cost-conscious standard of care to which a well-informed person of average income is willing to pay to ensure access; (2) makes this standard the approximation to the adequate level; and (3) includes everyone in a system delivering this standard, through a system of insurance premiums, regulation, and taxes and subsidies, with those whose incomes are above average taxed to subsidize those whose incomes are below average. How well do the British, Canadian and managed competition systems succeed in providing a uniform standard of care that is satisfactory to the average citizen and reflects the average citizen's trade-offs?

There are problems. In the British National Health Service, for example, attempts to eliminate regional inequalities in the distribution of health care personnel and facilities have not been completely successful. Criteria for obtaining treatment vary from one area to another; for example, the criteria for selection for kidney dialysis vary from place to another. Rationing of care falls disproportionately on care that requires expensive equipment, since it is easier to limit the supply of such equipment, thus constraining clinical decisions for its use, than it is to ration in other ways. There are queues for some procedures, resulting in lengthy waits for care for some patients.

Of more serious concern, government has severely limited the total resources allocated to the system, partly because of the general economic situation in Britain and partly because of an ideological shift in the political climate away from the basic commitment to a relatively egalitarian standard. The small size of the private sector in medicine over the first three decades of the NHS's existence attested to the acceptability to the average Briton of the standard of care provided; the private sector's spectacular recent growth suggests that the standard may no longer be as acceptable. Moreover, some critics have charged that British patients are not aware of the extent to which beneficial care is limited because physicians rationalize the failure to offer certain treatments as a result of resource constraints by redefining them as "not beneficial."[10]

In Canada, there is a high level of overall satisfaction with the health care system and a very small private sector. Nevertheless, the Canadian system also has its problems. There is a shortage of physicians in the remote northern areas. Constraints on rising costs are weak. There are too many specialists relative to primary care practitioners, and the fee for service reimbursement system, with minimal utilization control, encourages too much low benefit care. Hospital stays are believed to be longer than they need to be. As in Britain, the rationing of care falls disproportionately on care that requires expensive equipment. There is some queueing for certain high technology and specialty elective and diagnostic procedures (although the extent of it has been greatly exaggerated by certain American commentators).[11]

Managed competition has somewhat different problems.[12] There *are* financial incentives within the health plans to produce services efficiently and weigh benefits against costs in clinical decisions. Market pressure from consumers is supposed to make health plans respond to the incentives, without going too far in skimping on care, and thus produce an array of rationing strategies that matches consumer preferences.

However, consumers are likely to have difficulty judging the different rationing approaches and choosing among them. To do this, consumers must know both the stated policies and the degree to which the plan follows them before informed choices can be made. Managed competition reform plans give attention to this problem and provide for standardized information about the standard of care a plan provides. Nevertheless, given the many ways profit-oriented organizations can find to manipulate the standard of care unobtrusively, it is not clear how successfully this can be regulated. For example, all members of a plan may prefer that organ transplants, sophisticated perinatal care for defective newborns, or expensive rehabilitation services be available. The plan may make these part of its offered treatments but quietly ensure that very few patients are considered "medically suitable" for them. The patients' own families may not be aware that beneficial care has been denied, let alone the rest of the plan membership.

Regulatory mechanisms may also be unable to prevent plans from competing with one another by controlling the composition of their membership. There are strong financial incentives for a plan to avoid persons who use services intensively, by discouraging them from enrolling in the first place or inducing them to disenroll when their high utilization becomes apparent. These actions can be taken in subtle ways which are hard to control by regulation or market pressure. Health plans can use the geographic location of their facilities, waiting times, the quality level of particular departments, and a host of other variables to influence the composition of their patient populations.

Finally, health care is location-specific, and individual markets may not be large enough to support more than a few health plans.[13] These in turn may settle for a de facto sharing of the market and an inefficient but quiet life, rather than the vigorous competition on price and quality envisioned by competition advocates. Consumers may find that the range of choices actually available in the market is limited and not very responsive to their preferences, just as automobile buyers have found it difficult to get the American automobile industry to produce the kind of cars they want. Although we do not have much experience with "managed competition" in health care, we do have a great deal of experience with imperfect markets for other commodities, and the experience is not encouraging.

Thus, achieving a standard of care that reasonably approximates the "average well-informed middle-class person's trade-offs between costs and benefits" is not easy. But even if it could be achieved, how well would it approximate adequacy? Such a level is likely to have systematic biases in both directions, depending on the health condition and the type of care.

Setting the standard of care requires people to weigh probabilities. How much is it worth spending on hypertension treatment to lower the risk of cardiovascular disease? Should we guarantee the availability of a heart or liver transplant when the chances of needing one are very small? Studies have shown that people have great difficulty making decisions in the presence of uncertainty, especially when there is a small probability of a very adverse advent. Many decisions in health care are of this type. Moreover, the probability of experiencing many health conditions is unevenly distributed. Conditions that are unlikely to be experienced by the average person may receive far less consideration than more common conditions of lesser severity. Genetic and congenital conditions raise this problem in particularly clear form.

Thus, the standard of care acceptable to a person of average income can only be a rough approximation to an adequate level. People would undoubtedly differ in their assessments of the extent to which it should be modified and in which direction. Unfortunately, the conditions that this approach would not handle well—for example, preventive care, genetic and congenital conditions, organ transplants—are exactly the conditions about which the underlying philosophical theories differ. Even if a consensus about the amount of care required could be reached, it would not be easy to ensure the availability of care that is unlikely to be used by the average person, for the same practical reasons the level of public services provided to disadvantaged groups tends to erode.

Thus, there must be a process for scrutinizing the actual level of care and correcting it. A variety of institutional mechanisms could be developed to do this, including special congressional committees, NIH consensus panels, private charitable organizations, hospital ethics committees, even Oregon-style citizen discussion groups and committees. The debate would, however, be carried out in a context in which the broad outlines of the adequate level had already been determined. Questions about whether prenatal care would be provided and in what amounts, how much cancer screening should be provided to the general population and so on would be settled, and society could focus attention on questions such as how much care should be available for hemophiliacs.

In evaluating a method for approximating the adequate level, one should examine both its accuracy and its flexibility. Can we easily adjust the standard to make it morally acceptable? In a two-tier system in which those with political and economic power set a minimal level of care for the poor, believing they themselves are unlikely to use it, the approximation is likely to be biased downward and difficult difficult to adjust. A single tier system with some additional care available through a private market in which a publicly sponsored, cost-conscious but comprehensive standard of care is guaranteed to all and set at a level designed to satisfy the majority of the population—has advantages both in getting a good first approximation to an adequate level and in fine-tuning it, since the level available is explicitly the level to be guaranteed to all.

Under managed competition, much depends on the way the basic insurance package is specified. If, as in CCHP, it is defined in terms of a list of service categories and cost-sharing limits with the details of the standard of care set implicitly as the minimum of what individual middle class consumers decide they want over the near future based on their own personal risk profiles, rather than what they think should be available to all as a decent minimum, there is not even a conceptual framework for adjusting the resulting standard, let alone a set of practical institutions. If more structure is imposed, as in the Jackson Hole Initiative, there is a framework and institutions. The focus shifts to questions about the institutions and their missions. Do they see themselves as specifying an austere standard for the poor which the non-poor will naturally want to supplement or a cost-conscious standard of care which will satisfy the majority of Americans? How effectively are they able to ensure that the minimum standard of care they set actually prevails?

However the initial adequate level is set, adapting it requires collective decision-making and thus politics. This process may be formal and governmental (operating through regulation or other government decision-making and intervention) or informal and non-governmental (for example, providers, administrators and members of a health plan decide what the structure of coverage should be). It is not, however, *merely* political or economic. By asking what we owe one another as human beings and as members of a common society, this process will necessarily involve morality.

In a democratic society, difficult moral questions must often be handled through political procedures. Nonetheless, they remain moral questions, and it is appropriate and necessary that moral arguments figure in the debate. This point explains why so many Americans insist on casting the issue of access to health care in "rights" terms. They use "rights language" to signify their belief that deciding who gets what health care and how much is somehow a different kind of decision than what kind of cars automakers should put on the market, or which state gets a new highway or dam.

Implications for Health Care Reform

At last, Americans seem to have achieved a national consensus that whether or not there is a right to health care, access to health care cannot be unlimited. Unfortunately, the consensus is rather shaky. The public does not really understand *why* beneficial health care must be limited. It is not that advances in technology have suddenly made health care unaffordable, but rather that health insurance (whether private or public, voluntary or compulsory) is and always has been prohibitively expensive when contracts promise everything of benefit.

Failure to understand the efficiency reasons for limiting care is a major obstacle to achieving equity. Since even private insurance plans cannot afford to guarantee access to "medically necessary" care when the term means "everything beneficial," limits on care have always been a part of the American health care system, even for the well-insured. However, in the absence of public acceptance of the need for such limits, they have had to be imposed in concealed ways on the people least able to resist. This has led to inefficiency and inequity in the distribution of care and of its cost.

The alternative is not necessarily an Oregon-style process of convening citizens to assign benefit-cost rankings to treatment-condition pairs and decide which pairs constitute "basic care" that should be available to all and which do not. In other industrialized countries, when national health care systems were established, there was no explicit debate on what *not* to provide. Rather, universal access was introduced together with financing structures that included a variety of methods of restraining utilization and costs. There was an implicit shared understanding that health care was a social enterprise, funded by collective resources, and therefore no individual's claim on the system was absolute, but the emphasis was on extending access to all, not limiting benefits to some. Over time, the standard of care evolved, but always in a context of constrained resources. In this country, this understanding is absent. Americans hold inconsistent views on health care reform. They want universal access to health care at an affordable cost but without limits on the care they themselves receive. They give lip service to the desirability of a single-tier system with guaranteed access to quality care for everyone, yet are reluctant to vote the funds to pay for it. Pressure is building to resolve these contradictions.

The first step is understanding the need for a cost-conscious standard of care for those who can afford to pay for their own care. The second step is to reach a national consensus on whether the level of care guaranteed to the poor should be a cost-conscious standard of care that the average American finds satisfactory, or something lower.

All agree that there should be universal access to basic care, but there is ambiguity about how minimal basic care should be. Would the tension between distrust of a two-tier system and fear of the cost of providing mainstream care to the poor be resolved if the mainstream standard of care were made more affordable? Making the adequate level the same as the cost-conscious standard of care that is satisfactory to the average American has significant administrative and poltiical simplicity. It would be much simpler to educate physicians, supervise quality, and define and manage medical malpractice.

Some have argued that given the intense individualism of American society, it would be impossible to build a system around a single cost-conscious standard of care satisfactory to most Americans; a single payer, Canadian-style system, for example, would never work in the United States. Managed competition advocates, in particular, have argued that Americans value choice so much that there must be multiple standards of care. Historically, however, the American health care system has been organized around the concept of a single standard of "medically necessary care," and Americans have been willing to give physicians extremely wide discretion over the establishment of that standard. Americans have insisted on freedom of choice but they have defined it primarily in terms of the freedom to pick the providers who would be most skillful in applying the standard of medically necessary care to their own individual circumstances. Rather than demanding detailed evidence on differences in the standard of care provided by different providers, they have often seemed to prefer to believe that such differences do not exist (or rather, that when they do, they represent either "amenities" or malpractice). Thus it is interesting to note that the Canadian system provides people with extensive choice of provider in the context of a universal, cost-conscious standard of care.

A third necessary step is to acknowledge that the content and financing of universal access to an adequate level should be determined at the national level, for both philosophical and practical reasons. An individual member of society's moral claim on society should not vary with place of residence, nor should his or her share of the cost of meeting the societal moral obligation. Americans are a highly mobile population, many changing their geographic locations frequently over their lifetimes. To the extent that there are systematic differences in philosophical positions on the definition of adequacy and on how the cost of care should be distributed, they are correlated not with place of residence, but with other individual characteristics. Moreover, the resources available in a particular region to fund care for the poor are inversely related to the size of the need. Significant differences across states and localities in the guaranteed level of care and the way the cost is distributed would set up perverse incentives. In sum, it would be best to reach a broad national consensus on the level of care that is morally obligatory and on the distribution of the cost of providing it.

This conclusion is not incompatible with decentralization in the administration of the health care system, nor does it necessarily imply the elimination of regional differences in the distribution of providers and facilities. The definition of the adequate level could and should include some flexibility to respond to individual preferences. These might well produce geographic variations in the actual utilization of care, if individuals with similar preferences happened to be geographically concentrated.

Finally, societal resource availability is and ought to be a major factor in setting the adequate level. Nevertheless, health care should be seen as a basic social expense, with the level set in relation to long-term resource availability within a society and not subject to fluctuations from month to month or even year to year.

NOTES

1. The terms "decent minimum," "basic care," and "adequate level" are used interchangeably in this paper.

2. For discussion of the various arguments, see, for example, the references cited in Mary Ann Baily, "Rationing Medical Care: Processes for Defining Adequacy" in *The Price of Health*, G.J. Agich and C.E. Begley, eds. (Dordrecht, Holland: D. Reidel, 1986), pp. 165–84.

3. Also, in practice, no real health care system has been able to completely eliminate differences in the standard of care available in different geographical regions and to different socioeconomic groups.

4. The committee used various methods to obtain citizen input, but determined the final structure of the list itself.

5. Henry J. Aaron and William B. Schwartz, *The Painful Prescription: Rationing Hospital Care*. (Washington, D.C.: The Brookings Institution, 1984).

6. United States General Accounting Office, *Canadian Health Insurance: Lessons for the United States*. (Washington, DC: US Government Printing Office, GAO/HRD-91-90, June. General Accounting Office, 1991).

7. "Portable" means that people can move from one province to another and one job to another and still retain their coverage.

8. Alain Enthoven, *Health Plan: The Only Practical Solution to the Soaring Cost of Medical Care*. (Reading, MA: Addison-Wesley, 1980).

9. Paul M. Ellwood, Alain C. Enthoven and Lynn Etheredge, "The Jackson Hole Initiatives for a Twenty-first Century American Health Care System" 1 *Health Economics* 1 (1993) 149–168. The Jackson Hole Group is an informal group of health industry leaders, public officials and health services researchers that has been meeting since the mid-70's in Jackson Hole, Wyoming, to discuss health care issues.

10. See Aaron and Schwartz.

11. General Accounting Office, Canadian Health Insurance.

12. See, for example, Mary Ann Baily, "Policies for the 1990's: Rationing Health Care" in *Competitive Approaches to Health Care Reform*, eds. R.J. Arnould, R.F. Rich, and W.D. White (Washington, D.C.: Urban Institute Press, 1993), and the references cited therein.

13. See, for example, Richard Kronick, David C. Goodman, John Wennberg, and Edward Wagner, "The Marketplace in Health Care Reform: The Demographic Limitations of Managed Competition", *New England Journal of Medicine* 328(1993):148–52.

James Lindemann Nelson

Public Participation and the Adequate Standard of Care

My goals in this chapter are three-fold. First, I want to stress the nature of the job to which we've set our hand in defining a "minimum adequate standard of health care": it is essentially a task of moral reasoning, to which technical information concerning outcomes and costs is necessary but instrumental. My second goal is to discuss some of options available for productive moral reasoning about the basic package and then to further discuss some of the advantages and disadvantages of those options. Of particular interest in this connection are the various proposals to integrate the values (or preferences) of citizens (or consumers) in the process of package definition. Third, I want to highlight some questions about the terms in which the deliberation about basic packages are set: what, for example, is the scope of the package that we're talking about? Will it range over a community, a region or the country as a whole? How sustainable will the basic package be? Will it have the stability of an entitlement, or will it be so resource-sensitive that we can expect it to change its shape biennium by biennium?

What is a "Basic Package"?

In the sense in which we are concerned about the matter, a basic package is fundamentally an attempt to strike a defensible compromise among three mutually antagonistic moral values. The first of these values is that of *fair access to health care*. What counts as a fair shot at a good is generally thought to shift around a great deal with the nature of the good in question: fair access to schools and fair access to Alpha Romeos are rather different. For various reasons, a substantial number of Americans seem to regard health care as being rather more like schooling than like luxury cars. Norman Daniels, for example, has argued that some measure of health care must be available independently of ability to pay for reasons having to do with the moral commitment of our community to fair equality of opportunity, coupled with the significance of health care in allowing us to realize the range of opportunities natural to our species.[1] Others have made the case on other grounds. But the consensus seems to be that ability to pay is not a morally defensible ground for the distribution of at least some level of health care, as it may well be for the distribution of Italian sports cars or suede pumps. Thus, when somewhere between 35 and 40 million citizens lack health care insurance at any given time, and tens of millions more are significantly underinsured, the moral value of fair access of health care is not merely violated but massively outraged.

The second value is often just called *cost control*, but I prefer to refer to it as *prudent husbandry of social resources.* There is nothing crassly money-grubbing about viewing the amount of our GNP devoted to health care, and its rate of growth, with alarm. We do not need to go over the figures here in any detail; suffice it to say that the amount of money being spent on health care in this country is putting considerable pressure on our ability to achieve other ends of our common life together—decent education, affordable housing, invigorated commerce and industry—which also have moral claims upon our resources. If we allow one of our legitimate social goals to absorb resources to a point at which other goals are first stinted and then starved, we have on our hands a justice problem which is every bit as significant as the problem of fair access to health care, because the pursuit of more and more medicine amounts to a denial of access to other valued goods and services. In its quest to serve the interest of specific, identified individuals, medicine has reached a point where our joint life as a community is very vulnerable.

Thirdly, we value *excellence in health care.* Valuing excellence is of course a reasonable thing to do quite generally, but in health care, given its tendency rather directly to involve issues of life and death, and to subject its patients to risks and inconvenience, we seem particularly sensitive to quality. As a country, we have the rather curious inclination to think not only that health care should be universally available, but that such care should be the best available, Presidential-level medicine for everyone.

The problem is clear: we spend too much money on health care and simply must cut back, if not on absolute dollars, at least on the rate of spending growth; we have to make health care available to tens of millions of people who do not now have it (and, incidentally, have to do it within a country whose population is aging, and which is suffering from an epidemic disease); we have to maintain high standards of quality in the health care that is provided. The role of the basic package in all this is simple to articulate: the basic package is the modus vivendi among these jointly unruly values, a compromise struck between them which expresses itself in the amount and quality of health care services which we must make available to all members of our community, against the backdrop of the constraints of justice in the allocation of scarce resources. Less than the basic package is an injustice to the person denied care; more than the basic package threatens to be an injustice to the rest of us.

Facts, Values and Defining the Package

What is involved in striking the still point among these kinetic forces? The literature suggests that we need fundamentally two kinds of knowledge. The one kind is factual information concerning the outcomes of various health interventions on the course of people's lives and the costs of those interventions. This data is essential, but instrumental to the second kind of knowledge we need: ethical knowledge, well-defended, widely shared insights into what it is that we owe to one another in the name of justice.

The difficulty, of course, is that we don't have either kind of knowledge. Analysis of medical practice in recent years reveals that patterns of resource utilization vary wildly region to region, that doctors rely a great deal on anecdote to support how they treat patients, and that in many instances they really don't know what works or how well in contrast to other possible interventions. Systematic research and expert consensus concerning effectiveness and outcomes is ongoing but in its very early days. In a recent article, Eli Ginsberg attributes to Paul Ellwood the claim that it will be ten years before useful results emerge from outcomes research.[2]

I don't know whether to say that the situation with respect to ethical knowledge is worse or better. Philosophical inquiry into justice has a much longer history than outcomes research, but it is far from likely that within the next ten years we will have arrived at a social consensus that one or another of the grand theories of justice is clearly the best. Will Rawlsian social-contract theory strike a knockout blow against Nozick's libertarianism, particularly since Nozick no longer seems inclined to defend his view?[3] Will Walzer's "separate spheres" approach or Sandel's communitarianism decisively win the day?[4] The record of philosophical disputation suggests not. Will views about justice which have been explicitly developed in recent years to deal with allocation of health care resources, such as the work of Norman Daniels,[5] or Daniel Callahan,[6] fare any better? Possibly, but some skepticism seems prudent.

If theories that try to show people what they *should* value—from the top down, so to speak—don't seem promising, the natural alternative is to look to what people *do in fact* value—from the bottom up, as it were. And this seems to be just where most interest currently resides. Somehow, those who will ultimately bear the cost, enjoy the benefits, and suffer the limitations of the basic package must let policymakers know what it is they want put in and left out.

There are a number of suggestions about how to accomplish this in the literature. Taking a rough cut, I will divide the suggestions into two camps: one asks consumers what they are willing to buy (the marketplace model); the other asks citizens what they value (the commonweal model).

A sophisticated version of the marketplace model is nicely articulated in a series of articles by David Eddy in the *Journal of the American Medical Association*. Eddy insists that the origin of our cost-control problem is that the medical marketplace contains many mechanisms and informational gaps which obscure the consumer's grasp of the relationship of "value to cost." What we need, accordingly, is a perspicuous grasp of that relationship, and to get it, he suggests that practice guidelines be set up in a way which measures not only the relationship between medical benefit and medical harm, but also the relationship of that ratio to economic costs. Specialty societies and government agencies, such as OTA or HCFA, who are involved in setting such guidelines should explicitly incorporate the cost dimension.

But how should we make the normative decision concerning which kinds of services are "costworthy?" Eddy defends a position he calls "majority choice by Average Patients." Very roughly, he holds that a representative group (50–2000) of Patients (by which we means anyone who might come to need health care) ought to make the final decisions on whether given health care services were essential by considering their benefits against what they cost. In an important move which implicitly acknowledges his awareness of the value of universal access, Eddy allows that society must subvene health care costs. Health care costs are to be presented as a percentage of Patients' daily income, when this is indexed to the median. So, if some medical intervention costs $100, and if $100 represents 100% of the median income, it is presented to each average patient as costing one day's wage. To make this a bit less abstract, consider an example from Eddy:

> Suppose, for example, we are interested in a hypothetical drug that decreases the possibility of dying of a myocardial infarction from 9% to 8% [by 1 chance in 100] . . .and that costs $10,000. . . .A man or woman who has a 5 out of 1000 chance of having a heart attack in the coming year would pay $50.00 [5/1000 times $10,000] to buy coverage for the drug that would decrease his or her change of dying of a heart attack by [what amounts to] one in 20,000 [5/1000 times 1/100].[7]

On the assumptions above, this drug represents half a day's pay to the hypothetical Average Patient. If Patients are willing to pay for it, into the package it goes. If not, it stays out and if a real patient has a nonhypothetical heart attack, she will not get the drug (unless, of course, she happens to have $10,000 on hand, and someone thought that the drug was worth making even if not included in the basic package). If Average Patients disagree about whether a given service should be included, in general, majority decision-making rules.

A number of problems quickly spring to mind when we consider this strategy. Suppose we were to ask whether AZT for HIV infection ought to be a part of the basic package. It might well depend on which Representative Patient you ask. For Eddy, the cost of a procedure to a Patient is a function of the price of the intervention times the likelihood that it will be needed, indexed to the median income. Clearly, AZT coverage will be much more expensive for a young gay man than an elderly straight woman. Eddy calls for a broad representative sample of Americans to make up the Representative Patients, and perhaps the fairest way of informing their deliberation would be to present them with a figure for the cost of the intervention which reflects their "community" risk, rather than their individually stratified risk. Coverage for AZT would presumably cost fairly little presented in this fashion. Still it might be seen as costing too much—at least, for people who feel that the risk assigned statistically to them is not realistic, perhaps *because* it reflects nonstratified figures. The endemic human difficulties about probabilistic reasoning and risk, coupled with tendencies toward bias and bigotry, might compete for impact on consumer deliberations with the figures actually given them; this could well have the impact of disenfranchising certain stigmatized or ignored disease states, such as AIDS or schizophrenia.

Another problem is that indexing the cost of a service to the average daily income really does not put us on a level playing field economically. If my average daily income is $15.00, none of it is discretionary, and the impact of spending a day's pay for a particular kind of coverage will be much greater on me than on someone whose average daily income is $500.00; she'll pay more than I do, of course, but there's a great deal more flexibility in her economic position than in mine.

Perhaps there are changes in the system which would help here. Eddy points out that the parameters of his system are not graven in stone; we might, for example, index everything to 125% of the median, or to 85%, and we might do this differentially, in a way that took total net worth into account, as well as income, or that was sensitive to a certain "index of discretion" in higher incomes. Perhaps we could also fool around with different ways of figuring risk as well, trying to correct for "subjective epidemiologies" by expressing the risk of certain stigmatized conditions in a way that represents a studied deviation from the median risk, as well as the median income. But these considerations of whether and how to "fudge" the figures really reflect a general concern which many might feel about Eddy's approach. Eddy effectively asks the Average Patients to be self-interested in their deliberations, and he relies on the assumption that all the relevant moral values that should go into this part of the debate will be adequately represented by money. But perhaps monetary values are not quite so fungible as all that.

Another approach can be considered here. Suppose that the people deliberating about what should go into the basic package are not asking about what services cost what amount of money, and what they are willing to buy for themselves, but rather about what services they value the most as a contribution to the goodness of their own lives and for the good of their community overall. These people are citizens deliberating about the fate of their commonwealth, not consumers trying to make shrewd deals in the marketplace. Such deliberators might produced a ranked list of valued states or ends or even services, and then a group of experts might link those values to various diagnosis-treatment pairs, whose outcomes are expressed in ways that reflect the kinds of things valued by the citizenry, and which are accordingly ranked in a way that reflects the extent to which the intervention serves the values. Clearly, this would not be an algorithmic kind of procedure, but one that was highly value-laden, and which called for the exercise of prudent judgment; hence, the expert group ought to contain citizen representation. Then, the elected representatives of the deliberators could decide how far down the list of ranked health care services the public purse allowed us to go, in a process which explicitly and publicly weighed the goods of health care against other goods sought after by the community.

I am not likely to get away with claiming that I dreamt all this up myself; this thumbnail sketch is, of course, inspired by the Oregon experiment. That process has from its inception been the target of moral criticism, of course—particularly on the basis that it involved the well-off engaging in deliberations which harmed the prospects of those who were already much worse off then they were. (This may indeed by morally dubious, but Oregon certainly didn't represent anything new in this regard.) It was temporarily derailed by a (quite mistaken, in my view) claim that it involved invidious discrimination on the basis of handicap.[8] But it has also been hailed by many as an early experiment in the incorporation of democratic values into the process of priority-setting, an incorporation which both provides absolutely indispensable normative guidance and grants an inherently difficult, contentious and potentially divisive process an important degree of legitimacy. As my colleague Bruce Jennings has written, coming up with a defensible basic package requires citizens involved in deliberations which reflect an attempt to forge and grasp a view of the common good:

> the common good is defined and constituted by a process of active, common deliberation in which each citizen self-consciously attempts to grasp the shared needs and aspirations at work in his or her community of co-equals and fellow citizens.[9]

This proposal is not immune to problems. One would have to be wary about the extent to which the deliberators involved really acted out of a grasp of what was in the best interest of their community as a whole and to what extent they were simply acting in the spirit of liberal individualism. Perhaps a way of increasing the chances that deliberators will think of themselves as acting in the name of the community and not simply of their own interests is precisely not to ask them to think about their choices in economic terms, but rather in terms of what health outcomes most contribute to the social good. Information about those outcomes would presumably be required for a responsible discussion of these values, but information about health care costs might well be reserved to a different level, which would naturally be the legislature. Still, there is no guarantee that the deliberators might not end up reflecting social prejudices in their ranking of what kind of physical states they valued most. And some commentators have argued that certain kinds of health care benefits ought to be regarded as a matter of strict entitlement, quite independently of what the majority may decide. Even if general philosophical accounts cannot satisfactorily motivate the entire, specific content of the basic package or mandate the values we should try to realize in putting one together, they may be able to demonstrate that certain services are the "core of the core," as it were, and constitute a sort of "health care bill of rights" that must constrain the majoritarian deliberations of the populace. A possible example here is the special stress put on nonabandonment and basic caring by Callahan.[10]

Other Endemic Problems

Whoever makes decisions about what kind of care is costworthy enough to be a part of the basic package, she, he or they will have to consider the decision in some terms. What terms should those be? I've already touched on the problem of whether economic information ought to be a part of the direct citizen deliberation about the relevant values, but other questions arise as well. Clearly, the economic dimension must come up at some point in the process. But are the economic numbers immutable? It is well known that the health care system is bloated with economic waste. But it is less noted that the system as it now stands reflects certain social decisions which are the legacies of a history from which we may now want to free ourselves. To what extent are the price tags of the services we will consider in designing a basic package artifacts of a historical anomaly in which fee-for-service and third-party payment inflated costs beyond what the market should bear? To what extent do prices reflect a system that is based on a hierarchial model of medical care which puts overtrained, highly-paid physicians in place to provide services that might be done just as well, better, or only marginally worse by professionals with lesser amounts of training and expense? If our fundamental interest here is in achieving the most beneficial package of health services which can be made available to everyone at a price consistent with our other social duties and goals, is our present system—specialist heavy, and acute-care oriented—structurally capable of meeting that challenge?

The point about how we should frame the decision about the basic package can be put a different way: as we are now at a crisis point in health care delivery, is this perhaps not the golden opportunity to seize the time and offer bold ideas about structural changes that could release more resources to be used in the provision of health care? Should there be more primary care doctors, or more nurse practitioners and fewer primary docs? If a monopsonistic system could free more resources for inclusion into the basic package, do we have an obligation to go that way? Or must we content ourselves with "reformist" reforms, which accept the basic structure of the current system, distribute its benefits, pains and costs as equitably and efficiently as we can, and try to nudge it by small increments into new and more helpful directions?

Another general problem concerns the scope and stability of the basic package. The idea of universal access to care is based on the idea that human beings by their nature deserve such care, at least when it is possible to provide it. This line of thinking has an "entitlement" air about it, and entitlements, whether philosophically grounded or not, generate expectations. But the basic package is also a function of the general level of resources available in a given community at a given time. Those levels can shift quickly, as can the cost of services. How committed should we be to developing a sustainable package of health care benefits? In putting the package together, ought we to plan for a future in which we may have less economic productivity overall and larger health care needs, to say nothing of general social needs? If a sustainable basic package is a goal, then we may need to have a broad social dialogue about the nature of needs and wants, and the role of medicine within the range of visions of a good human life which can command allegiance in our society—in short, the sort of dialogue that theoreticians such as Callahan and Jennings in particular have called for. This further suggests that kind of role that the deliberations of philosophers and other ethicists interested in justice in the distribution of health care might have. Neither the power of their arguments nor the structure of our political system allows them to be relied on as philosopher kings, from whom we can get the real story about all this sort of thing. But their work might inform public deliberation in a manner that is in some ways analogous to the role of health care practitioners, economists, policy people and scientists in making the relevant facts public property.

At the same time, involving citizen values raises the possibility that different clusters of citizens, identifiable by geographical proximity, perhaps, or by religious tradition or political philosophies, might have distinctly different sets of values, different images of the good life, and the role of health care services in obtaining that life. Should the basic package be flexible to this kind of "value variation"? Contemporary theorists who are particularly interested in the moral significance of difference—people like Martha Minow[11] and Iris Marion Young[12]—might be useful both to getting clear about whether such variation ought to be something we take into account, and, if so, how we ought to do it.[13]

Conclusion

I have tried to stress that designing the basic package is an ethical task of mediating between important human values that are uneasy in each other's company. As difficult ethical questions of this kind cannot be solved by appeal to philosopher kings, the best we can do is to bring to bear what values we do have on the matter, as clearly and thoughtfully as possible. Hence, grassroots involvement in the fashioning of the package seems the only straw floating.

There are, however, different ways of thinking about how to involve people. We are impressed (perhaps overly so) with the power of economic value to go proxy for the whole range of our values; Eddy's "marketplace" approach takes advantage of this phenomenon. Or, we might ask citizens what kind of functional and dysfunctional states they value and disvalue, and, relatively speaking, how much? This approach, one could hope, might encourage citizens to take a wider, more commodious view of the relevant moral and social values involved in fashioning a mechanism for bringing harmony to the rather raucous cacophony we've got going now.

Finally, designing a basic package, while a whale of a job under any construal, can be seen more or less narrowly. We can simply take the present health care system as more-or-less given, and do the best we can with that, or we can ask what kind of health care service would really be of most benefit for the amount we can afford to spend. This would involve questioning the distinction that some writers—

Eddy, for instance—make between the content of the basic package and how those contents are delivered. If, in doing this, we take thought not just for ourselves, but for our children and their children, we may have to think not just about services and interventions, practice patterns and delivery systems, but about what medicine is and what role we want it to play in supporting our diverse but overlapping conceptions of the good life.[14]

NOTES

1. Norman Daniels, *Just Health Care* (Cambridge: Cambridge University Press, 1985).

2. Eli Ginsberg, "A Century of Health Reform," *Society*, 30 (1) (November/December 1992): 25.

3. The *locus classicus* for Rawls is, of course, *A Theory of Justice* (Cambridge: Harvard University Press, 1971), and for Nozick, *Anarchy, State and Utopia* (New York: Basic Books, 1974).

4. I have in mind here the Michael Walzer of *Spheres of Justice* (New York: Basic Books, 1983) and the Michael Sandel of *Liberalism and the Limits of Justice* (Cambridge: Cambridge University Press, 1982).

5. Daniels, *Just Health Care.*

6. Daniel Callahan, *What Kind of Life* (New York: Simon and Schuster, 1990).

7. David Eddy, "What Care is 'Essential'? What Services are 'Basic'?" *Journal of the American Medical Association* 265, no. 6 (February 13, 1991): 786.

8. See David Hadorn, "The Problem of Discrimination in Health Care Priority Setting," *Journal of the American Medical Association* 268 (September 16, 1992): 1454–1459. But see also Paul Menzel, "Oregon's Denial: Disabilities and Quality of Life," *Hastings Center Report* 22, 6 (1992): 21–25.

9. Bruce Jennings, "Democratic Values and Health Policy Reform," in H. M. Leichter, ed., *Health Policy Reform in America* (Armonk, NY: Sharpe, 1992).

10. Callahan, *What Kind of Life.*

11. Martha Minow, *Making All the Difference* (Ithaca: Cornell University Press, 1990).

12. Iris Marion Young, *Justice and the Politics of Difference* (Princeton: Princeton University Press, 1991).

13. Hilde Lindemann Nelson drew my attention to the significance of this point. It has been discussed at length in Ezekiel Emanuel, *The Ends of Human Life: Medical Ethics in a Liberal Polity* (Cambridge: Harvard University Press, 1991).

14. I'm grateful for the comments of my colleagues at The Hastings Center, Philip Boyle, Joseph Fins, Bruce Jennings and Hilde Lindemann Nelson on an earlier draft.

JANET WEINER

Towards a Uniform
Health Benefit Package

There is growing consensus that the U.S. health care system needs major reform to ensure access to health care for all Americans. Most proposals for reform call for a uniform, standard or minimum benefit package that delineates the scope of health care we will have. There is far less consensus on what that benefit package must include. To which services must we all have access? Within the universe of possible human interventions to improve health, which ones can we agree to assure to everyone? For now, we will call this subset "basic health care."

Basic health care can be discussed in three ways. We could articulate the *criteria* by which services are judged to be "basic." Alternately, we could describe a *process* for determining which services are basic. Lastly, we could generate a *list* of categories of services that constitute basic health care.[1] A list of health care services makes sense only within the context of explicit criteria by which to make decisions and a process that allows social consensus for doing so. Thus, this paper explores the medical and health values that could form justifiable criteria for deciding among health services and suggests a fair process for determining and updating a benefit package. While health care can be discussed in the absence of a determined infrastructure, ultimately the benefit package will involve considerations of the structure and financing of the delivery system. Further definition of basic health care will help elucidate values and decision rules to be followed in the social process of creating a benefit package within a reformed health system.

An Approach to Basic Health Care

Before we can define basic health care, we must articulate why health care is so important, and what we want health care to do for us. These values and goals will be benchmarks against which to measure the adequacy of the definition and the acceptability of a benefit package.

What do we mean by basic? Often this discussion gets bogged down in alternate definitions and connotations of "basic," "minimum" or "adequate." Operatively, the benefit package will be the minimum level of care that we assure to everyone; it will be the floor beneath which no one will fall. But this should not imply that the benefit package will provide only *minimal* care; in a fairly well-off society, the benefit package should be adequate to meet our health needs, and should be a level within which the vast majority of people can live.

And who decides what we "need," as opposed to what we "want" or would "like"? Simply put, we do. We do this not as individuals at the point of service but prospectively, as a community of citizens. This has moral validity only if we assume that almost everyone will have access to the same level of care. This assumption gives everyone a stake in the scope of the definition and prevents any one group (e.g. the poor or the unemployed) from being singled out for certain minimums of care. It avoids the problem of one group defining "need" for another group. Even if some level of health care beyond those services in the benefit package remains available to individuals who can pay for it, our approach is geared to widen the standard package and narrow the demand for additional services.

Our second assumption is that health care is most effective when it is highly individualized and matched to patient health status and outcomes. Our goal is a benefit package that allows this to happen. This assumption leads us to question any benefit package that imposes arbitrary or actuarial limits on extent of service (such as a set limit on hospital days or office visits). Given the wide range of individual health needs, such limitations do not allow health care to be distributed in the most effective manner.

Lastly, we assume that the definition of basic health care is not limited by traditional notions of "insurance" for costly, unpredictable events only. Some health care, especially preventive care, can and should be offered at predictable intervals and for predictable conditions. We assume that a national health plan will act both as "insurance" against unforeseen risks and as a pre-payment plan for predictable health care expenses.

"Basic health care" is a continuous interaction of people and technologies that takes place in a given context. The question, "Which services constitute basic health care?" cannot be answered without reference to the context within which health services are delivered. This context can be broken down into five interlocking components:

1. Type of practitioner. Who provides the service? Examples: psychologists, nurse-midwives, optometrists.
2. Practice setting. Where is the service provided? Examples: home, office, hospital, intermediate care facility, school.
3. Service category. What kind of service is provided? Examples: drugs, physical therapy, dental care, screening, transplants.
4. Clinical situation. For what conditions is the service provided? Examples: substance abuse, infertility, dental malocclusion.
5. Patient demographics/characteristics. Who receives the service? Examples: infants/children, people with risk factors, rural populations.

In health care, these components cannot be divorced from one another. However, as a first step, we examine each component individually, and describe relevant medical and social values within each component. We will then build upon these values and integrate them into criteria for basic health care.

1. Type of practitioner
   A. education/training
   B. knowledge/skills/certification
   C. availability/accessibility
   D. cost-effectiveness
   E. patient preference/choice

We see no inherent medical or social reason to limit basic health care to services provided by physicians or by those under physician guidance. From a social perspective, other professionals have been deemed qualified to provide certain medical services, as evidenced by accredited degree programs, certifications and licenses. From a medical perspective, competence guidelines would help to delineate the range of services each type of professional is qualified to provide.

A liberal practitioner policy will expand access to health care in poor and rural areas, where physicians may not be as available or accessible. The benefit package could conceivably limit patient choice of individual practitioner, but should limit choice of type of practitioner only because of qualifications and cost-effectiveness.

    2. Practice setting (locus of service)
        A. cost-effectiveness
        B. patient safety
        C. accessibility/convenience
        D. patient preference

One of the most important medical values here is that patient safety directly affects cost-effectiveness; basic health care should not weigh (A) and (B) against one another. There is no inherent reason to limit the practice setting to hospital and doctor's office; care should be delivered in the most cost-effective place accessible to the patient. As a rule, this will be a place in which the patient's independence is maintained to the greatest extent. The preference of the patient should be considered, but could be constrained by safety and cost-effectiveness concerns.

    3. Service category
        A. effectiveness and cost-effectiveness
        B. balance among prevention, palliation and cure
        C. distinctions between cognitive and procedural services

An ideal health system would cover all appropriate and effective health care services. However, finite resources dictate that basic health care might not include all beneficial services. As a nation, we need to determine how well services work, both in studies and in practice. Effectiveness is not a yes/no proposition, but rather a judgment based on a continuum of outcomes. Is the service effective enough to justify its cost? Opportunity costs should be considered: what services are excluded because others are included?

For medical, social and humane reasons, we believe that prevention is preferable to cure but not to the exclusion of treating the sick. We also believe that cognitive services —the communication skills involved in patient evaluation and management—are indispensable to the provider-patient encounter and should be emphasized in health care. In many instances, the outcome of a cognitive service, such as counselling or case management, is harder to quantify than that of a procedure or test; for example, assessing the effectiveness of a CT scan on a brain-injured patient may be simpler than assessing the value of a family conference for the same patient. But if the preferred outcomes of care include patient satisfaction and reduced burden on families (as they should), we can more readily gauge the effectiveness of these services and appreciate their value.

4. Clinical situation
   A. burden of disease/condition (e.g. morbidity, mortality)
   B. impact of intervention upon life prospects/opportunities
   C. quality of life considerations (e.g. functional status)
   D. multiple diagnoses/complications

The clinical situation forms the essence of why we value health care. We want health care to make a difference in the quality of people's lives, as measured by a range of desirable outcomes: reduced morbidity and mortality, maintained or improved function, decreased symptomatology, and reduced dependence on others.

We believe that basic health care should rarely exclude a clinical situation per se. Basic health care should address health needs, regardless of the etiology of the problem and without assessments of personal responsibility for the condition. For example, it should cover appropriate treatment for lung cancer, whether the condition is work-related, smoking-related or both. Basic health care should only exclude conditions that society deems not important, as judged by (A), (B) and (C). Thus we can see the possibility that surgeries for cosmetic reasons might be excluded or treatments for male-pattern baldness.

For the most part, basic health care should be broad enough to allow decisions based on (A)—(D) to be made in the clinical setting, as part of an individual's health care. This should include ongoing discussion between patients and providers about the cost, benefit and effectiveness of medical interventions, as judged by (A)—(D). We believe that this discussion, in the proper clinical context, can be a powerful and fair mechanism for controlling costs, because it informs and mobilizes patients' points of view. Living wills and advance directives are solid examples of formalized discussion and patient decision-making about critical care and end-of-life issues.

    5. Patient demographics/characteristics
      A. age
      B. socioeconomic status
      C. race
      D. sex
      E. residence
      F. risk factors (behavioral, historical, physical)

Basic health care will have to balance two often contradictory values: the importance of doing the most good for the greatest number and doing the most good for the neediest. Just as health care needs to balance prevention, palliation, and cure, it needs to balance the moderate health needs of the many with the severe health needs of the few. To the extent that demographics can predict differential health needs, and to the extent that health care can have a positive impact on those needs, we can justify differential coverage in the benefit package. For example, children might need more extensive preventive services; rural populations might need transportation assistance; people below a certain level of income might need more assistance in obtaining health services.

In sum, basic health care is provided by competent practitioners who are available in settings that are safe, cost-effective and accessible, and it consists of the most effective services that improve or maintain the health status of people with differing health needs.

Basic Health Care and the Benefit Package

Up to this point, we have discussed health care without reference to the structure or financing of the health care system. Translating the values of health care into an acceptable and affordable benefit package, however, will necessitate structural and financial considerations. Does it make sense to elucidate basic health care without first knowing how we will deliver and pay for it? Why not structure the system, set a budget and then pay for whatever services we can afford?

It is true that the basic benefit package is relative to society, in that poorer societies may not have the resources to meet many of the population's health needs. As Daniels notes, "Deciding which needs are to be met and what resources are to be devoted to doing so requires careful moral judgement and a wealth of empirical knowledge about the effects of alternative allocations."[2] But in the United States, this judgment should not be made primarily on budgetary and structural grounds; doing so only perpetuates the inequities of our present system, which has not benefitted from thoughtful health planning. We are especially wary of using present costs to determine future allocations, since these costs are themselves a function of the system we want to change. We believe it is crucial to discuss what we want the benefit package to accomplish before we talk about how to pay for it.

Generally, the benefit package in a system of universal access should cover those services that fit the criteria for basic health care but may omit those services that can be provided more efficiently through other channels. However, quality and accessibility should not be diminished by this mechanism. For example, eyeglasses might fit well within the criteria of basic health care. But it might make economic sense to leave such a limited expense to individuals, rather than to increase the expense with the administrative costs of a universal plan. In such a situation, the benefit package might only cover eyeglasses for people of low income.

Can this argument be made to justify major discrepancies between basic health care and the benefit package? We think not. Other channels have been unable to assure access to basic health care for all Americans. Furthermore, other mechanisms (such as market forces or charity care) lack the coordination required to encourage the use of effective services. All too often, this results in rationing of health services by income or location, which violates the goals of health care. The benefit package should not be used as a vehicle to contain costs. The purpose of the benefit package is to provide appropriate health care coverage, not to limit it.

The example of work-related illness and injury is instructive. It is excluded from traditional health insurance because it is, in principle, covered by a separate mechanism of state-run, no-fault worker's compensation programs. However, often this channel leaves workers uninsured because their claims are contested (60% of disease claims and 10% of injury claims) or because workers have accepted some compensation that then excludes them from medical treatment under the system.[3] This channel, in its present form, is clearly less efficient in addressing particular health needs than a universal benefit package would be and should not be used to justify exclusion of work-related conditions from the benefit package.

Practically speaking, the benefit package might need to phase in health care services over some determined period of time. In fact, there are many international precedents for an incremental approach to the benefit package. Canada's program began with hospital coverage in 1957, extended to physicians' services in 1966, and offered optional coverage for supportive and ancillary services in 1977.[4] Alternately, the package could phase in coverage for segments of the population (children or pregnant women, for example). In any incremental approach, however, it is important to avoid creating financial incentives for *inappropriate* usage; it should not result in shifting ambulatory care to hospital care, or home care to institutional care.

Principles of Determining Benefits

The process for determining the benefit package will be neither easy nor simple. Various clinical outcomes need to be considered and valued; decisions will need to be based on available data, expert opinion and value judgments. At this point, proposed services should be accompanied by cost estimates. An economic analysis should be performed, using cost-utility methodology defined as "a method by which to gauge the desirability of a health care intervention relative to the status quo, using the ratio of the aggregate costs of the intervention to a numerical valuation of the aggregate change in health outcomes that results from it. This ratio is . . . the cost-effectiveness ratio."[5] The content of the benefit package should reflect consistent use of marginal cost-effectiveness ratios across services and across conditions. In other words, the additional amount we are willing to pay per additional unit of value gained should be consistently applied in making decisions about the benefit package.

However, our knowledge base for obtaining individual and social values, for standardizing them and incorporating them in an economic analysis, is still fairly limited, and its application in the benefit process will be slow. Although cost-effectiveness analysis will provide important information for the process of determining the benefits package, it will not be sufficient to handle all the complexities of the process. Economic analysis does not replace judgment, values or responsibility in the decision-making process; rather, it can improve the quality and consistency of those decisions. Not all criteria for making decisions can be quantified in reliable and valid ways. The process will still need to use qualitative judgments when quantitative data are unavailable or incomplete and must factor in a fair distribution of benefits and burdens for different populations when reaching final decisions.

The process for determining benefits should clearly distinguish decisions best made at a societal level from those best made on a clinical level. The process should define broad categories of coverage without attempting to legislate individual provider-patient encounters. In effect, the process should produce national "formularies" that integrate types of covered services with covered providers and covered treatment settings. It may give broad indications for services, especially if the service is costly or scarce. For the most part, it should not specify under what circumstances to provide services to a given patient, which are clinical decisions.

For example, the process will consider cardiac catheterizations. In all likelihood, it will decide to cover them, but only when done by physicians. It might decide to cover them in both hospitals and free-standing centers. However, the decision about when to provide the service to an individual patient will remain a clinical one.

Consider also physical therapy. The decision might be to cover it, when provided by a physician, physical therapist or other certified health professional. It might be covered on both an inpatient and outpatient basis, and even possibly in the home. The specific clinical decision to use the service will be left to patient-provider judgments.

Routine dental services, as defined by dental professionals, provide another example. The process might decide to cover them, when performed by dentists in outpatient settings. However, it might be decided that the benefit package will only cover children and the elderly for routine dental care, if the case is made that the services are most effective in these age groups only.

Bone marrow transplants are a good example of an expensive procedure. The process might cover them, when performed by physicians on an inpatient basis. Because of the cost involved in this case, the process might specify clinical indications, based on evidence of effectiveness. Thus it might cover BMT for leukemia and exclude it for breast cancer.

By this process, the "art" of medical care remains in the clinical sphere, while the "instruments" are designated in the social realm. Like the colors of a palette and the surface of a canvas, the benefit package should be viewed as raw materials for individualized health care, as "painted" by patient-provider negotiation.

We are not suggesting a carte blanche approach in the clinical sphere; we believe that patients and providers have both rights and responsibilities within this negotiation. Patients should be presented with the probable outcomes of treatments and should have their reasonable preferences honored; providers should have a degree of clinical autonomy and should practice according to their morals and best medical judgment. These rights carry concomitant responsibilities: for patients, these include having reasonable expectations of their care and being active participants in their care; for providers, these include eliciting patient preferences, clearly discussing treatment options, and incorporating data into their decision-making.

A broad benefit package can work only if individualized care is negotiated reasonably and fully. This will mean reducing levels of inappropriate care, including the practice of "defensive medicine" and extreme variations in practice patterns. Clinical guidelines and peer review should be incorporated into daily practice voluntarily; providers should participate more fully in the development of guidelines and in the process of proactive peer review. Effective methods to enhance patient education and decision-making (such as advance directives and interactive videodiscs) should be promoted and utilized.

Although the benefit package ultimately will be a product of social consensus, we offer these suggestions for inclusion in the process:

Preventive services. This category includes primary prevention (health promotion, counselling, immunizations), secondary prevention (screening) and tertiary prevention (minimizing complications and disabilities from chronic disease). We believe that effective preventive services should be part of the benefit package, since they directly improve health status. The U.S. Preventive Services Task Force has completed the important analysis of how well interventions work and has made age-specific recommendations for appropriate preventive care.[6] A recent analysis provided estimates of the insurance costs of covering the task force recommendations for the general population; the study found that coverage would add less that 5% to current insurance premiums.[7]

Acute care. This category includes ambulatory, inpatient and home care. The benefit package should encourage timely use of primary care in settings that maximize patient independence. Since ill health is at first a self-perception, the benefit package must provide an initial avenue of recourse. The primary care provider should be responsible for rational health planning with the individual patient. Broad coverage for cognitive services will encourage patients and providers to negotiate carefully and may decrease the utilization of tertiary/high tech/expensive care.

Long-term care. This category includes medical care provided in skilled nursing facilities, intermediate care facilities, community centers and in the home. It is difficult to conceive of a benefits package that did not include some coverage for long-term care, although the actual and potential costs of such care may be daunting initially. An incremental approach to coverage in this category may help to offset the political disinclination to absorb very large expenditures at the outset of implementing a system of universal access.

Reproductive services. This category includes family planning, abortion, prenatal care, and labor and delivery services. Coverage in this category should be comprehensive enough to enable appropriate use of these services including transportation assistance to health care, or home visits by a wide variety of qualified practitioners.

The Process of Determining Benefits

Since determination of the benefit package requires a reasoned judgment of appropriate health care, the process should include a spectrum of interested parties; scientific, economic and medical knowledge should share the podium with consensus opinions and group value judgments. Citizen participation is vital to the success and integrity of this process. We recommend the establishment of a national health board with responsibilities for making these decisions. The board should be composed of representatives of broad constituencies and include a representative sampling of important demographic categories: those that represent children's interests, the elderly, women, minority groups, and rural and urban populations. The board should be supported by a number of advisory groups, which could be composed of providers, business and organized labor, economists, ethicists, and proprietary interests. These advisory groups could be organized in many ways; one way to maximize communication would be to combine representatives into service-specific groups that would make recommendations on one category of care: preventive, acute, long-term or reproductive care.

We anticipate that the board will analyze and categorize health services into three broad groups:

Clearly ineffective therapies

Therapies of unknown/unproven effectiveness

Therapies that are somewhat or clearly effective (relative to others).

The judgment of effectiveness must be based on explicit criteria and outcome measures. How effective is a therapy in achieving which outcomes? Effectiveness lies on a continuum, and must be judged relative to other therapies. Let us now turn to this continuum and examine how the board might deal with coverage decisions at discrete points.

Therapies that fall into the clearly ineffective realm will not be included in the benefit package. If a therapy cannot achieve a desired outcome, it should not be paid for by a system of universal access. People will be free to pay for these services themselves if they choose. In all likelihood, the board will also exclude therapies of unknown or unproven effectiveness. These therapies will become candidates for technology assessment. We recommend the formation of a national council to prioritize these assessments and to authorize sufficient funds to conduct effectiveness research on the ones chosen in any given year. The council will also identify emerging technologies and new uses for established technologies. Patients will gain access to these "experimental" therapies only through participation in research. By linking insurance coverage with the investigational setting, the payment mechanism will steer people into evaluative contexts. We believe this process balances the needs of society to use finite resources wisely with the value given to medical and technological innovation. It gives us a way to diffuse technology rationally and systematically.

That leaves the large category of health services that fall somewhere in the spectrum of relative effectiveness. The board will have to base its coverage decisions on both the value placed on an outcome and the effectiveness of each therapy in achieving that outcome. For example, a clearly effective therapy (polio vaccine) that achieves a valued outcome (prevention of polio) will be covered. A clearly effective therapy (face-lift) for an outcome that is not highly valued (temporary lifting of sagging skin due to normal aging) may not be covered.

A therapy that is somewhat effective (heart transplants) for a valued outcome (extending life in patients with end-stage cardiomyopathies) may be covered only in those people with the best likelihood for survival and quality of life. A therapy that is marginally effective (gamete intrafallopian transfer) in achieving an outcome that may be inconsistently valued (treating infertility) will have to be judged on its cost-effectiveness and justice criteria.

The benefit package should be subject to periodic review and change based on its performance in addressing the health needs of the population. The report by the Department of Health and Human Services *Healthy People 2000*[8] could help set the standards for this judgment and be a benchmark for how well the package is performing. New as well as possibly outdated technologies should be reviewed for inclusion and exclusion; assessments of targeted technologies and procedures should be ongoing and advisory to this process. The medical profession should take the lead in assessing procedures deemed "experimental" or "obsolete," and adequate funding should be allocated to make these assessments timely and informative.

Can We Get There from Here?

The benefits process described above will take time to implement. At the onset of a national health care program, it is likely that a temporary package will be used in the first year while a more elaborate process is put into place. The temporary package will be a political compromise and can be drawn from a number of present packages: average employee benefits, Medicare, Medicaid or standard HMO coverages. The specifics of the temporary package are less important than the mechanism by which it will be replaced by a more thoughtful, value-driven process.

The benefit package will not be achieved in a vacuum. At the same time that we begin the process of benefits determination, we must also begin work to organize and integrate technology assessment efforts, including expanding outcomes and effectiveness research, to develop mechanisms to determine societal values and preferences, to match our health care facilities, personnel and equipment to the needs of the population, and to control costs in ways that do not adversely affect quality of care.

We *can* get there from here, if we can evoke the political and popular will to make real change.

NOTES

1. Norman Daniels, *Just Health Care* (New York: Cambridge University Press, 1985).

2. *Ibid.*

3. Institute of Medicine, *Role of the Primary Care Physician in Occupational and Environmental Medicine* (Washington, DC: National Academy Press, 1988).

4. Milton I. Roemer, *National Health Systems of the World* (New York: Oxford University Press, 1991).

5. Mark Kamlet, *The Comparative Benefits Modeling Project: A Framework for Cost-Utility Analysis of Government Health Care Programs* (Washington, D.C.: U.S. Dept. of Health and Human Services, 1992).

6. U.S. Preventive Services Task Force, *The Guide to Clinical Preventive Sevices: An Assessment of the Effectiveness of 169 Interventions* (Baltimore, MD: Williams & Wilkins, 1989).

7. Rose Chu and Gordon Trapnell, "Costs of Insuring Preventive Care," *Inquiry* 27 (1990): 273–280.

8. Public Health Service, *Healthy People 2000: National Health Promotion and Disease Prevention Objectives* (Washington, DC: U.S. Department of Health and Human Services, 1991).

MICHAEL J. GARLAND

Oregon's Contribution to
Defining Adequate Health Care[1]

The people of the United States are on the verge of politically transforming their right to health care from a manifesto right to an effective,
enforceable right. Following Joel Feinberg's usage,[2] I mean by manifesto right a widely and intensely held ideal about entitlement that
contradicts current institutional and legal practices and consequently
is not enforceable despite its broad appeal. Universal coverage for
health care is just such a manifesto right in the United States, despite
its being an enforceable right in most other industrialized societies.
An enforceable right to health care, however, requires that everyone
be covered by third party payment systems for an identifiable set of
health care services. The reform of health care toward which we are
moving needs a solid foundation of social consensus on four crucial
issues as yet unsettled: what services to cover, how to accumulate
needed funds, how to assure equitable participation in financing coverage, and how to use health care resources more efficiently.

  Whether ten years from now the United States will have a single
payer system or a coordinated system of multiple payers is uncertain,
but universal coverage for health care clearly will be a reality by that
time. I discuss below a range of typical reform proposals. They all
take the goal of universal coverage as a given but differ on how
many payers will manage the system, who will finance the system
(employers, workers, taxpayers), and what criteria will define equity
between rich and poor. Attention to these issues in public debate
tends to overshadow the point I address in this chapter: by what
social process should the content of the basic benefit package be
determined? The Clinton administration will assign this task to a
National Board of Health and has already formed a task force of
technical experts to work on the content of the package. I argue that
the general public as well as experts should have an integral role in
making this determination and that Oregon has developed a model
that can be adapted to a national level. The black box of basic health

care needs to be opened for public inspection as we move forward with national health care reform in the next several years. What is to be the content of the universal guarantee? Which health services merit collective financing? What role should the general public's values play in determining the substance of the guarantee? What is the role for technical experts in realistically identifying which services contribute to the community's common good?

In an attempt to deal with the content of the right to health care, the people of the state of Oregon created a prioritized list of health services as a decision tool for the legislature to use in determining the budget for Medicaid.[3] In the Oregon Plan, setting the Medicaid budget based on service priorities also establishes a basic benefit level for two private insurance programs designed to make health insurance available to 450,000 currently uninsured citizens.[4]

I will summarize the system used in Oregon to build benefit packages around a prioritized list of health services and explore its potential for contributing to the task of transforming a manifesto right to health care into an enforceable right through a national system of universal coverage for health care. In this account, I will focus particularly on the public participation activities essential to developing and implementing the Oregon Plan.

Oregon's Plan for Establishing Health Service Priorities

As part of its effort to produce a rational system of coverage for those currently uninsured for health care, Oregon is testing a model for enhanced democratic process in complex health policy decision making. The plan has been widely debated in popular and professional media. I have elsewhere described the plan's methodology in relation to the criticism that it treats the poor unjustly.[5] These criticisms express skepticism about the ethics and wisdom of the Oregon Plan's focus on specifying priorities among health services for the poor. Justice, it is argued, cannot be served unless limitations on health services apply to everyone, not only to the poor.[6] I and others have argued that in fact the Oregon Plan actually will improve the circumstance of the poor and thus serves justice, even though a more perfect justice could be achieved if prioritization were used to define a basic minimum standard that would apply to everyone.[7]

In the context of transforming a manifesto right into a universal enforceable entitlement to health care coverage, the problem of prioritizing services only for the poorer members of society is no longer a special issue. The enforceable entitlement must deal directly with equity between rich and poor in a coordinated system. The Oregon Plan aimed at improving the circumstances of the poor of Oregon in a context where there was not sufficient control over the whole system to pursue the kind of reform that is now on the national agenda since we are clearly determined to transform a manifesto right into an enforceable legal right. I will argue for the importance in a democratic society of defining the basic minimum standard through a process driven by public values while also employing data from appropriate experts. The process of prioritizing health services offers a politically feasible and technically appropriate path for resolving the ethical problem of achieving equitable access for all to adequate health care.[8]

The Oregon plan is an example of political decision making about the allocation of collective resources for health care that employs two principles highly relevant to the development of a universal health care guarantee: first, that explicit political choice is preferable to the hidden rationing that now occurs and secondly, that decisions about what belongs in the universal guarantee should be based on both expert data and community values.[9]

A trio of laws passed in 1989 seek to bring every Oregonian into the security of third party coverage. Medicaid reform, new employer incentives for health insurance purchase and a high risk insurance pool coordinated by state government are the three ingredients of the plan. The principal stimulus for the plan was the desire to bring some relief to more than 450,000 Oregon citizens who are without health insurance, the majority of whom, although they are employed, do not receive health insurance as part of their employment benefit package. The cornerstone of the plan is a prioritized list of health services that serves as the basis for determining the basic benefits to which Medicaid clients and those insured through new small business plans will be entitled.

The political approach of the Oregon Plan creates an important division of labor carried out in a four stage process: first, a public commission, the "Health Services Commission" (HSC) generates a priority list of health services; second, legislators use the list to determine budget allocations for publicly financed health care programs; third, agencies plan for and administer services within budget constraints; fourth, agencies and community providers effect the delivery of services in the community and cooperate in the evaluation of the new service arrangements on the health of the population.

In the first stage of the process, the Health Services Commission developed a list of health service priorities based on community values about health care and on technical information about the effectiveness of various health services relative to the needs of the population to be served. The method for establishing priorities rests on the decision analysis principle of separating factual technical information and value judgments in preparation for a rational evaluation of a complex decision.[10] The Commission recognized that its task required it to blend community values and the best available technical data about the effectiveness of health services in order to produce a list of socially significant priorities. The iteration of the list that won approval from the federal government drew on values expressed at community meetings and public hearings and data provided by health care experts concerning effectiveness and costs of specific services.[11] The list is not a once and for all product, but is to be revised continuously by the Commission and reported biennially to the legislature. The first prioritized list was delivered to the Governor and the legislature in May 1991.

Delivery of the list triggered the second stage at which the full legislature, using the list and actuarial estimates of costs as a decision guide, had the task of setting the budget which established the specific benefit package to be offered by the new Oregon Medicaid Program and substantially contained in any private health insurance plan offered under the aegis of the small business and high risk insurance programs. The legislature completed step two at the end of June 1991. The third stage in the process provides the relevant agencies (Office of Medical Assistance Programs, Oregon Medical Insurance Pool Board and Insurance Pool Governing Board) with the budget decision that creates the benefit package for Medicaid and related private insurance packages. The first administrative task for the Office of Medical Assistance Programs (OMAP) was to request necessary waivers of several federal Medicaid regulations from the Health Care Financing Administration (HCFA). The waiver request went to HCFA in August 1991, and was denied in August 1992, resubmitted in November 1992, and finally granted in March 1993, on the condition that one more iteration of the prioritized list be produced without using data about symptoms to determine position on the list.[12]

At stage three the agencies must also put in place all the administrative and evaluation elements necessary to run a complex social program. Part of the concept of the Oregon Plan is for the agencies to use the priority list to guide administrative decisions so that the new programs will be a consistent expression of the values on which the priorities rest.

The fourth stage is the actual implementation of new service programs in the community. Medicaid will serve all persons at or below 100% of the Federal Poverty Level (e.g., an income of $964 per month for a family of three[13]). Newly developed private insurance programs focused on small business employees and persons whose risk status makes private insurance unavailable or unaffordable will serve persons with incomes above 100% Federal Poverty Level (unless already included in a Medicaid categorical program). At this stage, the ultimate goal of improved access to basic health care depends on the ability of agencies to maintain cooperative relations with direct care providers. The Oregon Medicaid agency has developed plans to implement the new Medicaid Program beginning in January 1994, while the private insurance programs have already begun to market products and work on small group insurance reform.

The division of tasks and responsibilities among the general public, the Commission, the legislature, and specific agencies is an essential and often overlooked characteristic of the Oregon Plan. The division of tasks makes possible the critically important separation of value considerations from technical facts at the outset of the process of setting priorities. Articulating values from the community uses democratic processes that serve to promote the sense of community responsibility for the fairness and common good dimensions of collectively financed health care. This process allows the legislature to use the priority list as a decision tool relatively free from political pressures and protects them from the temptation to fiddle with the list at the request of lobbyists for special interests, such as provider groups or specific disease oriented associations like those for cancer, transplantation or Alzheimer's Disease.

Structure of the Priority List

The Health Services Commission (HSC) began its work in September 1989. Although the law required the Commission to produce a priority list, it did not prescribe a method for accomplishing the task. Some early critics asserted that the task of setting health services priorities is too complex and that only nonsense could be produced in the short time frame and with the methods the Commission first tried.[14] Conscious of their role as social innovators the Commission paid attention to its critics and kept working on its methods and revising its deadlines until it was sufficiently satisfied that the list, despite its imperfections, would be reasonable and suitable for its intended use. The list, along with an actuarial estimate of the costs of implementing it,[15] was reported to the legislature in May 1991. In response to the waiver denial in August 1992, the Commission reordered the list without using data from the telephone survey. As a condition of the waiver approval in March 1993, the Commission reordered the list once more, this time without using data about symptom control. The content and ordering of the list remains the responsibility of the Commission. Legislators are not permitted to alter the list but are to use it as a decision tool in budgeting for Medicaid.

The entire list consists of 696 items, each item made up of a health condition or diagnosis paired with a treatment likely to be used in providing care to a person with the stated condition or diagnosis. An "integrated list (containing 745 items) which merges mental health and chemical dependency services with physical medicine" was also submitted to the legislature in April, 1993.[16] These condition-treatment pairs were developed from standard lists of diagnoses and medical procedures used for statistical and billing purposes.[17] The May 1991 list was structured by a system of seventeen categories which were abandoned in both the November 1992 and March 1993 reiterations of the list. Items on the final list were ranked based on (1) their potential to prevent death, (2) their potential to spare resources, and (3) their potential to serve one or more key values identified through the community meeting process. At any point on the list, every preceding line has a higher or equal potential to save lives and (if it has the same potential to save life) has an equal or lower cost or serves one or more community values judged by the Commission to be similar in effect to other services in the same section of the list.[18] Thus, maternity care and care of the newborn appear in the top tenth of the list, general preventive care and comfort care (when cure is not hoped for) appear in the upper quartile, family planning ranks in the top half, and treatment for self limiting diseases and cosmetic interventions fall within the lowest 15 percent of the items. The 1991

Oregon Legislature passed a budget for Medicaid that would fund 82% of the lines. In 1992, the November revision of the list was approved for a similar level of funding.[19]

Prioritization Method

The Oregon Plan's method assumes that the effort to define a basic standard for health care benefits requires two inputs: an articulation of relevant values from the community, and relevant technical data from experts. Using public hearings, structured community meetings, and a telephone survey, the HSC gathered two kinds of values data: individual values and community values.

The primary source of the individual value data was a random sample telephone survey of the Oregon population using an instrument adapted from Kaplan's Quality of Well-Being Scale.[20] The results of the survey were originally intended to provide the Commission with a set of weighted functional categories and symptoms that were then to be used by health care providers to characterize the probable outcomes of treatments for specific conditions. Both these data were then to provide quantitative data for a net benefit formula intended to establish priorities. However, in August 1992, the Department of Health and Human Services identified the telephone survey as the primary cause for denial of the waiver. Consequently, data from the survey has not been used in the two subsequent revisions of the list.[21]

Another variety of values information was generated at twelve public hearings the Commission held in seven different sites around the state. Those giving testimony represented either individual interests or special group interests. Participants made vigorous pleas for preventive services, mental health and chemical dependency services, universal health insurance, the use of alternative providers, dental services, prenatal care, health education and transplant services. Others spoke to the need for hearing, vision and nutrition services. Many used the opportunity to urge that government alter its general budgetary priorities. The Commission considered the public hearings helpful for "understanding the general tone of public needs and concerns" and brought the information to bear on the continuing process of shaping the prioritized list.[22]

A unique expression of community-oriented values was generated for the HSC by special arrangement with Oregon Health Decisions (OHD), a nonprofit organization that has existed since 1983 to facilitate public participation in the development of public policy involving ethical issues in health care.[23] The goal of the community meetings was to generate for the HSC publicly examined statements about what makes health care a common good. OHD asked participants to think and express themselves in the first person plural, namely as members of a statewide community for whom health care has a shared value. According to OHD philosophy, these meetings not only generate data but also stimulate the sense of community responsibility for the ethical dimension of health policy decisions.

A total of 1,048 citizens participated in forty-seven community meetings held throughout the state. Each meeting aimed at discovering local consensus about community values regarding health care. The method for these meetings produced a separation of facts and values through structured small group discussions which called for first, individual judgments about priorities among a list of nine categories of health services; second, discussion among participants to identify values underlying their priority judgments; and third, identification of key shared values about health care. The *fourth* step was to identify for the whole group principal values from each of the small groups and, through further discussion with the entire group, determine which value themes would constitute an "authentic message" to the HSC from the particular geographic community. Reports from these community meetings were collated and reported to the HSC by OHD staff.

The community meetings are a distinctive feature of the Oregon Plan and were instrumental in bringing several important values into the HSC's deliberation. The meetings identified a constellation of thirteen community value themes about health care. These themes exhibit the richness of community values about health care. The value themes were not prioritized either by the communities or by the OHD staff. Without implying any priority order or weight the following themes summarize the "message from the communities" to the HSC.

Prevention: avoiding harm and suffering, improving quality of life, exercising wisdom and personal choice.

Quality of Life: attending to emotional well-being, pain and suffering, independence, functional capacity.

Cost Effectiveness: seeking wise investments in health.

Ability to function: restoring emotional well-being, productivity, independence, and general quality of life.

Equity: contributing to the fairness of community life.

Effectiveness of treatment: preferring to fund treatments known to work ahead of doubtfully effective interventions.

Benefits many: seeking to treat problems that affect a large proportion of the community.

Mental health and chemical dependency: connecting mental and physical health, supporting functional ability, and productivity.

Personal choice: preserving autonomy and personal dignity.

Community compassion: seeking to assure humane response to the terminally ill and other vulnerable persons.

Impact on society: attending to effects on others from treating (or not treating) certain health problems.

Length of life: acknowledging that continued life is necessary to realize any personal values.

Personal responsibility: encouraging individual autonomy and control over one's own health status.

These values became increasingly significant for the ranking of the line items as the Commission's methods evolved. In the March 1993 iteration of the list (which complied with the conditions attached to the waiver approval) values expressed in the community meetings and at the twelve public hearings presided over by the Commissioners explain the positioning of several special groups of services (e.g., maternity and newborn services, preventive services, dental care, comfort care) and "hand adjustment" decisions by the Commission to move particular items from section to section on the list.[24]

The Role of Technical Experts

Reasonable priorities require good facts as well as authentic values. From fifty-four panels of health care providers, the HSC solicited outcome-of-treatment information in order to connect its carefully gathered value information to reliable data about the effectiveness of specific health services. Since treatment occurs in response to a condition, the information was solicited in terms of condition-treatment pairs developed from diagnoses listed in the ICD-9 (*International*

Classification of Disease) or DSM-III-R *(Diagnostic and Statistical Manual of Mental Disorders)* which were linked to procedures listed in CPT-4 *(Current Physician's Terminology)* or ADA (American Dental Association) codes for treatments. Providers were requested to indicate: (1) median age at onset of diagnosis; (2) probability that the designated treatment would be used; (3) expected duration of benefits from the treatment; (4) outcome probabilities with and without treatment; (5) cost to payer with and without treatment. Outcomes were to be identified as *Death; Residual Effects;* (major symptoms, activity impairments and mobility restrictions) or *Asymptomatic Cure*. Each identified outcome was to have a probability estimate of its occurrence given the condition-treatment pair under consideration. Providers responded in terms of a reference list of twenty four symptoms and six measures of activity (two each for mobility, physical activity, and social activity) taken from the QWB scale. Eventually, in response to the federal government's concern over potential violation of the Americans with Disabilities Act, the Commission discarded all use of symptom related data from its prioritization method, keeping only (1) data about probability of preventing death, (2) cost of treatment, and (3) medical effectiveness.

The other technical data associated with the prioritized list were the estimates by actuaries of the expected costs of providing services down to and including each line of the list.[25] The estimates were revised each time the Commission significantly reordered the list (in November 1992 and March 1993). The actuarial estimates did not affect the prioritization but allowed the legislature to know what costs would be associated with the inclusion of more or fewer services at the margin.

Originally, the Commission used the value weights (QWB) and the outcomes data from providers in a net benefit formula. The formula, however, disappeared by stages from the Commission's methodology. At first, it was a cost-benefit formula and intended to be the primary methodological instrument for prioritization. For the May 1991 list, however, the formula became a secondary element, being used to establish an ordering within the categories that were themselves placed into a priority order using a unique category ranking method.[26] In the May 1991 application, only a net-benefit ratio was used with consideration given to cost information only when items in the same category had the same score or when the Commissioners had doubts about the reasonableness of an item's location on the list.

For the November 1992 list, the Commissioners dropped the categories and determined the ranking only on the basis of a treatment's probability of preventing death, probability of controlling symptoms, costs of services, or relation to specific community values derived from public hearings and community meetings. For the last revision (March 1993), the Commission eliminated the criterion of symptom control and added consideration of medical effectiveness.

In each iteration of the list, after the computer had ranked line items in terms of quantifiable elements, such as priorities for preventing death and cost of treatment, the Commissioners went through the entire list line by line to identify any items that intuitively seemed "out of place." Commissioners who wanted to move an item on the list held themselves to a consensus rule and argued for movement on the basis of several considerations (derived from Public Hearings and Community Meetings):[27] (1) prefer services that prevent disease or avoid deterioration of current health status of affected persons; (2) resolve conflicts when multiple values affect line placement; (3) give priority to groups of health services based on values identified by the public;[28] (4) give priority to treatments that reduce public health risks; (5) rank cancer treatments based on rates of treatment effectiveness expected for different stages in the progression of the cancer; (6) give priority to symptom relief that improves functioning when treatment for a self-limiting condition would otherwise have low priority; (7) merge lines where significant symptom relief serves ancillary purposes or the items involved constitute a continuum of care.

In summary, the Oregon Plan is an application of basic democratic principles to the complex field of health care. It stimulates active participation by the general citizenry in declaring the values on which new political choices should be based. It maintains a role for experts in describing the probable outcomes of specific health care interventions that in the aggregate make up a package of benefits. It requires legislators to conduct an open and accountable budget-making process that finally delivers to human services agencies the resources necessary to organize and administer a valued set of health services.

The Oregon prioritization process was designed first and foremost as an instrument for more rational budget management of Medicaid and for defining a basic benefit package for small business health insurance programs. The approach, however, has great applicability to the pursuit of a nationwide universal health care guarantee. The coming reform demands a socially acceptable definition of a basic benefit level on which the guarantee rests. A key element of the Clinton administration's health care reform is the definition of a uniform benefit package, a principle task of the proposed National Health Board.[29] The Oregon approach offers an innovative model for involving both experts and the general public in this task.

Prioritization and Universal Guarantees

Movement from the present situation in health care to a system of universal coverage for all citizens requires a clear definition of the basic benefit package. The uniform benefit package gives society the capacity to settle important questions about duties and entitlements regarding access to health care. The content of the guarantee is of crucial importance for the next stage of health care reform. Of all the proposals for health care reform that have emerged in recent years, only the Oregon Plan has given the question of the content of the guarantee the level of attention it deserves. The reform path on which the Clinton administration has embarked will be one of compromise, seeking some balance of preferred elements from a wide spectrum of proposals that have multiplied in recent years as the need for significant change became increasingly apparent. New proposals for universal coverage range from government run health insurance systems[30] through a variety of mixed public-private systems.[31] Blendon and Edwards have devised a typology of mixed public-private proposals into three basic forms: (1) those that call for compulsory, employment based private insurance, with government insuring non-workers and the poor; (2) those that require employers either to provide insurance or to pay an equivalent tax that will be used to buy health insurance for uninsured workers, with government insuring non-workers and the poor; (3) the use of tax credits and vouchers to purchase private health insurance.[32]

Common to all of these proposals is the assumption that the new program will define a "basic" or "standard" or "comprehensive" or "minimum" set of health care benefits which any private insurer or government program must contain. Linda Bergthold describes four different ways of approaching this problem of basic benefit package design: some emphasize primary care, some emphasize catastrophic coverage, some emphasize a broadly comprehensive indemnity approach (often assuming fee for service medical practice), and some emphasize a comprehensive benefit approach within an HMO framework.[33] These different approaches yield significantly different benefit packages. The challenge of movement toward an enforceable right to health care is to define one standard set of benefits which can be claimed and which society is obligated to provide for everyone. This determination, which the Clinton proposal assigns to the National Health Board, is a crucial step toward justice in a new health care system. The following list shows the ways in which these typical proposals identify the requisite content of the guaranteed level of health care their authors envision.

PROPOSAL	CONTENT OF GUARANTEE
AMA Health Access	"Minimum Benefits"—broadly defined by AMA
Pepper Commission	"Adequate minimum Standard"
"Physicians Who Care"	"Catastrophic coverage for major illness"—not defined
Medical Schools Section (AMA)	"Medically Necessary Services"
Karen Davis	"Current Medicare coverage"—plus other categories
Kansas Employer Coalition	"Broad, minimum plan"—like HMO Act (1973) or Medicare
Enthoven and Kronick	"Federal Standards"
Urban Institute	"Minimum Standards"
Heritage Foundation	"Basic package"—federally defined
USHealth (Roybal)	"Broad coverage"
Physicians' for NHP	"Medically Necessary Services"—national standards
Committee for NHI (Fein)	"Core Benefits"—federally defined (state option)

This list illustrates that several different words carrying different assumptions are being used by those who have recently stepped forward in the name of universal access to health care. Architects of the Clinton Proposal used the words *benchmark, standard, comprehensive, uniform, mainstream, and broadly acceptable to the public* to refer to the content of the basic guarantee.[34] Debates tend to focus on differences in ideology about the role of government and private insurance in the transition to a universally guaranteed system of access. The issue of how to control total expenditures in the new system is much discussed. Too little attention has been paid to the task of defining the content of the guarantee—what is it that we should all have access to? Except for the work done for the Oregon Plan, public discussion to date has done little to prepare the way for the proposed National Health Board's first major task, defining a standard benefit package as the cornerstone of equity in the new health care system.

The need for such a definition was identified as a critical social task by the 1983 report on access to health care produced by the President's Commission for the Study of Ethical Issues in Medicine and Biomedical and Behavioral Research.[35] The Commission's report made two significant conceptual moves in the then languishing debate about "National Health Insurance." First, they side-stepped the question whether health care should be viewed as a moral or human right. Because such a right could not be clearly grounded, its limits could not be clearly set and the correlative duties could not be appropriately assigned. Second, they introduced two key words into the customary formula about access to health care: *equitable* access and *adequate* care. "Society has a moral obligation to ensure that everyone has access to *adequate* care without being subject to *excessive burdens*."[36] The report urged that the concept of "adequate health care" should be used to guide social efforts to arrive at mutual guarantees of a level of care that should be available to all, allowing that some persons may have the resources to privately purchase services in excess of the basic standard. Equity demands only that an adequate level be available to all, not that every kind of care be equally available to all. The Commission openly endorsed the concept of a two or more tiered system, provided that the bottom tier could meet some standard of equity.

The President's Commission pointed to an array of four values for which health care is deemed important: it contributes to equality of opportunity in the society, it can reduce pain and suffering, it can inform persons about their life prospects, and it is associated with many central symbols of human existence.[37] Through its community meeting process the Oregon approach evoked an even richer articulation of "what makes health care important to us" from members of the general community, resulting in an even broader base of values by which to judge the scope of "adequate" health care, the thirteen value themes discussed above.

The President's Commission did not offer a definition of adequate care but discussed factors that require consideration: which conditions merit guaranteed access to treatment, health conditions in relation to treatment options, the costs and effectiveness of such treatments, and the quality of guaranteed treatments. Several approaches were suggested by the President's Commission for defining criteria of adequacy, such as professional judgment, average current use, or compiling comprehensive lists of services. Two caveats run through the President's Commission's remarks on adequacy. First, care must be taken to keep the definition dynamic and not an uncritical endorsement of the status quo. Second, recognizing that the definition of *adequate* is not objective, the ultimate source of value determinations should be the public. "In a democracy, the appropriate values to be assigned to the consequences of policies must ultimately be determined by people expressing their values through social and political processes as well as in the marketplace."[38]

One principal equity issue is embedded in the concept of adequate care. Fairness in a two-tiered system rests on the content of the universally guaranteed level of service. Where will this basic benefit package come from? Who will define it? What values will it encompass? By what process will it be reviewed for adequacy? I believe that it is in answering these questions that the Oregon Plan has its most interesting and nationally useful feature. The relevant values according to the Oregon method are to be identified through face-to-face discussion with members of the community that experiences health care as a feature of its common good.

A concerted effort over time with a broad selection of American citizens could contribute important information to the national task of defining the content of the guaranteed basic health care benefits; such definition will make it possible to judge equitable access to adequate health care. Since the virtual demise of the Health Planning Agencies created in the 1970s to provide a national network for citizen input into the health care system, any current effort along the lines of the Oregon Plan would require some coalition building among civic groups such as the American Health Decisions groups[39] (a coalition of statewide organizations similar to Oregon Health Decisions), League of Women Voters, AARP, and the like. A model around which such a nationwide outreach could be constructed has been developed by the Public Agenda Foundation, California Health Decisions, and New Jersey Citizens' Committee on Bioethics. These groups mounted the first large scale effort to use mass media and the face-to-face dialogue of the health decisions method in the spring of 1992.[40]

A second equity issue is that of the level of burden, especially financial, required of someone seeking access to adequate care. Most of the current universal access proposals pay a great deal of attention to this issue of financial burden, both on the part of those seeking care and on those called upon to contribute resources that would lighten the burden of those in need. As used in Oregon, the community meetings did not shed light on this dimension of equity, but there is no reason to believe that a community meeting process might not be able to shed light on the values in the community that underlie its choices of the distribution of financial burden. The greatest challenge for such a search for consensus is how to keep the discussion from being overwhelmed with deeply ingrained feelings about taxes independent of their capacity to serve equity. This discussion, though difficult and sensitive, is an essential element in moving forward with the universal access project.

The Oregon plan takes the position that the content of the "basic benefit" package should result from an open, democratic process in which public values and technical expertise play complementary roles. This approach is important for dealing with questions of justice and fairness, especially in terms of access to socially guaranteed benefits. It also contributes to the exercise of social responsibility for the content of the common good and the fairness of the burdens of sustaining the common good in a democratic community.

Most of the universal access proposals described above concern themselves so much with financing their programs that they treat the content of the basic benefit package as if it were a minor problem. The status quo is highly variable among the different parts of the U.S. health care system. In the public sector we have fifty different Medicaid programs, Medicare, Veterans Administration, Department of Defense Medical Programs, the Native American Health Service, state and local welfare programs. Private insurance plans have enormous variability in services covered. The system as a whole tends to define benefits broadly, deferring as far as possible to professional autonomy. All the proposals address the need for some uniformity in national standards for benefit packages. Uniformity in the lower tier—the universally guaranteed tier—is seen as a prerequisite for fairness and equity in the system. If this is the case, then at some point it is necessary to say what is and what is not guaranteed as a basic benefit.

The Oregon approach assumes that defining the basic benefit requires expertise and political choice. The determination of adequate health care is partly technical and should not be done without serious input from health care experts, both providers of service and those who are technically skilled in organizing and financing the endeavor itself. There is also a role for the public whose wants, needs, and expectations the health care system is supposed to serve. The Oregon approach highlights as well that the synthesis of public values and technical knowledge requires a visible point of political accountability. The dedication of public resources to health care rather than some other use is an important political accomplishment. The Oregon approach seeks to keep that act out in the open with its decision making rationale accessible to public scrutiny.

In addition to universal access, the other major pieces of the national health care puzzle are cost containment, quality assurance, and the capacity of the political system to assess the relative value of health care among other uses of collective resources. Defining the basic benefit package using a public involving method like Oregon's does not solve these other dimensions of the national puzzle but does establish a frame of reference for approaching them as integrated problems. Cost containment goals derive from community values about the good of health care. Efficiency in health care is not an absolute concept, but one which gets its definition from the health care goals of society. Quality is not objective but subjective and should be determined by a community's sense of acceptable levels of hardship, inconvenience, and difficulty associated with the pursuit of health and health care.

Political assessment of the relative worth of health care in comparison with other uses of collective resources is intensely dependent in a democracy on the capacity of members of the political community to make their serious and stable values accessible to those who manage public resources both at the legislative and the executive level. Through openness and public involvement, the Oregon Plan strives against the alienation and cynicism about politics that is pervasive in the United States. If there is much that is wrong, unfair, and perverse in the way those with political power behave, it is not likely to be corrected by further isolating them from scrutiny and accountability to the community they are, at least nominally, supposed to be serving. In a technologically complex society such as ours, a romantic call to populist solutions seems doomed to fail. The system needs experts. But the experts need to understand the community's values.

Oregon is creating an environment where experts and the public can collaborate in politically and technically complex decision making. As we move into a universal access system during the next decade, the need for such collaboration will become more rather than less persistent. As we seek ways to slow the rate of growth in total expenditures for health care, we need to draw into the picture public values and public accountability and community responsibility. As we seek to identify for ourselves what hardships, inconveniences, and difficulties are compatible with our expectations of quality in health care, the voice and values of the community are even more important. As we seek to decide which "other uses" of collective resources we are willing to trade for more health care or which health care services we are willing to forgo in return for some other use of scarce resources, we need to find our political voices.

As a participating observer, I have come to understand the unfolding Oregon plan as a revitalization of democratic processes in health care. As such, health care reform is and always will be a dangerous and unfinished project. Movement from a manifesto right to an enforceable right to health care challenges us to understand the consequences of our solidarity, or lack of it, in the face of common threats from death, disability, pain, suffering, and loss of vigor. Solidarity in health care is always unfinished work because the source of the threats change. Consider how the HIV epidemic has placed new challenges before patients, providers, and policy makers. It is dangerous work because solidarity makes unsettling demands on our sense of "what is mine and not yours." A manifesto right does not become an enforceable right without vision, sacrifice, and commitment.

NOTES

1.   This chapter revises an article entitled "Light on the Black Box of Basic Health Care: Oregon's Contribution to the National Movement Toward Universal Health Care" previously published in the *Yale Law and Policy Review* 10 (1992), 409–430.

2. Joel Feinberg, "The Nature and Value of Rights," The *Journal of Value Inquiry* 4, no. 4 (Winter, 1970): 243–257.

3. The primary documentation of the Oregon prioritization process is found in Oregon Health Services Commission, *Prioritization of Health Services: A Report to the Governor and Legislature* (1991).

4. Three statutes passed in 1989 define the scope of the Oregon Plan. One created the Medicaid reform process with the prioritized list of health services as the cornerstone. The second provided funding for a previously established but unfunded high risk pool for persons unable to purchase health insurance in the free market. The third established a "play or pay" incentive system to make health insurance more available to employees in small businesses. The legislative intent was to achieve virtually universal coverage for persons most likely to be without health insurance.

5. See Michael J. Garland and Romana Hasnain, "Community Responsibility and the Development of Oregon's Health Care Priorities," *Business and Professional Ethics Journal* 9 (1990): 181–200; see also my discussion of the justice and common good issues when the plan is viewed as a form of rationing: "Rationing in Public: Oregon's Priority Setting Methodology," in *Rationing America's Health Care: The Oregon Plan and Beyond*, eds. Joshua M. Wiener, Martin A. Strosberg, Robert Baker and I. Alan Fein (Washington, DC: The Brookings Institution, 1992) and "Justice, Politics and Community: Expanding Access and Rationing Health Services in Oregon," *Law, Medicine and Health Care* 20: 1–2 (Spring–Summer 1992): 67–81. Parts of the present article are revisions of material describing the Oregon Plan published in these previous articles.

6. See Norman Daniels, "Is the Oregon Rationing Plan Fair?" *Journal of the American Medical Association* 265 (1991): 2232–2235. Daniels provides the most carefully articulated version of the justice arguments against the Oregon Plan. His criticism goes beyond that of requiring that everyone's health care be subject to the "basic care" limited guarantee. He makes several process criticisms as well.

7. See Garland, "Justice, Politics and Community;" also see Leonard M. Fleck, "The Oregon Medicaid Experiment: Is it Just Enough?" *Business & Professional Ethics Journal* 9 (Fall–Winter 1990): 201–217; and David M. Eddy, "Oregon's Plan, Should it Be Approved?" *Journal of the American Medical Association* 266: (1991) 2439–2445.

8. This is the formulation of the goal of universally guaranteed health care proposed by the President's Commission for the Study of Ethical Problems in Medicine and Biomedical and Behavioral Research, *Securing Access to Health Care: A Report on the Ethical Implications of Differences in the Availability Health Services* (Washington, DC: U.S. Government Printing Office, 1983).

9. The primary documentation of the Oregon Plan is found in *Prioritization of Health Services, A Report to the Governor and Legislature*. (Salem, Oregon: Oregon Health Services Commission, 1991). Available from the Office of Medical Assistance Programs, Department of Human Resources, 203 Public Service Building. Salem, OR 97310.

10. See generally Howard Raiffa, *Decision Analysis* (Reading, Mass.: Addison Wesley, 1968) and Milton C. Weinstein et al., *Clinical Decision Analysis* (Philadelphia, W.B. Saunders, 1980).

11. Data derived from a random sample telephone survey of Oregon citizens had to be dropped from the prioritization methodology after the waiver denial issued in August 1992.

12. Terms and conditions attached to the waiver approval are contained in a letter dated March 19, 1993 from William Toby, Jr., Acting Administrator of the Health Care Financing Administration addressed to Kevin W. Concannon, Director of the Oregon Department of Human Resources.

13. See Notice 57 *Federal Register*, 5456 (1992).

14. See for example, William B. Schwartz and Henry J. Aaron, "The Achilles Heel of Health Care Rationing" *New York Times*, July 9, 1990, at A 17.

15. Health Services Commission, *Prioritization of Health Services*, Appendix I: Actuarial Analysis.

16. Report of the Health Services Commission, April 22, 1993.

17. The Commission used *International Classification of Disease*, 9th edition; *Diagnostic and Statistical Manual of Mental Disorders; Current Physicians" Terminology*, 4th edition; and the American Dental Association codes for treatments.

18. See elsewhere detailed account by Harvey Klevitt of the Commission's process for bringing these judgments to bear on the list.

19. At the time of writing the legislature had not established a funding line for the March 1993 revision. It is unlikely that the legislature would significantly alter its funding commitment to the program.

20. Robert M. Kaplan and J. P. Anderson, "A General Health Policy Model: Update and Applications," *Health Services Research*, 23 (1988) 203–235.

21. See also Paul Menzel, "Oregon's Denial: Disabilities and Quality of Life" *Hastings Center Report* 22, 6 (November–December, 1992): 21–25; in the same issue, see also Alexander Capron, "Oregon's Disability: Principles or Politics?": 18–20.

22. Oregon Health Services Commission, *Prioritization of Health Services*, Appendix C, pp. C-7 and C-8.

23. Romana Hasnain and Michael Garland, *Health Care in Common: Report of the Oregon Health Decisions Community Meetings Process* (Portland: Oregon Health Decisions, 1990). The report is included in the Oregon Health Services Commission, *Prioritization of Health Services*, Appendix F. See also the discussion of this process in Michael J. Garland and Romana Hasnain, "Health Care in Common: Setting Priorities in Oregon", *Hastings Center Report*, 20(September/October 1990):16–18.

24. Personal communication on March 30, 1993, from Paige Sipes-Metzler, Executive Director of the Health Services Commission. See also Commission document dated November 16, 1992 which published the October 1992 revision of the list. The same effect of the community meeting values was carried forward in the latest revision completed by the Commission on March 29, 1993 and sent to the Department of Health and Human Services in April, 1993.

25. Oregon Health Services Commission, *Prioritization of Health Services,* Appendix E.

26. See, Oregon Health Services Commission, *Prioritization of Health Services,* pp. 69–71.

27. Oregon Health Services Commission, *Prioritization of Health Services,* pp. 18–22 and Appendix G. See also Harvey D. Klevitt and others, "Prioritization of Health Care Services: A Progress Report by the Health Services Commission," *Archives of Internal Medicine,* 151 (1991): 912–916. Information on the hand placing process for the March 1993 iteration was provided in a personal communication from Paige Sipes-Metzler, Executive Director of the Health Services Commission on March 30, 1993.

28. For example, maternity care should appear in the 50–74 range; general preventive care of proven effectiveness should appear in the 125–174 range; comfort care should appear in the 150–174 range; family planning services should appear in the 250–274 range; symptomatic treatments for self-limited diseases should appear in the 600–624 range; cosmetic services should appear in the 650–700 range. The numbers in parenthese identify the range in the list where the Commission decided to "hand place" the particular item. The total number of line items on the complete list is 688. See Oregon Health Services Document dated November 16, 1992, which gives the November iteration of the list and explains its process.

29. Starr, Paul and Walter A. Zelman, "Bridge to Compromise: Competition under a Budget." *Health Affairs* 12 (Supplement 1993): 7–23. See also in the same issue, Bergthold, Linda A., "Benefit Design Choices under Managed Competition": 99–109.

30. See, for example, D. Himmelstein and S. Woolhandler, "A National Health Program for the United States: a Physicians' Proposal" *New England Journal of Medicine* 320 (1989): 102–108; E. Roybal, "The 'US Health Act': Comprehensive Reform for a Caring America" *Journal of the American Medical Association* 265 (1991): 2545–2548; and R. Fein, "The Health Security Partnership: A Federal-State Universal Insurance and Cost-Containment Program", *Journal of the American Medical Association* 265 (1991): 2555–2558.

31. See, for example, *A Call for Action: Final Report of the Pepper Commission* (Washington, DC: United States Government Printing Office, 1990); Ronald S. Bronow, Robert A. Beltran, Stephen C. Cohen, and others, "The Physicians Who Care Plan: Preserving Quality and Equitability in American Medicine" *Journal of the American Medical Association* 265 (1991): 2511–2515; *Health Access America: The AMA Proposal to Improve Access to Affordable, Quality Health Care.* (Chicago: American Medical Association, 1990); Donald O. Nutter, Charles M. Helms, Michael E. Whitcomb and W. Donald Weston, "Restructuring Health Care in the United States: a Proposal for the 1990s," *Journal of the American Medical Association* 265 (1991): 2516–2520; Karen Davis, "Expanding Medicare and Employer Plans to Achieve Universal Health Insurance," *Journal of the American Medical Association* 265 (1991): 2525–2528; The Kansas Employer Coalition of Health, Task Force on Long Term Solutions, "A Framework for Reform of the US Health Care Financing and Provision System," *Journal of the American Medical Association* 265 (1991): 2529–2531; Alain C. Enthoven and Richard Kronick, "A Consumer Choice Health Plan for the 1990s," *New England Journal of Medicine* 320 (1989): 29–37, 94–101; John Holahan, Marilyn Moon, W. Pete Welch and Stephen Zuckerman, "An American Approach to Health System Reform," *Journal of the American Medical Association* 265 (1991): 2537–2540; Stuart M. Butler, "A Tax Reform Strategy to Deal with the Uninsured," *Journal of the American Medical Association* 265 (1991): 2541–2544; National Leadership Coalition for Health Care Reform, *Excellent Health Care for All Americans At a Reasonable Cost: A Proposal for Three-Dimensional Health Care Reform* (1991); Rashi Fein, "The Health Security Partnership: A Federal-State Universal Insurance and Cost-Containment Program," *Journal of the American Medical Association* 265 (1991): 2555.

32. Robert J. Blendon and Jennifer N. Edwards, "Caring for the Uninsured: Choices for Reform," *Journal of the American Medical Association* 265 (1991): 2563–2565.

33. Bergthold, "Benefit Design Choices," 101–103.

34. See Paul Starr and Walter A. Zelman, "Bridge to Compromise: Competition under a Budget", 10, 13.

35. President's Commission for the Study of Ethical Problems in Medicine and Biomedical and Behavioral Research, *Securing Access to Health Care: A Report on the Ethical Implications of Differences in the Availability of Health Services*, Volume One: *Report* (Washington: United States Government Printing Office, 1983).

36. *Securing Access*, 22 (emphasis mine).

37. *Securing Access*, 16–17. See in this regard, Norman Daniels, *Just Health Care* (New York: Cambridge University Press, 1985), pp. 81–83. Daniels argues for a narrow rationale, maintaining conditions for equality of opportunity, as the basis for claiming a societal duty to secure access to health care for everyone. The more narrow rationale, Daniels argues, more clearly establishes a basis in justice for the social obligation. Other rationales are less forceful and less likely to sustain a critical perspective on the current structure of the health care system. The Oregon approach of asking the community to help define what they believe makes health care a significant common good is even more broad than the President's Commission four point basis. I believe that is a strength rather than a weakness.

38. *Securing Access*, 37.

39. See Bruce Jennings, "A Grassroots Movement in Bioethics—Community Health Decisions," *Hastings Center Report* 18 (June 1988) 1–15.

40. Material for this project, *Condition Critical: The American Health Care Forum*, is available from the Public Agenda Foundation, Six East 39th Street, Suite 900, New York, NY 10016.

Thomas B. Jabine

Indicators for Monitoring Access to Basic Health Care as a Human Right

As a statistically advanced country,[1] the United States has a wealth of statistical data about the health status of its people, their use of health care services and their health related behaviors (e.g., exercise and smoking habits). These data are used by units of government at all levels and by nongovernmental organizations (NGOs) and individuals to assess and monitor the effectiveness of the American health care system. Health indicators derived from the data are an important part of the process.

Examination of these health indicators has made it quite clear, in recent years, that there are serious defects in the American health care system. Comparisons with other developed countries show that Americans are spending more and getting less. Under any reasonable definition of basic health care services, many people are being left out. One particular indicator, the number or proportion of persons without health insurance coverage has become a symbol, for policy makers and the public, of the shortcomings of our health care system.[2] Wide awareness of the plight of the uninsured may have contributed more than any other factor to the demand for health care reform.

There is no constitutional provision or law which gives every person in the United States the right of access to basic health care services. Constitutions of several other countries in the Americas specify rights to health protection.[3] The International Covenant on Economic, Social and Cultural Rights, to which 122 countries have subscribed, commits those countries to "recognize the right of everyone to the enjoyment of the highest attainable standard of physical and mental health" and to take steps toward the full realization of that right.[4] The United States has not yet ratified the Covenant but may give it serious consideration in the near future. In January 1993, Congressman Pastor of Arizona introduced a draft resolution stating that "it is the sense of the Congress that access to basic health care services is a fundamental human right'' and that legislative proposals for national health care reform should be based on the recognition of that right.[5]

Realizing a right to health care requires developing objective indicators that can be used to track the effectiveness of measures designed to implement that right. Adequate standards cannot be developed by one person, nor can they be developed before substantial agreement has been reached on what should be included in a package of basic health care services. The goal of this paper is to suggest some strategies than can contribute to the process of developing appropriate indicators of the right to health care in the United States. *Underlying all other strategies to be discussed is that of making good use of what already exists.* The work on indicators reflected in the recent Institute of Medicine report on access to health care,[6] is directly relevant. Work on health indicators by other groups, including the World Health Organization,[7] the United States Public Health Service in its Healthy People initiatives[8] and the American Public Health Association in its state-by-state Public Health Report Card[9], can also contribute useful ideas about strategies to follow in the selection of indicators.

The principle of making good use of what already exists also applies to the selection of data sources for the indicators. In a data-rich country, it should be possible to develop a useful set of indicators by relying largely on existing data sources. American health data systems that are presently in operation and some of their advantages and disadvantages for indicators use will be discussed in this paper. Health data systems can and should be improved and modified to reflect changes in the health care system, but the effects of the initial phases of health care reform will have to be tracked largely with indicators based on existing surveys and other data sources.

The next section of this paper looks at the special features of statistical indicators that are used to monitor the attainment of defined human rights, as opposed to those that are used for other purposes like guiding public policy. The following section provides a brief description of three major health indicator systems. Following these introductory sections, the main part of the paper discusses general strategy issues in the selection and use of indicators of access to basic health care as a human right and several considerations in the selection of specific indicators for that purpose.

Statistical Indicators for Human Rights

Regardless of the particular category of human rights to be monitored, three aspects of proposed indicators require special attention:
disaggregation, the measurement of change, and comprehensibility
to non-experts. These features are of particular importance when indicators are used for human rights monitoring rather than for other
purposes, such as policy analysis.

Human rights are meant to be enjoyed equally by all persons.
Article 2 of the Universal Declaration of Human Rights says:

> Everyone is entitled to all the rights and freedoms set forth in
> this Declaration, without distinction of any kind, such as race,
> colour, sex, language, religion, political or other opinion,
> national or social origin, property, birth or other status.[10]

Thus, a single national value of an indicator, such as the infant mortality rate in the United States or the overall proportion of persons
with health insurance, is inadequate. Some level of *disaggregation* is
essential, whether it be by race, gender, income or other defining
characteristics of subgroups of the population. Human rights advocates believe that the most vulnerable sectors of the population, like
migrant workers and their families and disabled and homeless persons, deserve special consideration. Mainline existing health data systems do not readily provide data for some of these groups, but indicators of their status, both in absolute terms and relative to other groups,
are necessary for human rights monitoring.

Most economic and social indicators are used to *measure changes*
in society. Change has special significance in monitoring economic and
social rights because most of these rights, as defined in international
human rights instruments, are not immediately achievable, with existing resources, for all persons in every country. Article 2 of the International Covenant on Economic, Social and Cultural Rights commits
countries to take steps, to the maximum of their available resources,
". . . with a view to achieving progressively the full realization of the
rights recognized in the present Covenant . . . ."[11] No one expects
that universal health care coverage can be achieved in the United
States instantaneously. Indicators of the right to basic health care,
however defined, must be designed to track progress toward the
progressive realization of goals related to that right.

The most effective indicators are *transparent*, that is, they are readily understood by people who are not policy wonks. Transparency is especially important for human rights indicators because so much of the impetus for progress in the realization of human rights comes from the bottom up, through the efforts of NGOs and individuals, rather than from the top down, i.e., from governments and international bodies. A major strategy of human rights advocates is to inform the general public about rights that are not being realized by everyone, thereby generating pressures on governments to take action. Readily understood indicators, such as the proportion of persons without health care insurance, can direct public attention to inequities in the provision of basic needs for all members of society and generate support for change. They may prove to be the single most effective tool of advocates for the right to basic health care services.

Recent Work on Health Indicators

Much can be learned from the recent development and use of health indicators by two United States organizations, even though their sets of indicators were not selected specifically for the purpose of measuring health care as a human right. These indicator systems are described here and their features will be referred to as needed in subsequent sections.

In 1979, the United States Public Health Service launched its Healthy People initiative, setting specific goals for achievement by 1990 in the areas of health promotion, health protection and clinical preventive services. After broad consultations with interested groups, 15 goals and 226 measurable objectives were established. Most of the objectives had measurable targets, for example, to reduce infant mortality to 9 deaths per 1,000 live births by 1990 (note the distinction between the indicator—the infant mortality rate—and the target or objective, which is a specific value of the indicator). Progress toward achieving the objectives was evaluated continuously during the decade and the final results were widely examined at the end of the decade.

For the decade of the 1990s, a similar process was undertaken, with the title *Healthy People 2000*. A new set of 300 objectives was established, with emphasis on ". . . more participation, stronger focus on the needs of special populations, and assurance of data availability to track each objective."[12] The first of these criteria moves at least part way toward the bottom-up approach which is important for the realization of human rights, and the second provides for greater disaggregation of the indicators or objectives, which is critical. The third criterion points to the possible need for some compromises between indicators that would be ideal from a conceptual point of view and those for which data are more readily available. The final evaluation of the 1980s exercise had shown that 23 percent of the objectives ". . . had inadequate data for a valid assessment of progress."[13]

The more than 300 objectives in *Healthy People 2000* were grouped into 22 "priority areas," the last of which was Surveillance and Data Systems. One of the objectives in this area was to "develop and implement common health status indicators for use by federal/state/ local health agencies." A committee formed under the auspices of the United States Public Health Service developed a consensus set of 18 indicators. It also identified 16 topics for which it found that measures did not exist or were incomplete but ". . . could be obtained with minor modifications to existing data systems."[14]

Although the Healthy People initiatives have included some objectives relating to access to health care, mainly for preventive services, their major emphasis has been on health status and outcomes. The National Institute of Medicine (IOM) has recently completed a study that focused much more directly on indicators of access to personal health services.[15] The IOM study committee defined access as "the timely use of personal health services to achieve the best possible health outcomes."[16] The study report proposes an initial set of 15 indicators that can be used to track success in achieving 5 broad objectives: promoting successful birth outcomes; reducing the incidence of vaccine-preventable diseases; early detection and diagnosis of treatable diseases; reducing the effects of chronic disease and prolonging life; and reducing morbidity and pain through timely and appropriate treatment. To monitor progress in achieving each of these objectives, both utilization and outcome indicators have been recommended.

The IOM study paid careful attention to the development of a conceptual framework for monitoring access and to the methodological and data availability aspects of proposed indicators. As part of the study, the proposed indicators were tested by using them to examine changes in access during the 1980s. Where possible, indicators for different population groups were developed, using variables like age, race/ethnicity (mainly restricted to black/white comparisons), income, education and location of residence (e.g., central city, other metropolitan area and outside metropolitan area). Appendices to the report discuss possible access indicators for special population groups: persons with HIV disease, drug abusers, homeless persons, and migrant workers and their families.

In the international sphere, the World Health Organization (WHO) has developed indicators for use in its program of *Health for All by the Year 2000*. Recognizing the disparities among member countries with respect to the structure of their health care systems and the availability of data, WHO does not prescribe a large set of specific indicators. However, it does recommend that every country develop indicators to monitor progress in achieving health for all in each of four categories: health policy, social and economic indicators related to health, provision of health care, and health status. Countries are asked to make periodic evaluations of the strategies they have adopted, based on analysis of the indicators they have selected, and to submit their findings to WHO.

WHO has identified a set of 12 "global indicators" which are used to evaluate the worldwide progress of the Health for All program and for which all countries are urged to provide information. Initially, all of the 12 global indicators were defined in terms of the number of countries that had achieved specified goals. For example, indicator number 10 was the *number of countries* with life expectancy at birth of more than 60 years. However, in 1990 the global indicators were reformulated so that many of them are now more like conventional indicators for individual countries. Indicator number 10 became Life expectancy at birth, by sex, in all identifiable subgroups. Disaggregation was recommended for several of the indicators, including those covering access to primary health care. The dimensions suggested for disaggregation include sex, location of residence (urban/rural), geographical or administrative subdivisions and defined socioeconomic groups.

The WHO global indicators have the broadest substantive scope of the three sets of indicators examined in this section. They cover resource availability (the per capita GNP) and allocation (the percentage of the GNP spent on health), as well as the adult literacy rate. The larger set of indicators, from which countries may select those most suitable to their needs, includes measures of other external factors that can influence progress in achieving health for all, such as population growth and internal migration, working conditions, housing and food availability.

Most of WHO's global indicators have been adopted more or less directly in the General Reporting Guidelines for the periodic reports that are required of countries that have ratified the International Covenant on Economic, Social and Cultural Rights.[17] Where appropriate, these Guidelines call for breakdowns by urban/rural and socioeconomic groups, and they also ask countries to identify geographical areas that ". . . are worse off with regard to the health of their population."[18]

Many other organizations and individuals have proposed and, in some instances published, health indicators for a variety of purposes. The American Public Health Association has issued a *1992 Public Health Report Card*[19] that presents indicators for each state in five categories: medical care access, healthy environment, healthy neighborhoods, healthy behavior and community health service. For each of these categories, averages of the relevant indicators are used to identify states as belonging to one of four quartiles. Stoto[20] cites several other efforts to develop indicators for assessment of public health programs and indicators of health status, some of which may be useful in efforts to develop indicators for access to basic health care as a human right.

Strategic Questions in Selecting Indicators

Check List A contains a series of questions that should be answered as an initial step in planning to develop a set of statistical indicators. In this section the check list will be discussed in the context of constructing indicators for monitoring achievement of the right to basic health care in the United States.

CHECK LIST A: Strategic Questions

(1) Who will be responsible for the selection, compilation, analysis and dissemination of the indicators?
(2) What purposes are the indicators meant to serve?
(3) What should be the general scope of the indicators and what types of indicators are appropriate?
(4) How many indicators are needed or desirable?

(5)   How often should the indicators be compiled and presented?

(6)   What should be the general approach to disaggregation?

(7)   To what extent should the indicator set be modified over time?

(1) Who should select the indicators?   No one has the exclusive right to decide which indicators should be used for a particular subject. This is especially true for indicators of human rights, where a bottom-up approach, involving NGOs, can be most effective in promoting full realization of specified rights. Nevertheless, the selection, compilation and analysis of a useful set of indicators will unquestionably benefit from participation by subject matter experts and by statisticians who are familiar with the major sources of health data, the desirable properties of statistical indicators and the most effective ways of presenting them to policymakers and the general public. A set of indicators of the right of access to basic health care, developed by a team with the necessary skills and knowledge, could serve the needs of many NGOs and acquire widespread public acceptance.

Looking at the first of the three indicator systems discussed in the preceding section, the Healthy People initiatives were undertaken by a federal agency, with widespread inputs from other public and private sector organizations. The agency in question, the United States Public Health Service, was able to draw on substantial health policy and statistical expertise within its component units. For the 1990s round a consortium, with participation from the Institute of Medicine and various organizations and professionals across the country, was formed to establish the objectives for the year 2000.[21] As noted earlier, a committee representing several public health organizations developed a consensus set of 18 health status indicators ". . . to assist communities in assessing their general health status and in focusing local, state, and national efforts in tracking the year 2000 objectives."[22]

The IOM Study on Access to Health Care in America, unlike many activities of that body, was self-initiated. The members of the committee that undertook the study, aided by a small staff, were selected from several disciplines relevant to the project goals. The proposed indicators resulting from the study are available and intended for use by anyone. The report includes a recommendation that federal, state and local governments all take an active role in monitoring access to personal health care services and suggests ways in which state and local governments can modify the indicators to suit their own special needs and data availability. The report also suggests that private foundations can play an important role in stimulating government action and funding research and demonstration activities.[23] The Robert Wood Johnson Foundation has already funded some follow-up activities.

The global indicators developed by the WHO and adopted for use by its member countries are an integral part of the Health for All by the Year 2000 program. The indicators were defined and subsequently revised with extensive participation from member countries, regional committees, the Executive Board, the World Health Assembly and WHO staff. As noted above, most of these indicators have been adopted by a United Nations human rights treaty-monitoring body, the Committee on Economic, Social and Cultural Rights.

(2) What purposes? In planning and designing a statistical survey, the most essential and often the most difficult step is to formulate a clear statement of purpose. How and by whom will the survey data be used? Good answers to these questions are a prerequisite to the determination of specific survey content. Without such a focus, the content may turn out to be largely irrelevant. The same considerations apply to the selection of a set of statistical indicators.

The IOM Study provides a good model of how to approach the process. As noted earlier, the committee defined what it meant by access to personal health care services and developed a conceptual framework relating access to outcomes. American health care policymakers at all levels of government were identified as the primary audience for the indicators. The indicator data would allow them to monitor access to services over time and guide their choices with respect to access, quality and cost of health care services. The data would inform them of the status of access to services by vulnerable population groups. In a broader arena, ". . . the expectation of routinely available reports would stimulate national debate about needed policy actions and the consequences of actions taken."[24]

What might be different about the users and uses of indicators of access to health care as a human right? Hopefully, policymakers in all branches and levels of government would still be an important user group, but one would expect greater interest by NGOs with interests in health care issues or in the rights of particular population groups. Indicators revealing the status of vulnerable groups would take on additional importance. Depending on how the right of access might be formally defined in statutes or other legal instruments, the indicators could become relevant to legal actions by individuals or groups that believe they have been denied their rights. Such uses would inevitably lead to greater scrutiny of the conceptual bases for the indicators and the quality of the source data.

One possible use of indicators is to establish goals and track progress toward their achievement, as has been done in the Healthy People initiatives. If measurable goals are set for a variety of health care indicators, advocates and policymakers can then focus their attention on those components of the health care system falling short of goals. Another use is to permit comparison of achievements with those of other countries. One frequently sees current levels of infant and child mortality in the United States and other indicators of maternal and child health compared unfavorably with those of other countries.[25]

(3) Scope and types of indicators.   Suppose that a right of access to basic health care services has been established and that, by some appropriate process, a "package" defining these services has been agreed on. What is the universe of potential indicators from which a selection should be made?

A highly focused set of indicators might be limited in scope to indicators of actual utilization and barriers to utilization. Utilization indicators might show, for appropriate groups of the population, the proportion of persons requiring selected services who have actually used those services. Possible barriers to utilization might be monitored by presenting the utilization indicators for population subgroups defined by characteristics such as insurance status, income, education, sex, race/ethnic category and location of residence (e.g., state and whether or not in underserved areas).

Further reflection and a review of the IOM Study, however, might suggest the inclusion of some outcome indicators that provide direct or indirect information about the effectiveness of basic health care services. As stated in the IOM Study:

> Carefully selected outcome indicators, based on such measures as death rates, disease incidence, and conditions that require hospitalization, indirectly provide clues about access barriers that may be impeding appropriate care.[26]

The definition of the basic package of health care services is not likely to remain constant, nor should it. Continuous assessment and adjustment of its content will be necessary in order to maximize equitable and effective allocation of resources, to keep up with advances in medical knowledge and technology and to take account of changes in the structure of the health care system. Outcome indicators can guide the assessment and adjustment of the basic package.

The possible relevance of other broad categories of health indicators, such as those covering behavior related to health (e.g., exercise, diet, use of alcohol and tobacco, use of seat belts) and health knowledge and attitudes, should also be considered. Allocation of resources to measures designed to improve knowledge and reduce risky behavior may, in some instances, reduce the future cost of providing health care services that are part of the basic package.

(4) How many indicators? Considering the limited attention that policymakers, the media and the public can give to any particular issue, even one as important as the right to basic health care services, it would probably be wise to identify a small set of indicators that non-specialists can easily track on a regular basis. The WHO suggests that ". . . it is particularly important to select a small number of national indicators that have social and political punch in the sense that people and policy makers will be incited to action by them."[27] As noted previously, a special "consensus set" of 18 health status indicators was developed for widespread use in connection with the Healthy People 2000 initiative. Stoto and Durch, in a review of the Healthy People 2000 objectives, pointed to the need for a short list of "sentinel objectives."[28] In a subsequent article Stoto proposed a set of 23 health status indicators, organized by 5 age groups.[29] Although not precluding future additions to its list, the IOM Study committee selected only a total of 15 indicators.

The use of a short list or core of indicators does not preclude the identification of a much longer list for use by health policy analysts and researchers. In fact, it would be desirable to start with a long list of candidates as the basis for the selection of a short list. The short list can be regarded as a representative sample (not a random or probability sample) from the longer list, selected to provide a coherent view of the major issues related to basic health care as a human right. Since health care requirements vary considerably by sex and age, it makes good sense to be sure, as did both Stoto and the IOM Study, that all groups are covered. Starting with a longer list, it is also possible to consider the desirable properties of indicators, such as relevance, data availability and transparency, in making the selection of a core set.

Even with a short list, it may develop that one or two indicators stand out among the rest and capture the public imagination as bellwether indicators. The number or proportion of uninsured persons certainly falls in this category, although if health care reform succeeds in meeting one of its major goals, this particular indicator will become obsolete.

(5) How often should the indicators be published? Several considerations weigh on decisions about how often indicators should be published. There can be no hard and fast rule about what is best. Rights advocates will want to keep the issues in the public eye and therefore may want to publish some indicators at least annually. Data availability is a major determining factor. Indicators derived from the National Center for Health Statistics (NCHS) National Health Interview Survey could be published annually or even quarterly, with some time lag following the end of the reference period. Indicators based on the American vital statistics system could be published annually. Indicators based on other national surveys, like the National Health Examination and Nutrition Surveys[30] and the series of National Medical Expenditure Surveys conducted during the two past decades would not be available on an annual basis.

Some health indicators are subject to considerable change over time, while others are more stable. For some of the indicators selected by the IOM Study Committee, there were fairly dramatic changes from one year to the next. For example, the incidence of congenital syphilis increased significantly during the latter half of the 1980s and the rate for 1990 was about 3 times that of the preceding year. The incidence of measles (rubella) increased dramatically between 1988 and 1989. Other indicators, like the percentage of low-birthweight infants changed only moderately during the 1970s and hardly at all in the 1980s. The percentage of women receiving early prenatal care showed a similar pattern.[31] Thus, in an ongoing program to compile and disseminate indicators, some expert judgment will be needed to decide which ones to present annually and which to present less frequently. One should also be aware that observed patterns in the counts of reportable diseases sometimes reflect changes in reporting practices rather actual changes.

Closely related to frequency is the question of timeliness. Anyone who looks carefully at the dates and source notes in periodic indicator publications will find that the reference dates or periods are seldom the same for all of the indicators presented. This variation is due partly to the fact that some kinds of source data are not collected annually and partly to the time required to process data from national surveys and other key data sources. Gaps and delays in data availability are a fact of life. Organizations that compile and disseminate indicators, unless they have unusually large resources to devote to direct data collection and processing, will have to adapt their publication formats and timing to the schedules of the organizations that produce the data.

What can be learned from other major health indicators programs? The WHO regards monitoring and evaluation at the national level as a continuing activity which, in most instances, will be undertaken at least annually. The reporting of monitoring data to the WHO by the member states is periodic and there have been four global evaluation exercises since the Common Framework and Format for collecting and analyzing relevant information was developed in 1982.

In the United States, the original Healthy People initiative included essentially continuous review at the federal level, a formal mid-course review and publication of a Prevention Profile every three years during the decade. Results for the decade were compiled by the National Center for Health Statistics and published in a Prevention Profile and in *Health, United States, 1991.*[32] Tracking data for the Healthy People 2000 objectives will be published annually in *Health, United States.* As part of these programs, most states have developed and begun tracking objectives that were modelled after the national ones but tailored to their own needs and resources. The report of the IOM Study was released in March 1993 and the author has been informed that the Robert Wood Johnson Foundation, which has had a continuing interest in access to health care, plans to present at least some of the indicators each year in its annual report.

(6) Disaggregation of indicators. As has already been emphasized, a human rights perspective on health care access requires that indicators be presented and monitored separately for subgroups of the total population. For some defining characteristics, this is easy to do. Many

data sources for indicators provide separate data by age and sex and for the five standard race/ethnic groups as defined by the Office of Management and Budget.[33] At the other extreme, source data for indicators of health access by homeless persons are practically nonexistent. There are three main sources of limitations on the ability to disaggregate indicators: limited sample sizes, failure to identify the subgroup separately in the source data system and failure to cover the subgroup in the data system. The IOM Study report does an excellent job of describing the effects of these limitations on the utility of major American health data sources for access indicators.[34] The following summary draws from that report.

Sample size, of course, only comes into play when the source data come from a sample survey or other type of data system based on sample data. Mortality data are based on all death certificates, so the level of detail to which they can be tabulated is limited only by the classification variables included on the certificates. The National Health Interview Survey, a major annual source of health indicator data, is typically based on a sample of about 50,000 households with over 100,000 persons. Since 1985, the black population has been over-sampled to ensure better reliability of estimates for that subgroup.[35] In spite of the large overall sample sizes, there are limits to the levels of disaggregation that it can support, especially if the subgroups are defined by multiple characteristics, including geographic location.

Sample size limitations depend both on the number of subgroups and their distribution by population size. If all households or persons are sampled at the same rate, estimates for smaller racial groups, like the category American Indians, Eskimos and Aleuts, will have substantially larger sampling errors. One option is to use a design that oversamples households or persons in these categories. Another method of "buying" additional sample size is to aggregate data over more than one year, trading off the ability to monitor annual changes against more reliable estimates over a longer period.

Birth and death certificates, which are an important source of data (with no sampling errors) for both utilization and outcome indicators, do not include all of the data items that might be desired for purposes of disaggregation. There are no direct measures of income or health insurance status. Death certificates do not identify persons who were homeless before they died. To some extent, such problems might be overcome by linking birth and death certificates with other data sets containing the desired information or, as the National Center for Health Statistics has done, by conducting followup surveys, using birth and death certificates as a sampling frame. However, such solutions reintroduce the problem of sampling error, as well as other difficulties associated with costs and with legal and policy barriers to record linkage studies.

Some of the most vulnerable groups, like homeless or institutionalized persons, are not covered in the National Health Interview Survey and most other major national health surveys. Migrant workers and their families are not excluded by definition from such surveys, but their migrant status is generally not identified and because of their mobility they may be missed in surveys more often than members of other population groups. Some data on access to health care by these groups can be obtained from clinics and other facilities that serve them, but these would be primarily numerator data and would not by themselves support calculation of rates that could be used for comparisons with other population groups. An appendix to the IOM Study report suggests several ways in which more adequate indicator data could be obtained for migrants and the homeless.[36]

Disaggregation of data for race/ethnic groups presents special problems. The Office of Management and Budget's Directive No. 15 requires that all federal agencies sponsoring surveys or maintaining program records that classify persons by race and ethnicity collect information that will permit classification into a minimum of five prescribed categories. With minor exceptions, all reported deaths can be classified into the same categories and births can be similarly classified on the basis of the parents' race/ethnic status. Consequently, any indicators based on these sources (including the Census of Population, which is used to provide denominators for some indicators) can be presented separately for these five groups, subject only to sample size limitations.

However, this level of disaggregation may not be adequate for tracking differences by race and ethnicity in access to basic health care. There may be wide variations within, for example, the group of persons classified as Asian and Pacific Islanders, depending on specific countries of origin. Many of the data sources mentioned do provide more race/ethnic detail for persons not classified as black or white, but the specific classifications used vary from one source to another. Thus, it may not be possible to use the same classifications for all indicators.

In the face of these data limitations, what strategies for disaggregation should be followed in the construction of a set of indicators for access to basic health care services as a human right? An obvious conclusion is that not every indicator can be presented for the same set of subgroups: what is possible will depend on the source of the indicator data. Sampling error should not be ignored. Even if sample data are available for a particular group, indicators for that group should not be presented if the sample sizes are insufficient for meaningful comparisons with other groups or for tracking moderate changes over time.

In the short run, the choice of indicators for vulnerable and other subgroups of the population will be limited by the coverage, content and other characteristics of existing data sources. In the longer term, gaps can be filled to some extent by adding to the content and coverage of existing data systems and, with more difficulty and delay, by creating new ones. A few NGOs may be able to fill some of the gaps by mounting their own data collection efforts, but for most, the more effective strategy would probably be to point to the gaps in the indicators and advocate appropriate modification and expansion of existing federal, state and local data systems.

(7) Changes in the set of indicators. A major use of human rights indicators is to track the progressive realization of rights over time, for the population as a whole and for different subgroups. For this purpose, it is necessary that at least some of the indicators be retained for long periods and that changes in definition and methods of compilation be kept to a minimum. But the health care system in the United States is in flux and some of the key indicators of the past are losing much of their relevance. The health insurance status indicator is of major interest now and will continue to be as health care reform proceeds, but if the goal of universal coverage is met, that particular indicator would need to be replaced by some measure of the adequacy of coverage.

There may also be important changes in the availability of source data for utilization indicators. At present, the complex structure of health care financing arrangements involving government programs (primarily Medicare and Medicaid) and numerous private insurers has made it difficult to use program records of health care encounters and services as the basis for broad statistical analyses of utilization of health care services by the general population. However, serious efforts are underway to promote standardization and computerization of health care records[37] and are likely to be accelerated as the expected reforms occur. From a human rights perspective, it is important both that the confidentiality of such health records be protected and that their potential value as a new data source for indicators of access to health care be realized.

Experience with changes in two of the three major health indicator systems that were described at the start of this paper is instructive. The WHO's 12 global indicators were revised about 10 years after their initial issuance. The purpose of the revision was ". . . to improve, where possible, the relevance, sensitivity and specificity of the indicators and the feasibility of obtaining the information required for them."[38] Most of the indicators which had initially been formulated in terms of the number of countries achieving certain target values, such as life expectancy over 60 years, were changed to present values of the same variables for each country. This new approach greatly increased the amount of information in the system, making it possible, among other things, for countries to compare their own achievements with those of other countries. A few new items were added, such as maternal and child mortality rates, but the revision was primarily in the whole approach to the compilation and presentation of indicators.

As noted earlier, the goals for the second decade of the United States Healthy People initiative were different from those selected for the first decade. The number of objectives increased from 226 to 300, and they were selected with ". . . stronger focus on the needs of special populations, and assurance of data availability to track each objective."[39] The indicators recommended in the IOM Study report are too new to have undergone revision, but the report includes a chapter on "Future Indicators" which lists nine topics that the study committee considered worthy of coverage by the access indicator system. They were not included in the initial set of fifteen indicators because ". . . the state of the art of measuring them as an access problem is underdeveloped or because it is unclear whether routine data related to them will be available to track utilization or outcomes."[40]

The lesson to be drawn from these experiences is clear. For a new indicator system to have maximum value, there should be a plan for systematic reviews of its content, concepts and methodology. Efforts should be made to fill significant gaps and to take advantage of new data sources. Analysis of changes in existing indicators may suggest the need for new ones. For access to basic health care services as a human right, the basic package of services is likely to be modified periodically, perhaps in response to analysis of the indicators. Ideally, there should be a strong interaction between the basic health care system and the indicator system used to track its effectiveness.

The Selection Process

The purpose of this section is to outline a specific process that any organization might follow in selecting a set of statistical indicators for the right of access to basic health care services. Check List B lists the seven steps in the process.

CHECK LIST B: *Steps in Selecting Indicators*

(1) Decide on general strategies.
(2) Develop a candidate list of indicators.
(3) Divide (stratify) the candidate list into major categories.
(4) Decide on the number of indicators to be selected and their allocation among the major categories.
(5) Evaluate the relevant properties of each candidate indicator, including availability, quality and transparency.
(6) Make the final selection.
(7) Make provisions for periodic review and modification.

(1) Decide on general strategies.   Before developing a candidate list of indicators, tentative decisions must be reached on general strategies, as discussed at length in the preceding section. To determine which of the available indicators can reasonably be considered, one needs to know the purpose and scope of the proposed indicators, the frequency with which the indicators will be compiled and presented, and the specific subgroups of the total population for which indicators are needed.

(2) Develop a list of candidate indicators.   This and the following steps in selecting a set of indicators are in some ways analogous to the procedures that are followed in selecting a sample for a survey. This step is equivalent to the development of a sampling frame, a list of units in the target population from which the sample is to be

selected. It is not necessary—indeed it would be impossible—to identify all possible indicators. Instead, we need a list of indicators that are relevant to monitoring access to basic health care services by all persons.

One might begin by ignoring previous work entirely and listing a large number of possible indicators of access to those services included in the basic health care package. Having done this, one could then compare the result with other lists of indicators and take account of the availability of source data. A reverse approach would be to start with all of the indicators identified by the WHO, the Healthy People 1990 and 2000 programs, the IOM study and other organizations and identify those believed to have some relevance to monitoring access to health care in the United States as a human right. The resulting list would then be reviewed for gaps and additional candidate indicators would be proposed to fill the gaps. Probably some combination of the two approaches would be best. Although one would expect many of the final list of candidate indicators to be used in other contexts, the de novo approach may identify critical measures that have been overlooked.

The process of developing a list of candidate indicators will be aided by a knowledge of existing sources of health data. There is a wealth of material that describes such sources with information on their respective strengths and weaknesses. A useful discussion at the international level is provided by the WHO,[41] which identifies six primary sources: vital events registers, population and housing censuses, routine health service records, epidemiological surveillance data, sample surveys and disease registers.

For the United States, the IOM Study, with its relatively narrow focus on access to personal health services, identifies five major sources: vital statistics, surveys, hospital discharge data, notifiable diseases and disease registries. For each of the sources used for one or more of its fifteen indicators, it describes limitations related to coverage, frequency, timeliness and quality of the data. In several instances enhancements and improvements of the data sources are recommended. Publications associated with the Healthy People program provide substantial information on United States health data sources. Appendix I to *Health United States 1991* describes fifty sources of health data and lists publications and other sources of additional information for each one.

What information should be listed for each candidate indicator? At a minimum, one would want to have a reasonably precise definition of the indicator and information about source data availability and quality and about the kinds of disaggregation that would be feasible with available data. It might also be useful to classify indicators by type, perhaps using the IOM split between utilization and outcome indicators, or by broad categories of basic health care services.

(3) Divide the list into major categories.   The purpose of this step (which is equivalent to stratification in selecting a sample) is to select a final set of indicators that is representative in that all major topics and population subgroups of importance are covered. Audrey Chapman has suggested that the basic standard of care might cover seven components: preventive care, primary care, acute care, long-term care, mental health services, health-related social services and ancillary services, such as medical equipment and prescriptions.[42] This classification might be a good basis for grouping indicators relating to use of health care services. Following the access model used in the IOM study, separate categories could be established for indicators of structural, financial and personal barriers to health care and health status outcomes, such as mortality, morbidity, well-being and functioning.

The total number of categories should not exceed the total number of indicators to be selected for the final set. If inclusiveness along other dimensions, such as age and gender, is a goal, then the number of major categories should probably be smaller, even though it would not be absolutely necessary to have an indicator that could be disaggregated by gender or age group in every major category.

(4) Decide on the number of indicators and their allocation among categories.   The number of indicators to be selected will depend largely on who will be using them and for what purposes. It will also be a function of the interests of and the resources available to the organization that will compile and disseminate them. A hierarchic approach might be desirable if the indicators are to be used both for advocacy (suggesting a small number) and to guide analytical research (suggesting a larger number). The larger set could be selected first and a subset of these selected for use as sentinel or core indicators. Whatever number is decided on (no specific targets are suggested here), it would seem reasonable to spread them fairly evenly across the major groups established in the previous step.

(5) *Evaluate each candidate indicator.* A systematic procedure for assigning ratings to each of the candidate indicators is highly recommended as a preliminary to the final selection of one or more sets. A list of rating factors might include (a) the availability of source data including frequency, timeliness, and cost; (b) conceptual suitability including relevance to the right of access, sensitivity to changes in what is being monitored, and specificity or resistance to the influence of extraneous factors; (c) potential for disaggregation; (d) quality including sampling error, coverage error, and other nonsampling errors; and (e) transparency.

For rating each indicator on these factors, one might use a five-point scale with ratings from zero to four, with four being the highest (most suitable) rating on each factor and with a rating of zero indicating that the indicator is disqualified on the basis of that factor. To assure the reliability of the rating process, ratings could be assigned independently by two or more persons with appropriate qualifications. For categories (2) and (5) above, persons who are experts on health policy and health economics might be best qualified. For the remaining categories, one might look for raters who are knowledgeable about health statistics. All of these five factors have been discussed earlier, so they will be discussed only briefly here:

(a) *Availability.* Potential indicators for which no source data are currently available or in prospect can be given a rating of 0 and placed on a separate list. Indicators on that list could be examined to determine whether they are of sufficient importance to advocate or recommend the development of new data sources. For a proposed indicator to receive a top rating on availability, it should be possible to present annual values of the indicator and the data should be available fairly soon after the year to which they refer. Some data sources, such as the vital statistics system, provide provisional or preliminary estimates, followed later by definitive data. "Cost" refers to the costs of actually acquiring the data from the sources and of any processing operations that might be necessary to compile specific indicators from the source data.

(b) *Conceptual suitability.* Each indicator must be *relevant* in some way to the right of access. This does not mean that each one must be a direct measure of access, however that may be defined. It can be an outcome measure, such as mortality or morbidity rates that are likely to be influenced by access or an indicator of barriers to health care, such as health insurance coverage or physical access to basic health care facilities. *Sensitivity*, which would apply primarily to indirect indicators, means that the indicator is likely to be affected by changes in what is being monitored, in this instance, access to basic health care services. *Specificity* means that the indicator is not likely to be strongly influenced by factors that are extraneous to what is being monitored. One example of an indicator lacking specificity might be the total amount spent on basic health care services, which could be influenced by inflation and by changes in the size and age structure of the population and advances in medical technology. Of course it would be possible to adjust for some of these effects.[43]

(c) *Potential for disaggregation.* This issue has been discussed in previous sections. A high rating should be given to indicators which can be used for vulnerable and difficult to measure populations, such as homeless persons and migrant workers and their families. Indicators that would have to be based on sample data would generally receive a lower rating than those, such as mortality rates, based on data for the entire population. Data collected by states, especially vital statistics, do not always provide uniform treatment of racial and ethnic population groups.

(d) *Quality.* Indicators based on small samples will be subject to large sampling errors, which can obscure the size and even the direction of changes over time. Coverage error refers to failure of the data sources to cover the entire population of interest, either by design or for other reasons. Some amount of undercoverage may be tolerated if the other properties of an indicator are good. For example, as of 1988, information on births of Hispanic parentage were available only for 30 states and the District of Columbia; however, about 95 percent of the total Hispanic population of the United States lived in these states.[44] Some data sources may be affected significantly by other kinds of nonsampling or measurement errors. Measures of acute and chronic conditions, which might be useful as indicators of the need for health care, are frequently underreported or misidentified in household sample surveys; indeed, people often are not aware of some conditions until they obtain care. Primary causes of death are not always reported correctly on death certificates. For each candidate indicator, one should review any information available, from publications of statistical agencies, about the limitations of the source data.

(e) *Transparency.* Some indicators, like those relating to mortality, preschool immunization and health insurance coverage, are relatively easy for the general public to understand. Poor performance, either in an absolute sense or in comparison with other countries that have comparable resources, is likely to be a matter for public concern. Indicators that have these qualities should receive a high rating and may be considered for inclusion in a small set of sentinel indicators.

(6) Make the final selection. A first approximation to the final selection might be achieved by ranking candidate indicators in each major group according their overall ratings (a sum, weighted or unweighted, of their ratings on each of the five rating factors) and selecting the required number from the top of the list. However, the chances are that the resulting list would show a lack of balance or diversity with respect to subtopics within each major group and across groups. The initial list may not provide adequate coverage of vulnerable subgroups of the population or it may fail to include a sufficient number of indicators that have suitable properties for inclusion in a core group of sentinel indicators. At this stage, the list will have to be revised by making trade-offs among the multiple goals of the selection process.

Making the final selection should be a group effort. Several persons might be asked to make independent selections, all using the same general selection criteria and instructions for the number of indicators to be selected from each major category. Lists would then be compared and reconciled through group discussions.

(7) Make provisions for review and modification. The need for periodic review and modification of the indicator set was discussed under item (7) in the section on "General strategies." Additions and deletions will be needed in order to maintain the focus of the indicator set on components of the basic health care package for which access is less widespread and on access by the most vulnerable and underserved groups of the population. For each of the indicators, those who compile the indicator set each year, or at some other interval, should pay close attention to current documentation of the source data, watching for conceptual or operational changes that may affect the comparability of the indicator values over time, and make necessary adjustments.

Conclusion

Indicators by themselves cannot pinpoint the exact nature and causes of problems in the American health care system, but they can provide valuable clues as to what the main problems are and which groups of the population are most affected. A necessary first step in developing a set of indicators for access to basic health care services as a human right is to define the components of a package of services to which everyone should have access. Once this is done, various organizations may want to use indicators to monitor progress toward the realization of this right. This paper has suggested some specific strategies and steps that could be followed in developing sets of indicators for this purpose.

Major efforts have been devoted to the development of health indicators and goals over the past two decades by the United States Public Health Service and the WHO. More recently, the IOM has completed an excellent study on indicators of access to health care in the United States. The work of these groups provides valuable background on the conceptual issues related to health indicators and the sources of data for constructing them. Their lists of indicators could provide a starting point for the selection of indicator sets for monitoring the right of access to health care.

However, there are some special requirements for indicators of access to health care *as a human right*. The most important of these is that the indicators must measure, directly or indirectly, access by subgroups of the population as defined by gender, age, race/ethnic status, income, location of residence and other characteristics. It is especially important that these subgroups include the population groups that are vulnerable and most likely to be underserved. For indicators based on survey data, this *disaggregation* requirement presents some practical problems related to sample sizes and to the operational difficulties of obtaining any data at all for groups like homeless persons and migrant workers. One goal of developing indicator sets should be to identify the data gaps, so that human rights organizations can advocate appropriate steps to eliminate them.

The health indicators developed by the Public Health Service, WHO and IOM have been intended mainly for use by policy analysts and policymakers to help them monitor the success of current policies and suggest ways in which they might be made more effective. For indicators of access to health care as a human right, however, the main users are likely to be NGOs that follow a bottom-up approach to the realization of the right by all persons. For such organizations, a major activity will be to inform both the public and the policy makers about those areas in which the right is not being fully realized and thereby to generate pressure for change. For this purpose it is important that the indicators be simple and understandable and, as the WHO put it, in refreshingly non-bureaucratic terms, that they have "punch." Meeting these two requirements—disaggregation and transparency—without sacrificing professional standards will be a major challenge.

NOTES

1. Moriguti proposes a classification of countries according to 4 levels of development of their statistical systems: rudimentary, basic, intermediate and advanced. See S. Moriguti, "The Role of Statisticians," *International Statistical Review* 60 (1992), 227–246.

2. There are, of course, many possible ways to define indicators relating to health insurance coverage. An indicator could reflect the number of persons without coverage at a particular time or the number without coverage during all or part of a specified time period. Careful attention should be given to what constitutes coverage; alternatively, indicators might be established for various levels of coverage.

3. Hernan Fuenzalida-Puelma and Susan Scholle Connor, eds., *The Right to Health in the Americas: A Comparative Constitutional Study* (Washington, D.C.: Pan American Health Organization, 1989).

4. International Covenant on Economic, Social and Cultural Rights, in *Human Rights: A Compilation of International Instruments* (New York: United Nations, 1983), p. 3.

5. Concurrent Resolution No. 58, introduced in the 103rd Congress, 1st Session, by Congressman Ed Pastor, Arizona, January 1993.

6. Michael Millman, ed., *Access to Health Care in America* (Washington, D.C.: National Academy Press, 1993).

7. See *The Development of Indicators for Monitoring Progress Towards Health for all by the Year 2000* (Geneva: World Health Organization, 1981) and *Evaluating the Strategies for Health for All by the Year 2000*, WHO/HST/90.1, (Geneva: World Health Organization, 1990).

8. A recent summary of the initiatives for 1990 and 2000 is given by J. Michael McGinnis, Julius B. Richmond, Edward N. Brandt, Jr., Robert E. Windom and James O. Mason, "Health Progress in the United States: Results of the 1990 Objectives for the Nation," *Journal of the American Medical Association* 268 (1992): 2545–2552. See also Michael Stoto, "Public Health Assessment in the 1990s," *Annual Review of Public Health* 13 (1992): 59–78, and National Center for Health Statistics, *Health United States, 1991,*(Hyattsville, MD: U.S. Public Health Service, 1992).

9. *America's Public Health Report Card: A State-by-State Report on the Health of the Public* (Washington D.C.: American Public Health Association, 1992).

10.   Universal Declaration of Human Rights, *Human Rights: A Compilation of International Instruments* (New York: United Nations, 1983).

11.   See "International Covenant."

12.   McGinnis, *et al.*.

13.   *Ibid.*, Table 6.

14.   Centers for Disease Control, U.S. Public Health Service, "Health Objectives for the Nation: Consensus Set of Health Status Indicators for the General Assessment of Community Health Status," *Morbidity and Mortality Weekly Report* 40 (1991): 449–451.

15.   See Millman.

16.   *Ibid.*, p. 4.

17.   Committee on Economic, Social and Cultural Rights, *Report on the Fifth Session*, UN Doc. E/1991/23, Annex IV, "Revised guidelines regarding the form and contents of reports to be submitted by States parties under articles 16 and 17 of the International Covenant on Economic, Social and Cultural Rights," (1991).

18.   *Ibid.*, p. 105.

19.   See American Public Health Report Card.

20.   Stoto, "Public Health Assessment," 60.

21.   McGinnis *et al.*.

22.   Centers for Disease Control, p. 449.

23.   Millman, ed., p. 139.

24.   *Ibid.*, p. 1.

25.   See, for example, *The State of America's Children: 1992* (Washington, D.C.: Children's Defense Fund, 1992).

26.   Millman, ed., p. 37.

27.   World Health Organization, The Development of Indicators, p. 13.

28.   Michael A. Stoto and Jane S. Durch, "Healthy People 2000: National Priorities for Health?" in *Analyses of Healthy People 2000* (Washington, D.C.: Institute of Medicine, 1991).

29.   Michael Stoto, "Public Health Assessment."

30.   Until now, these surveys have been conducted on a three to six year cycle. In the future, it is hoped that a two-year cycle will be possible.

31.   The results cited in this paragraph are from Millman, ed., Tables 3-9, 3-12, 3-7 and 3-3, respectively.

32.   National Center for Health Statistics.

33.   *Race and Ethnic Standards for Federal Statistics and Administrative Reporting*, Statistical Policy Directive No. 15, (Washington: U.S. Office of Management and Budget, 1989).

34.   Millman, ed., pp. 23–29.

35.   National Center for Health Statistics, Appendix I, p. 308.

36.   Millman, ed., Appendix C.

37.   See, for example, Workgroup for Electronic Data Interchange, *Report to Secretary of U.S. Department of Health and Human Services*, July 1992.

38.   World Health Organization, Evaluating the Indicators, p. 3.

39.   McGinnis *et al.*

40.   Millman, ed., p. 130.

41. World Health Organization, The Development of Indicators, pp. 15–17.

42. Audrey Chapman, "Conceptualizing the Right to Health Care: Reflections on a Series of Consultations," presented at the Annual Meeting of the American Association for the Advancement of Science, Boston, February 1993.

43. The definitions of sensitivity and specificity given here may differ from those used in other contexts. They are based on a recent United Nations report, *Social Statistics and Indicators*, Twenty-sixth session of the Statistical Commission, UN Doc. E/CN.3/1991/20, (New York: United Nations Economic and Social Council, 1991).

44. National Center for Health Statistics, Appendix I, p. 306.

Managed Competition and the Future of Health Care in the United States

Daniel Wikler

Privatization and Human Rights in Health Care

Health care has not been officially recognized as a human right in the United States, which alone among the major industrialized nations has had no comprehensive system of health care delivery and insurance. Moreover, the vast majority of Americans other than present and past soldiers have obtained their health care from private hospitals, clinics, and physicians. In the strict sense of the term, therefore, the American health care system has not been "privatized," since it has been private from its beginnings.

Nevertheless, something akin to privatization indeed occurred in the United States since the beginning of the past decade. Since other nations seem to be interested in adopting some of the American model for their own health care systems, the implications of such reforms for human rights should be taken into account. The present paper relates both scholarly and informal observations of the American "privatization" strategy in health care in light of the conception of health care as a human right, closing with a note on current attempts to reconcile human rights to health care with privatization in current proposals in health care reform.[1]

Health Care as a Human Right

A growing philosophical literature in the United States examines the issue of whether health care is a human right.[2] American bioethicists have led the way in this work perhaps because the status of health care is an open question only in the United States. Citizens of the other wealthy states believe that health care is their birthright. Indeed, until the Reagan era a consensus existed even in the United States supporting the right to health care as a moral ideal, even if not yet a legal one. In the wake of the rightist trend in American politics, heralded in philosophy by the publication of Robert Nozick's libertar-

263

ian work,[3] writers on health care topics for the first time focused on the property rights of investors and liberties of physicians as fundamental, even if entitlements to care on the part of the sick were ruled out as a result.[4] In this social vision, the just society need not attempt to determine the health needs of the population, nor does it organize health services in the manner most propitious for meeting these needs. Instead, the just society simply guarantees rights of property and liberty and permits individuals to make the best deals they can.

This libertarian outlook, however, remained a marginal view in health policy. In mainstream academic writing, in government documents, and in the public statements of officials, the ultimate criterion for success in health care delivery continues to be whether the system meets the public's health care needs. Interests of investors and providers, while politically and administratively impossible to ignore, have been viewed as morally secondary. It was not clear, however, that this humane philosophy could coexist indefinitely with an increasingly harsh reality. The spirit of privatization imposed changes that threatened to undermine the nation's basic commitment to its morally ideal of health care. Those nations which are looking to the American experience of the last decade as a model for health care financing must be alerted to the possibility that the organizational initiatives carry a moral and philosophical virus, the effect of which will not become apparent until after the model has been adopted.

"Privatization" in the American Health Care Context

Before the late 1960's, government involvement in health care, aside from the military, was small. This era ended with the passage of Medicare and Medicaid, government health insurance for the elderly and the poor, respectively. These steps in the direction of national health insurance, however, were partly responsible for a rocketing medical inflation rate which has never abated. An era of regulation, intended to curb over-building and other inflationary excesses, soon followed, only to be defeated politically by the providers. As conservative, Republican rule came to Washington in the early 1980's, the search for cost controls led to a reemphasis on the market in health care delivery.

Despite the important differences noted above, American public and private initiatives in the era of competition have enough in common with classical privatization, understood as transferring public functions to private hands, to warrant the use of the term. It is true that few publicly-owned hospitals went private; and government health care expenditures increased rather than decreased during this period. What has been privatized is not so much the actual delivery of care but the mission of care for the deliverers. For the first time, investor-owned hospital chains became an important player in American health care, fueled by capital in search of margins rather than by communities seeking health care or charitable and religious orders in pursuit of good works.[5] In response to the market challenges of these for-profit institutions, and more generally in competition with each other, the long-dominant nonprofit hospitals abandoned community planning for institutional strategy. Before long, they ceased to apologize for raiding their competitors market base, signing exclusive contracts with referring physicians, paying bounties for patients, and exhibiting other market behavior once considered unseemly. Some public hospitals, including even some military ones (serving veterans), began to recruit well-insured patients to fill beds denied to uninsured patients in their traditional constituencies.

The "private", or institutional, mission of each of these organizations was, of course, to prosper through selling services (fee-for-service providers), insurance (health insurance companies), or both (Health Maintenance Organizations and other hybrids). The optimistic expectation was that these units would have to offer greater customer satisfaction, lower prices, and more efficient operation to attract the patients needed for revenue and the capital needed for expansion and modernization. Thus, the best would be rewarded, care would improve, costs would moderate, and the need for regulation—a blunt instrument at best—would be minimized. Competition did not work. It utterly failed to restrain prices; physicians' morale lowered; access deteriorated; and one important element in patient satisfaction, the ability to choose one's physician, was threatened with extinction. Americans voiced greater dissatisfaction with their health care system than did the citizens of any comparable country.

The reasons for the failure of the competition/privatization strategy to accomplish its primary mission of cost control are complex and need not concern us here. The source of the threat to health care as a human right comes from the central mechanism of the strategy itself. In what follows, I briefly survey some of the symptoms of this destructive tendency, proceeding afterward to some philosophical conclusions.

Privatization as National Health Care Policy

Once individual health care providers are released from their community mission and encouraged to pursue private ends, some will find their welfare enhanced by improving services, lowering prices, and becoming more efficient, as the theory promises. Some of these gains may be ephemeral. Some clinics have allocated revenues to hiring "smile" consultants from the airline industry to teach flight attendant's manners to gruff surgeons, but even this source of patient satisfaction counts as an improvement in service.

It took no time at all, however, for providers to learn that a quicker, surer road to profit detoured entirely around how health care was delivered; the real money lay in careful selection of patients. Insurers did well by identifying patients likely to need care, especially expensive care, and barring them from risk pools (and employers and other payers achieved lower insurance costs by refusing to hire these people). Clinics and physicians who were not in the insurance business, on the other hand, found it important to identify those who had insurance. The hybrid insurer-provider organizations (prepaid health plans) had to manage both winnowing tasks, a feat made more difficult when the interests of the constituent parties (doctors versus investors) were in tension.

Which patients represented the "cream," then depended on one's position in the health care game, but throughout, the profit-maximizing strategy was the same: skim off the cream (before your competitors did), dump the rest (onto your competitors if possible, to reduce their ability to compete; or onto the street, if no one else would take them).

To be sure, the health care system before competition and privatization was by no means perfect. The United States lagged behind comparable countries in its reluctance to erect a substantial social safety net. Still, the health care system had been an island of relative security. Though access to care was far from assured, a tradition of cross-subsidization had permitted providers to offer some care to the uninsured at the expense of the better-off. During the privatization era, this tradition faded. A hospital which provided charity care funded by its general revenues had to charge higher prices, or suffer a narrower margin, than competitors who turned these patients away; this drove away the very patients who were funding the charity care and dissuaded bankers from loaning the money for the modernization needed to lure the wealthier patients back.

Just as American's heart toward the poorest was hardening in other sectors, with middle-class urbanites literally stepping over the bodies of homeless families living on city sidewalks, so too reports of heartlessness began to appear and then become routine. In one celebrated instance, a man was refused care in a St. Louis emergency room for want of insurance even though he had a knife in his back up to the handle, and religious hospitals in Texas turned away rural women minutes away from childbirth. This "economic patient dumping"[6] has become pandemic, doubling annually in many cities.[7] On one estimate, a million patients are denied care for economic reasons annually,[8] and up to a quarter million in need of emergency care are transferred each year for economic reasons.[9]

These practices have made the "wallet biopsy" (pre-admission financial screening) as familiar a part of health care as the doctor's stethoscope. Ironically, the same competitive health policy which motivates this behavior also creates needless duplication of services, as each clinic and hospital strives to offer the most and the best to attract the cream of patients. The hospitals turning away patients are often half-empty.

Refusing care to emergency patients presenting themselves at the hospital door is offensive to the community, and statutes have been enacted in many states to prevent it. In 1986, the United States Congress enacted the Emergency Medical Treatment and Active Labor Act, which forbad these practices throughout the country. Compliance has been questionable. Only 150 violations were found by government investigators in the first four years after the legislation; based on the best estimates, a million instances of patient "dumping" would have occurred during this time, at least before the legislation went into effect. Only nineteen hospitals were penalized.[10]

However well-intended these laws may be, they treat a symptom rather than the underlying source of distress. Even if hospitals and other providers complied with the letter of the law, the institutional self-preservation and self-enhancement mission now deemed suitable in health care dictates a host of practices which deny care just as effectively but far less visibly. In skimming as in medical care itself, an ounce of prevention is worth many pounds of cure; the trick is to ensure that the wrong patients never come to the door in first place.

Hospitals can change their patient mix and compete more effectively even before they physically exist. For-profit hospital chains often choose a site which is located near affluent neighborhoods, as one might expect. But since the poor in American tend to congregate in the center of cities, the profit-maximizing hospital will be located on the outer edge of these neighborhoods. This decision both makes them inaccessible to the urban poor and draws the well-insured patients away from inner-city hospitals which had cross-subsidized in the past, reducing their ability to modernize and thus driving still more of the richer patients to the new suburban facility. The ultimate financial woes, or even bankruptcy, of the older hospital do not show up on the new hospital's balance sheet.

A managed-care plan can offer services which appeal to healthy young families, such as excellent obstetrical care, including champagne breakfasts following childbirth, and sports medicine clinics which advise enrollees on choosing running shoes; and it can permit its reputation in chronic care and mental health to sag. Through information obtained from market research consultants, it can send information about its offerings only to the most desirable individuals and families. Other patients may find it difficult to get information about the plan, or to enroll. In these ways the plan draws enrollees who are less likely to get sick, or to have long, expensive illnesses, and visits these uneconomic patients on competitors who do try to provide first-rate care for these patients. The latter, once again, take a financial beating, and must offer less to the desirable patients, who abandon them in ever greater numbers.

Hospitals can also prosper by carefully choosing the doctors to whom admitting privileges will be granted. For example, an applicant's patient list can be given an instantaneous analysis by computer to determine whether a large number of patients live in postal code areas marked by poverty and lack of insurance. These doctors can be (and have been) denied privileges. One hospital found their wards swamped with illegal aliens who had no money or insurance; by spreading the word that the hospital was cooperating with immigration authorities to permit daily sweeps, the problem was handled at the source. Another hospital was unfortunately placed near a main traffic artery which passed through the center of the city; cars carrying poor emergency patients filled beds with nonpaying patients. The solution was to physically remove the hospital's sign so that the hospital could not be found by passers-by.

The American Hospital Association, which promulgates ethical guidelines to maintain high moral standards among its member institutions, assembled a working group to address the problem of emergency rooms which draw the wrong kind of sick people. Among the group's recommendations:[11]

> Provide little or no parking for emergency department patients;
>
> Provide an unlisted number for the emergency department;
>
> Segregate waiting areas for paying and nonpaying patients; in the area for nonpaying patients provide few seats, poor lighting, few signs, and no food or drink;
>
> Segregate treatment areas, providing fewer staff and less equipment in areas for nonpaying patients.

Though these suggestions have not been officially endorsed by the American Hospital Association, they are indicative of a frame of mind which undermines the right of health care at a point of entry into the system. In the United States, with one seventh of the population uninsured, many patients have no personal physician and wait until symptoms are unbearable before seeking help. Twelve-hour waits, which drive many of the sickest patients back home in pain and despair, are satisfactory neither to the patients or to the hospitals.

Rescuing the Right To Health Care

While readers from many countries, especially poorer ones, may recognize some of these same practices from their own health care experiences, it must be kept in mind that these incidents occurred in a nation which spends over $600,000,000,000 per year on health care. The system is awash in money. No other nation spends so lavishly on health care. Yet each provider who demarkets, dumps, or skims will say, in all sincerity, that they would like to offer the care needed by the patients but lack the funds to do so.

The picture of care denied by underutilized facilities points to a basic, even trite, moral truth in health care: the system should cater to human need, not to provider profit. To be sure, many backers of privatizing the health care mission viewed the strategy as a means to the higher end. Through the efficiencies and consumer sovereignty of the market, health care would be provided with greater sensitivity to patients and at lower cost.

In practice, however, too few patients have realized these benefits. The regulations which would have required providers to compete on the basis of price and service rather than on ability to skim and dump were never enacted, though the architects of the strategy urged their passage.[12] The providers and payers who opposed them succeeded in staving off their subsequent imposition.

As denying care came to seem normal, how long could the residual moral commitment to a right to health care persist? Would the hospitals and clinics which heeded the nation's call to follow Adam Smith someday forget, if they ever knew, that privatization in health care was intended to serve the interests of the community as a whole? Doctors and nurses who work in these organizations have been instructed to keep their organization's interests foremost in mind; could these allegiances coexist with professional commitment to health care as a human right? Would the patients themselves have to adjust their expectations. Having been denied care while in obvious need, having found responsibility for their care fragmented and dumped from one provider to the next, and sometimes back again ("reverse dumping"), how long can one maintain a sense of entitlement?

The Problems of Managed Competition

The rapidly increasing insecurity of middle-class Americans in the health care system finally put health care delivery reform at the center of political debate. The new Democratic President took office with a mandate to extend access to care to every citizen by legislating a right to health care for the first time in American history. Yet the President's proposal puts privatization at the core of the proposed system of managed competition.

The President's proposed reforms exist at the time of this writing only as a submission to the Congress, and they are certain to be revised extensively before enactment if, indeed, they survive the legislative process in any form. Even so, they are an important case study for those who are concerned with the potential role of privatization, in the particular sense used in this essay, in the fulfillment of a public mission to provide health care. In effect, the President attempts to reconcile what in light of the above must be considered natural opposites. Urged on by a group of insurance industry executives and market-oriented academics, the President's version of managed competition regulates the market heavily to force private, mostly profit-making insurer-providers to compete on the basis of quality and price. On its face, any success it would enjoy would present an argument against the view expressed here. But a closer look at the plan removes this impression. It is not clear that managed competition amounts to privatization. If the plan turns out to be privatization, human rights are still at risk. If human rights are respected, the plan will not constitute privatization. And the plan is probably at risk for conflict between the two tendencies.

Will the President's plan respect human rights? The concept of managed competition which the President has embraced in his new plan, has not only been tried; it is in fact responsible for many of the indignities and inequities in American health care which have made it such a moral scandal. The competition era in American health care was in part inspired by the work of the same theorist, Alain Enthoven of the Stanford Business School, whose latest work was taken to heart by the Clinton team (though Enthoven has since rejected the Clinton plan entirely). In its earlier incarnation, Enthoven relied only in part on private initiatives in the market.[13] He called for safeguards for patient-consumers who were at a disadvantage in information and bargaining power relative to insurers and providers, and he urged protection, in the form of vouchers, of those too poor to buy into the market. By the time the proposal became policy, these had been removed. Time will tell whether these safeguards will remain in the new version, should it be enacted into law. If not, the effects on health care as a human right could be even worse, since the health care system would be more thoroughly remade along market lines and the ideology of competive advantage would be further normalized in the thinking of health care providers and insurers.

Will the President's plan constitute privatization? If the provisions for fairness and human rights remain in the plan, one ought not conclude that privatization is consistent with human rights, for the result would only in part be privatized. The heavy regulations involved (each plan must offer precisely the same generous benefits; no plan could turn customers away, regardlesss of health status; all insureds pay the same; plans can differ in price only within a narrow band; and so on) take most of the key market decisions away from the competitors and leave them to seek advantage only on the narrowest playing field. This, indeed, is the point of managed competition: to make the adversaries compete only on the basis of price and quality. What is called a regulated market in this instance has some market-like qualities but in other ways can be read as a series of governmental initiatives in a politically protected disguise. The requirements that each insurer take all customers and charge the same rates is nearly equivalent to a social transfer scheme subsidizing the care of the sick at the expense of the well, at least to the extent that health status can be predicted before enrollment. The insistence that competing health plans offer the same and charge nearly the same forces the well-to-do to participate in the same plans as others, helping to prevent a segmentation of the market which genuine privatization entails, to the enrichment of those who succeed in skimming the cream. In a political climate that abhors taxes labeled as taxes and which champions the prerogatives of the well-off, it is politically attractive and feasible to try to accomplish these social ends through what are fashioned as regulations on private enterprise rather than launching them as government social welfare initiatives.

Even if we cast the managed competition plan as a scheme to respect health care as a human right while wearing the clothing of the marketplace, the two tendencies are bound to conflict. For example, competing plans will attempt to skim the cream of healthy clients and dump or avoid unhealthy ones; their task will be to defeat the many regulations which seek to prevent this kind of market behavior. Selective promotion and subtle methods of de-marketing to undesirables can alter the mix of patients, even if the plans must enroll all who choose to buy. The Clinton plan calls for insurers who succeed in enrolling healthier patients to subsidize their competitors, but the regulators must document the skimming and the industry will look for ways to avoid unfavorable audits. Similarly, insurers aiming to enroll wealthier clients will try to find ways to offer benefits which distinguish their plans as superior, perhaps in ease of access to services in addition to the differences explicitly permitted and envisioned by the President, such as amenities and greater choice of physicians.

To the extent that managed competition tends toward a genuinely privatized system, therefore, its recognition of health care as a human right is undermined. The basic thesis of this paper—that competition and privatization in health care delivery tends toward the antisocial rather than toward social goals—suggests that privatization is and will remain an improbable vehicle for achieving a right to health care.

NOTES

1.   This paper is adapted from a contribution to Kathleen E. Mahoney and Paul Mahoney, eds., *Human Rights in the Twenty-First Century: A Global Challenge* (Dordrecht: Martinus Nijhoff Publishers 1993).

2. President's Commission for the Study of Ethical Problems in Medicine and Biomedical and Behavioral Research. 1983. *Securing Access to Health Care.* Vol.1, *Report;* Vols. 2 and 3, *Appendices.* (Washington, D.C.: Government Printing Office. 1983); Norman Daniels, *Just Health Care* (Cambridge: Cambridge University Press, 1984); C. J. Dougherty, *American Health Care: Realities, Rights, and Reforms* (Oxford: Oxford University Press, 1990).

3. Robert Nozick, *Anarchy, State and Utopia* (New York: Basic Books, 1974).

4. L. Lomasky, "Medical Progress and National Health Care", *Philosophy and Public Affairs* 10 (1981): 65–88.

5. Bradford Gray, ed. *For-Profit Enterprise in Health Care.* (Washington, D.C.: National Academy Press, 1989).

6. L. M. Beitsch, "Economic Patient Dumping: Whose Life is it Anyway?" *The Journal of Legal Medicine* 10 (1989): 433–478.

7. L. Uzych, "Patient Dumping", *Journal of the Florida Medical Association* 77 (1990): 97–100.

8. R. J. Blendon, "What should be done about the uninsured poor?" *Journal of the American Medical Association* 260 (1988): 3176–7.

9. Uzych.

10. Sidey Wolfe, "Hospitals Named for Patient Dumping Violations." *Public Citizen Health Research Group Health Letter* 7, no. 5 (May 1991): 1–7.

11. L. A. Burns, "Hospital Initiatives in Response to Ambulatory Care Programs". Working paper, (Chicago, American Hospital Association, 1981). Quoted in R. Schulz, and A.C. Johnson, *Management of Hospitals and Health Services: Strategic Issues and Performance.* (St.Louis: C.V. Mosby Company, 1990).

12. Allan Enthoven, *Health Plan* (Reading: Addison-Wesley, 1980).

13. Enthoven.

AUDREY R. CHAPMAN

Assessing the Clinton Administration's Health Security Act

One of the major purposes of this volume is to develop human rights standards for formulating and evaluating proposals for health care reform. While a wide range of such proposals have been put forward, the Clinton's administration's Health Security Act is setting the agenda for debate and is likely to provide the framework for the restructuring of the health care sector. Therefore this chapter turns to the task of assessing the managed competition model as embodied in the text of the Health Security Act bill submitted to the 103rd Congress. To analyze the proposal from a human rights perspective, it will use the ten criteria identified in the earlier chapter, "A Human Rights Approach to Health Care Reform."

Initial Questions

For a number of reasons the assessment in this chapter can only be considered, however, to be provisional. First, the Clinton administration's proposal is still evolving and key features are as yet unclear. At the time of writing, this author has reviewed three different versions of managed competition—"Health Security: Preliminary Plan Summary,"[1] an official document made available shortly after President Bill Clinton's September address to the nation putting forward his proposal; a book entitled *The President's Health Security Act* published by *The New York Times* and described as "put out by The House Domestic Policy Council based on a test of The Working Group Draft dated September 7, 1993;"[2] and a 1342 page Health Security Act bill published in October, 1993.[3] There are likely to be further revisions as the bill passes through Congress. Moreover, any legislation that reconstructs the health care sector will need ongoing monitoring, with the flexibility to make further adjustments to be able to achieve its stated goals.

Second, despite the length and complexity of the proposed bill, significant details are either unclear or undecided, some of which have major implications for a human rights evaluation. One issue to be determined, for example, is the precise nature of the subsidies that will be given to offset the costs of participation to the poor and those with low incomes. Another is the degree of autonomy that states will be accorded in implementing standards and guidelines set by the federal government, particularly whether states will have the freedom to opt for a financial mechanism other than the managed competition system outlined in the bill. Several states are interested in a "single-payer" system similar to Canada's in which the government finances health care by directly imposing and collecting taxes and controls health care expenditures by setting payment rates for private doctors and hospitals and then prepaying or reimbursing them for their services. If the White House revises its plan to make it easier for states to adopt a single-payer system, as reported in the press,[4] and a number of states select this option, they will have a very different framework than those states operating under managed competition.

Third, the complex and novel features of the proposed managed competition system make it difficult to assess in advance of its implementation. Managed competition has never been tried to date by any national or subnational government so there are no models from which to extrapolate. A managed competition model would involve new relations between the federal government and the states, between the private and public sectors, and between health care financers and health care deliverers,[5] all of which are likely to bring many unanticipated as well as anticipated consequences. Currently there are major disagreements, even among proponents of managed competition, as to how the system will operate. A fundamental assumption in the managed competition model is that competition among private health insurers for contracts with the regional health alliances (health insurance purchasing cooperatives representing all consumers in their jurisdictions) will restructure the market for health care services by giving insurance providers incentives to offer the guaranteed national benefit package mandated by government at the lowest possible cost. Yet proponents disagree as to whether the goals of achieving universal coverage while constraining costs also require global budgets to impose ceilings on total health care expenditures. Alain Enthoven, the principal theoretician of managed competition, argues that blending competition and regulatory strategies would succeed in controlling health care expenditures without global budgets. Paul Starr and Walter Zelman, key staff members of the President's health care reform inter-departmental group, claim that capping the mandated corp of spending and setting a target of out-of-pocket expenditures is essential.[6] Other health care economists concur with Starr and Zelman that competitive mechanisms by themselves will not generate the right level or mix of health care spending,[7] while still others conclude that managed competition, even with global budgets, will not be able in the long-term to slow the rate or increase in medical costs.[8]

Fourth, the segmented design and presentation present yet another problem in assessing the Health Security Plan. As with other proposals put together by a series of independent task forces, the various sections of the proposals are not integrated into a consistent whole. Several sections, such as the provisions on public health initiatives, seem tacked on to the plan and unrelated to its major thrust. The dilemma in undertaking an assessment is whether to consider the parts or the basic design of the whole. For example, the task force which drafted the ethical foundations of health reform worked independently of the groups which designed the framework and mechanisms. The latter apparently had made most of their key decisions about the managed competition system before the ethicists even convened. Under such circumstances it is questionable what role, if any, the stated ethical foundations had in shaping the reform proposal.

While the Clinton administration's proposal has many admirable features, managed competition also presents major problems from a human rights perspective. From that point of view, other proposals, particularly the single-payer system, seem preferable. Nevertheless, if a health care reform bill is to be adopted—and the many failed efforts attest to the fundamental difficulties of achieving this goal in the United States—it may be necessary for those who believe health care is a human right to accept the framework of managed competition while seeking appropriate modifications to it. Accordingly, this evaluation of the Clinton proposal will be followed by a chapter recommending changes in the Health Security Plan that would make it more consistent with a human rights approach.

Evaluating the Proposed Health Security Act

1. A right to health care requires that a basic and adequate standard of health care be guaranteed to all citizens and residents.

The proposed Health Security Act articulates the goal of ensuring individual and family security through health care coverage for all Americans, but it does not fully conform with the human rights principle of universality. On balance, the Health Security Act would provide security and comprehensive coverage for the middle class but falls short in offering a secure and meaningful right to health for those who currently lack health insurance coverage and/or access to health care.

A. A secure entitlement requires legal recognition. One of the greatest weaknesses of the proposed bill is its lack of legal recognition of a right to health care. Much like the 1983 report of the President's Commission for the Study of Ethical Problems in Medicine and Biomedical and Behavioral Research, universality is framed as an ethical principle, not as a right. Moreover, the language of the "Working Group Draft" that "every American citizen and legal resident should have access to health care without financial or other barriers"[9] is even weaker than the conclusion in the 1983 report on *Securing Access to Health Care for All* that "society has an ethical obligation to ensure equitable access to health care to all without undue burden."[10] To assert that every American citizen and legal resident should have access to health care is to assign no one or government agency a specific responsibility to provide such health care. Moreover, the actual provisions of the bill amount to considerably less than a guarantee. It merely states that "each eligible individual is entitled to the comprehensive benefit package under subtitle B through the applicable plan in which the individual is enrolled consistent with this title."[11] This falls far short of the recognition that the government has the legal obligation to assure that every eligible person have access to health care. The bill's formulation also precludes legal recourse to eligible individuals and groups whose rights are denied, particularly in situations where there are financial and structural barriers. Most important, the absence of a legal right raises the possibility that the government can renege on its commitment to universal coverage. Since the bill does not propose to extend coverage to those who currently lack health insurance until January, 1998, it leaves nearly thirty nine million persons hostage to the outcome of the next presidential election. If Bill Clinton is displaced by a more conservative opponent, it is likely that the commitment to universality will be indefinitely postponed. Moreover, the achievement of universality is implicitly linked to achievement of projected cost savings in the Medicare and Medicaid that may not materialize. A government which is reluctant to impose new taxes may not be able to extend health care coverage to all Americans.

B. A secure and meaningful right to health care requires elimination of all grounds for exclusion. For those who are eligible, the Health Security Act seeks to assure that there will be no grounds for exclusion. An individual obtains coverage by enrolling in a plan through a regional or corporate health alliance. These alliances have to accept all participants and cannot turn down any patients on the grounds of preexisting conditions, lack of employment, differences in financial status, or insufficient residence. It is also illegal for an alliance to drop any member. Coverage is portable and has no lifetime limit. Under certain conditions an individual may receive coverage for necessary medical service outside the geographic area served by his or her regional or corporate alliance. An individual will not lose coverage even if he or she changes jobs, becomes unemployed, retires, moves, graduates from college, gets divorced, or starts a business.

C. A legal entitlement to basic health care must be provided to all citizens and residents, including undocumented or illegal aliens. Coverage under the Health Security Act is limited to citizens and legal residents. Although employers are required to pay health insurance premiums for all their employees, regardless of their immigration status, undocumented or illegal aliens will not be eligible for guaranteed benefits. Individuals living in the United States without proper documentation may purchase coverage from a private insurance plan, which they are unlikely to be able to afford, or use emergency health services, whose financing will be severely cut back under the proposed reform. Excluding undocumented aliens is both a violation of the principle of universality and detrimental to public health, making it more difficult to undertake health prevention measures and to control communicable diseases, particularly in areas where there is a large concentration of nonlegal immigrants. Moreover, many of those who are excluded from preventive and primary health services will eventually be treated less effectively in hospital emergency rooms at a much higher cost. Also, distinguishing between legal and illegal residents is likely to have adverse effects on all immigrants and foreign-looking people.[12]

D. The standard package of benefits guaranteed to all citizens and residents should be set at a generous and comprehensive level. For those who are eligible, the Health Security Act proposes to provide a very comprehensive standard package, with more generous benefits than most current health insurance policies. Benefits are subject to cost sharing requirements and some exclusions and phase-in provisions. Because there is no legal guarantee, benefits would also be subject to future curtailment, particularly if found too costly. The following are included in the proposed package:

hospital services (inpatient, outpatient, and emergency services, not including treatment of a mental or substance abuse disorder)

services of health professionals (nearly all medical and surgical treatments, with the exception of cosmetic and sex-change surgery)

emergency and ambulatory medical and surgical services

clinical preventive services (physical checkups at prescribed intervals, immunizations targeted to specific age groups, pap smears, some mammograms, cholesterol screening, well baby care)

mental health and substance abuse services (to be phased-in with coverage limited prior to January 1, 2001)

family planning services and services for pregnant women (excluding in vitro fertilization)

hospice care (benefits limited to the terminally ill)

home health care (focused on persons with severe disabilities)

extended care services (limited to 100 days each year as an alternative to hospital care after an illness or injury)

ambulance services

outpatient laboratory, radiology, and diagnostic services

outpatient prescription drugs and biologicals

outpatient rehabilitation services

durable medical equipment and prosthetic and orthotic devices

vision care (eyeglasses and contact lenses are covered only for those under eighteen years of age)

dental care (services for those under eighteen years of age) health education classes

investigational treatments.[13]

2. A rights approach emphasizes the equality of all persons and their inherent right to health care as the framework for health care reform.

Equality or nondiscrimination is a fundamental human rights principle. The Clinton reform proposal constitutes a considerable improvement over the current health care system, but some of its features would be problematic. While conferring a qualified equal status on participants, it would establish a three-tier health care system that stratifies access to quality health care services. Under such a system, the poor would be denied equality of access to quality medical care.

A. All citizens and residents need to have equal status and receive equal entitlements without distinctions between the employed or umemployed, young or old, able-bodied or disabled.   Under the Health Security Act all citizens and legal residents would in principle be treated alike. They would receive the same health security card. They would be eligible to enroll in any of the health plans. All would receive the same comprehensive health benefits package. In setting premiums, regional and corporate alliance health plans would be required to use community ratings that would not vary the premium charged to residents of an alliance area, except with respect to different types of individual and family coverage under the plan. Alliances would then adjust premium payments to health plans to reflect the level of risk assumed for patients enrolled as compared with the average population in the area. The risk adjustment would take into account factors such as age, gender, health status, and services to disadvantaged populations.[14]

Despite these admirable features, the proposed system would likely result in inequality of treatment. Three problems have been identified. Firstly, as discussed below, the Health Security Act establishes a three-tier health care system in which the poor are likely to have access to lower quality and more limited health care. Secondly, the boundaries of the regional alliances may be drawn in such a way as to segregate certain types of population groups. Although the

Health Security Act states that "in establishing boundaries for alliance areas, the State may not discriminate on the basis of or otherwise take into account race, ethnicity, language, religion, national origin, socioeconomic status, disability, or perceived health status,"[15] there are few effective controls on gerrymandering. Although the Health Security Act envisions a series of relatively equal regional health alliances, each with a diversity of groups, they may in fact be stratified. Thirdly, regulatory features in the act do not appear to be sufficiently stringent to offset the types of practices, described by Daniel Wikler in his article in this volume, designed to "skim" off the most preferable patients and ensure that the wrong patients never come to the door in the first place.[16] Such practices as citing facilities to make them inaccessible to the poor and to attract more of the richer patients, developing services which appeal to healthy young families and neglecting others required by chronic care patients, and establishing admission procedures too complex for someone who is poorly educated are likely to continue under managed competition.

B. Health care requires a national standard set by the federal government that does not vary according to the resources of specific states or subdivisions of states.   Currently health care spending varies greatly by state and by region. Per capita outlays for hospital care, doctors' services, and prescription drugs in 1991 ranged from $2,402 in Massachusetts to $1,234 in Idaho.[17] The Health Security Act does set national standards that would reduce these disparities. It creates a National Health Board responsible for setting national standards and overseeing the establishment and administration of the new health system by states. The Board would interpret and update the guaranteed benefit package, issue binding regulations concerning implementation of the national budget for health care spending and enforce the budget, and establish and manage a performance-based system of quality management and improvement.[18]

C. To promote equality, there should be a single-tier medical system not a dual-tier system in which the poor are given a different standard of health care than the middle class.   The proposal mandates that each health alliance offer three kinds of plans. Premiums would vary depending on the plan and according to family type. Employer contributions would finance 80 percent of the average priced plan in the alliance for each family type and families and individuals would pay the difference between 80 percent of the average priced premium and the actual cost of the plan selected. The three plans are:

(1)   a lower cost sharing plan based solely on the basic benefits package.
(2)   fee-for-service/giving patients freedom to use any health provider without seeking approval through a gatekeeper.
(3)   a combination cost sharing plan in which patients pay $10 per office visit to make use of affiliated doctors and hospitals in Health Maintenance type Organizations (HMOs). The premiums for this plan would be higher than the lower cost sharing plan but less than a fee-for-service plan.[19]

In this proposed three-tier system of health care, there would be differences in the standard of care. Poorer people are likely to receive inferior and lower quality services, with the result that the health care system will perpetuate and reinforce inequities among individuals and groups. Although all three plans will offer the same package of benefits, quality and accessibility are likely to vary considerably. Benefiting from higher revenues and driven by more sophisticated and educated consumers, fee-for-service plans, and to a somewhat lesser extent combination plans, are likely to offer better facilities and more sophisticated equipment, more experienced physicians, a greater proportion of whom are specialists, and shorter waiting times. Poorer individuals are unlikely to receive subsidies that will enable them to choose any but the most basic plans. The risk is that such plans to be competitive may operate like Medicaid mills which hold down costs by requiring that doctors see a much higher volume of patients and discouraging them from prescribing expensive diagnostic tests and treatments.[20] More affluent individuals and families would also be able to purchase supplemental insurance, covering a wider range of benefits than the basic package.

3. By employing rights language, the provision of health care would be understood as a fundamentally important social good to be considered differently from other goods and services.

As a hybrid, the Clinton reform proposal treats health care as both a social good and a commodity. Managed competition seeks to combine market principles with a regulatory framework that protects the public's interest. The Health Security Act proposes to restructure the market for health care services into competing prepaid plans that offer the comprehensive benefits package and serve both high-risk and low-risk populations. Regional health alliances, which are envisioned as health insurance purchasing cooperatives representing the interests of consumers and purchasers of health care services, would contract with varied private health plans, including health maintenance organizations (HMOs), preferred provider organizations (PPOs), and free-choice-of provider option, to offer their plans to members of the alliance. According to rules for competition derived from microeconomic principles, providers will purportedly have incentives to improve quality, cut costs, and satisfy patients to gain more subscribers and revenues. In relying on market principles, cost containment appears to have greater priority than achieving true universal access and redressing historical inequities in the health care system. Moreover, as the analysis below indicates, managed competition does not comfortably meet a social or community standard.

A. In applying a rights designation, a society assigns priority to a particular human or social attribute and accepts responsibility for its promotion and protection.   The stated purpose of the Health Security Act is "to ensure individual and family security through health care coverage for all Americans in a manner that contains the rate of growth in health care costs and promotes responsible health insurance practices, to promote choice in health care, and to ensure and protect the health care of All Americans."[21] This language is less than a ringing endorsement of health care as a social good which should be distributed in accordance with principles of justice. The section of the bill dealing with universal coverage and individual responsibility does not even repeat the weak formulation of the ethical principle contained in the "Working Group Draft" that "every American citizen and legal resident should have access to health care without financial or other barriers."[22] The bill lacks a clear acknowledgement that health care is a high priority social good to which all persons are entitled either as a matter of right, or an acceptance that the federal/state governments bear the ultimate responsibility to assure that all eligible persons have access to quality health services.

B. A logical corollary of health care being a fundamentally important social good is that the health care system should be evaluated

by a social or community standard. Of the various proposals that
have been put forward, managed competition does not seem best able
to meet the goal of fostering the common good and collective health
of the society. The decision to go forward with the plan appears to
reflect a political calculus that it is not feasible to craft a more equitable
system that would come at the expense of powerful economic beneficiaries of the current order. In this equation, the interests of most
Americans have been sacrificed to the health insurance industry, pharmaceutical manufacturers, and health care providers. It is also quite
incredible that a country is willing to risk one-sixth of its economy
on a model that is completely untested and about which reputable
analysts disagree as to its likely impact.

Independent sources, such as the Congressional Budget Office,
have concluded that, of the proposals under consideration by Congress, the single-payer system would show the greatest overall cost
savings, and it would be the only one in which all Americans would be
able to have health care coverage immediately upon implementation.[23]
The Congressional Budget Office has determined that a Canadian-
style system would reduce annual medical spending by \$114 billion
by 2003.[24] Because a single-payer system would provide a central
role for the government, its opponents claim that it would create
unwarranted interference in the practice of medicine, intruding the
government in the doctor-patient relationship. Yet a managed competition system would impose even greater restrictions. Under the
single-payer system, the government would set prices for medical
services, limit annual price increases to the rate of overall economic
growth, and collect taxes to finance health care; the same arrangement,
however, would also give patients greater flexibility in choosing their
providers than would a managed care situation. The single-payer
system would also be less likely to prescribe specific care practices on
providers.

Because market solutions have contributed to the crisis of health
care, more of the same appears to be a poor candidate for shaping
solutions. Market applications to health care have been identified as
a major factor in leading to high costs, widespread overuse of medical
resources, overemphasis on expensive technology, neglect of less
profitable primary care, and dumping of high risk patients.[25] Although
the regulatory mechanisms in the proposed bill would mitigate some
of these problems, the single-payer system would do so more effectively. As analysis below will amplify, the Health Security Act does

not effectively deal with many of the factors contributing to high costs, particularly the uncontrolled introduction and diffusion of expensive technologies, which some economists believe is the most important source of cost inflation in health care. The bill's efforts to reorient the health care system more toward primary care offered by general practitioners are inadequate to achieve this goal. Also its regulatory mechanisms do not appear able to prevent "gerrymandering" or manipulation of the boundaries of regional health alliances so as to insulate relatively healthy middle class populations from higher risk or higher cost groups.

C. *A health care reform initiative designed to assure a meaningful and secure health care entitlement requires a new paradigm that places a greater emphasis on health protection, prevention of disease, and community-based and oriented primary medical services.* The Health Security Act, however, basically leaves the current curative care paradigm in place, supplementing it with some public health measures and preventive health services. Like most of the current proposals before Congress, the Clinton plan would restructure the financing of health care but would mandate very few changes in the practice or delivery of health services. Managed competition would probably push more consumers and providers into health maintenance organizations which would still be oriented toward curative care; they would not function as primary health care centers. In the bill, the core functions of public health programs are conceptualized more as monitoring and controlling disease rather than as major initiatives at health protection. The bill seeks to strengthen the capacity of state and local public health agencies to do the following: (1) to monitor and protect the health of communities against communicable diseases and exposure to toxic environmental pollutants, occupational hazards, harmful products, and poor quality health care; (2) to identify and control outbreaks of infectious disease: (3) to inform and educate health care consumers and providers about their roles in preventing and controlling disease; and (4) to develop and test new prevention and public health control interventions.[26] However, the program is significantly underfunded. National initiatives regarding health promotion and disease prevention are to be appropriated at levels ranging from $175 million to $200 million.[27] Moreover, the proposal lacks and does not even identify a need for comprehensive health protections measures to improve air quality, significantly reduce exposure to toxic substances, assure greater workplace safety, discourage substance abuse, control the availability of guns and weapons, and cleanup water supplies. While the Health Security Act does propose to cover some clinical preventive services, including childhood immunizations, it does not envision extensive new initiatives and limits access to several of the clinical tests to population groups deemed to be high risk.[28]

4. A human rights approach focuses particularly on the needs of the most disadvantaged and vulnerable communities.

The Clinton health care proposal is disappointing because it is geared primarily to addressing the health security of the middle class and not focusing on the needs of the most disadvantaged and vulnerable groups. Earlier drafts of the plan acknowledged the problems and proposed some measures to rectify historical inequities, but the bill is more reticent in this regard. Because the bill postpones extending coverage to the nearly 39 million Americans who are currently uninsured until January 1998, the Health Security Act may never achieve its stated goal of universality. As noted, this phase-in makes the achievement of universality hostage both to the outcome of the next presidential election and to implicit cost savings. From a human rights perspective, the Health Security Act has the wrong focus and priorities. To be consistent with a human rights approach, health care reform should give the greatest emphasis, with commensurate investment, on low-income, ethnic and racial minorities, and groups with disabilities. By virtue of its great complexity, the Clinton proposal may also establish unintended hurdles for groups unable to understand or negotiate within the new system. This would particularly be a problem for those with little education and poor command of English. The analysis below considers other provisions as set forth in the bill and the subsequent explanations and revisions suggested by the Clinton administration.

A. A human rights approach implies both nondiscrimination and affirmative action to rectify historical inequities in access to health care. The Health Security Act does not provide acceptable standards of either nondiscrimination or affirmative action. In defining the problems to be addressed and the goals of the Health Security Act, the bill does not specifically mention the need to provide meaningful access to health care for the 38.9 million Americans who currently lack insurance. Although the "Working Group Draft" has a chapter on "Health Care Access Initiatives" that identifies and addresses some of the financial and non-financial barriers that reduce access for a number of population groups in American society,[29] there is no comparable section in the Health Security Act. Nor does the bill assign states, which have the major responsibility for implementing the health care reform, the mandate of assuring that health plans enroll vulnerable populations and meet their personal health care needs. The Health Security Act proposes to provide funds for improving access to health services for medically underserved populations, but these initiatives are both underfinanced and conceptualized more like small business grants than affirmative action measures. These measures include grants to community and migrant health centers (at a level of $100 million for each of the fiscal years 1995 through 2000), grants to qualified community health plans that provide health services in areas where there are health professional shortages or a significant number of individuals who are members of a medically underserved population ($200 million for fiscal year 1996, $300 million for each of fiscal years 1997-1999, and $100 million for 2000), payments to hospitals serving vulnerable populations who do not have coverage under the Act, such as undocumented aliens ($800 million per year).[30]

Rather than fashioning a proposal that energetically addresses financial and nonfinancial barriers to health care access, the Health Security Act has the potential of making an already bad situation worse for some groups. In fact, one of its major financing mechanisms would take from the poor and vulnerable to improve the coverage of the middle class. According to figures made available by the administration, it calculates that under the Clinton proposal that Medicare and Medicaid would save $65.7 billion over five years by eliminating Medicaid payments and reducing Medicare payments to hospitals that serve disproportionate numbers of poor people. Administration spokespersons justify doing so by claiming that they would no longer be needed if all Americans had insurance coverage. However, the bill does not provide such universal coverage—for eligible uninsured Americans until 1998 and for undocumented aliens at all, and until now hospital emergency rooms have been the only source of medical care for many in this group. Speaking on behalf of the 4,000 hospitals represented by his organization, Richard Davidson, president of the American Hospital Association, has been very critical of the proposal noting that "those payments have made the difference in our ability to care for the poor." The administration also proposes to save $79.5 billion over five years by not underwriting the cost of insurance for low-income people under 65 who are now on Medicaid but not on welfare.[31]

B. Because a human right is a universal entitlement, its implementation is measured particularly by the degree to which it benefits those who hitherto have been the most disadvantaged and vulnerable and brings them up to mainstream standards. There are two major unknowns that will influence whether the Health Security Act will improve the status of poor and underserved individuals and communities. The first question is whether the phase-in of coverage to these groups will in fact occur as scheduled—by January 1998—or if not then, whether it will ever take place. The second issue is the financial arrangements for these groups, particularly the nature of the subsidies and the manner in which eligibility for subsidies will be determined. The Clinton plan envisions individuals and families contributing twenty percent of their health care premiums. Those with incomes of less than 150 percent of the poverty ceiling (about $15,000 for a family of three) would receive a subsidy on a sliding scale, the amount of which is as yet unspecified. Ideally the subsidy would be sufficiently generous (perhaps 120 to 130 percent of the basic plan) to permit poorer individuals to be able elect the medium cost and high cost plans, but the reluctance to levy new taxes to finance health care reform effectively eliminates such an option. Quite the contrary, the administration is proposing to place limits on subsidies to small businesses and low-income people, requiring action by Congress if funds run out in a given year.

Proposed funding arrangements may impose unfair financial burdens on the poor, even for participation in the lowest cost plan. In Congressional testimony, Diane Rowland, executive director of the Kaiser Commission on the Future of Medicaid, a private bipartisan study group, observed that "the Clinton plan would require significant cost sharing by most low-income Americans," and expressed doubt that it would be possible for them to meet such "onerous financial obligations."[32] While the Health Security Act proposes to provide federal subsidies to help low-income persons pay their insurance premiums, with the exception of welfare recipients, it would not cover their share of the charges for medical services. It is estimated, for example, that a family of four with income of $8,500 and average health costs will pay $265 a year in copayments alone.[33] The amount that low-income employees will have to pay for premiums would be capped at 3.9 percent of income, but even so, for some it would be a hardship. Critics believe that these charges could deter poor people from getting timely medical care. The Clinton administration acknowledges that the plan would make demands on this category of welfare recipient but seeks to justify it as necessary to finance the plan fully. Charges by some critics that the plan would punish poor people who work have some validity.[34]

Although proponents claim that provisions of the Clinton plan would be a boost for the 3 million Americans who are very disabled, if the plan becomes law without changes, unlike Medicare, it would not automatically provide services to these individuals. Under the plan, disabled persons would be entitled to an assessment but services would be provided according to the availability of funds. Each state would decide what services to give its disabled residents and the level of funding it would contribute. To be even eligible for assistance for home or community-based services, a person would have to either be substantially mentally impaired (for example, victims of Alzheimer's disease), or very disabled physically (unable to perform without assistance three activities of daily living). Thus many disabled Americans who could use long-term care services will not get them under the Health Security Act because the government won't judge them sufficiently impaired to qualify.[35]

For the 51.7 million Americans suffering from a mental disorder or substance use disorder, the Clinton plan has been compared with a sweater on a frigid winter day: "It won't entirely do the job, but it is better than nothing." [36] While the Clinton plan goes further in broadening the scope of mental health services than most existing insurance benefits and some alternative health reform proposals, mental health advocates have been critical that it puts an unfair and singular burden on the mentally ill to prove that they are really sick.[37] The plan will provide good coverage for those who need intensive outpatient care, covering up to 180 days a year of intensive nonresidential services. However, severely ill patients who are not poor enough to quality for Social Security disability or Medicaid benefits but who may need long-term institutional care (for example a person with severe schizophrenia), are limited to sixty days of hospitalization coverage each year. Mental health benefits would be phased in gradually until the year 2001.

Another special population group, older Americans, would fare relatively well under the Clinton proposal. The Medicare system would be retained, apparently so as not to frighten elderly Americans, with its benefits expanded to cover prescription drugs for the elderly and disabled.[38] Older persons would also benefit from the provisions for coverage of some long-term care. In its first full response, the board of directors of the American Association for Retired Persons (AARP) gave the proposal higher marks than any of the alternatives emerging in Congress. The AARP commended the plan for "vital provisions," including home and community based long-term care for all Americans, prescription drug coverage for Medicare beneficiaries, and health coverage subsidies for early retirees not yet age 65. AARP's President also, however, expressed reservations about the advisability of financing new benefits through savings from Medicare and Medicaid and the reliability of the financing planned for the long-term care program. AARP has also been critical of the administration's decision to keep the Medicare program separate, because it would create a two-tier system in which older persons would receive less generous benefits than those available to younger participants enrolled in the regional health alliances.[39] The standard package provided by the regional health alliances, for example, would cover far more preventive care and would have lower out-of-pocket costs. While the Clinton plan would allow states to request permission to integrate Medicare beneficiaries into the health alliances, states doing so must provide current Medicare beneficiaries only access to the same or higher level of benefits as standard Medicare. Representatives of AARP have pointed out that this standard would still allow less generous benefits for elderly and disabled people than for younger people in the same alliance. Others, including many governors and administration officials, also prefer that elderly people be integrated into the new health alliances in order to be able to control costs.[40]

5. By establishing clear individual entitlements to health care, a rights approach would empower individuals and groups to assert their claims.

Empowerment of individuals and groups to make claims is an important consideration where there are historical inequities in access to care. While the Health Security Act has a good appeals process, it does not empower individuals or groups to assert their claims. The failure to use rights language strips the bill of a normative vocabulary that facilitates the framing of claims and the identification of rights holders. This is not an accident. Conversations with members of the ethics task force suggest that awareness that using a rights formulation would give rise to such claims was a major factor precluding recognizing a right to basic health care. Empowerment obviously requires more than the legal recognition of a right to health care, but establishing an entitlement is a prerequisite. Moreover, the Health Security Act also lacks an educational component to inform and facilitate underserved populations claiming their entitlements. The bill also does not place a priority on improving the accessibility of health services through such measures as using vans, expanding and relocating primary care sites to local neighborhoods, or providing health services in schools.

6. A meaningful and secure right requires that health care be affordable and publicly financed.

The Clinton administration proposes to finance its health care reform package through four principal means: an employer mandate requiring payment of eighty percent of the costs of employees' health care premiums; individuals assuming responsibility for twenty percent of the cost of their insurance and contributing a variety of deductibles, copayments, and coinsurance fees; a projected savings on Medicare and Medicaid; and selected "sin" taxes, primarily a seventy-five percent increase in the federal excise tax on cigarettes. It would provide subsidies to two groups, small businesses and low income persons, to underwrite part of the costs of coverage. Critics have raised a series of questions, some of which are already noted, as to whether the financial mechanisms are equitable and fair, whether the projected costs and revenues are realistic, and whether managed competition can effectively restrain cost increases. On balance, the financial provisions do not conform to a human rights approach. If enacted, there is likely to be a net reduction in funding for programs that underwrite the health care costs of the most vulnerable groups. In addition, the bill does not propose a progressive source of financing that links contributions to the ability to pay.

A. Recognition of a right to health care requires that society remove financial barriers to basic and adequate health care. If adopted, the Health Security Act would reduce but not remove finan-

cial barriers. Although the Clinton proposal would offset some of the costs of participation for the poor, the subsidies envisioned would purchase the lowest cost plan and may be inadequate to cover copayments and other costs for health services and prescriptions. The working poor currently eligible for Medicaid will be worse off in the realignment of fees and benefits because they will also have to contribute up to 3.9 percent of income towards premiums, which for them may be a substantial amount. The proposal to set a cap or limits on the cost of subsidies that can only be exceeded by congressional authorization suggests that the likely increased costs will be met by a decrease in the level of subsidy support rather than by the identification of a new source of income. In December, 1993, Lewin-VHI, a respected nonpartisan consulting concern, reported its analysis of the Clinton health care plan which indicated that subsidies to small businesses and low income people would cost the Government $153 billion in the first six years, about one-third more than the White House had estimated.[41] And the elimination of federal payments to hospitals serving substantial numbers of persons ineligible for benefits under the current and the future system is an affront to human rights.

B. A human rights approach assumes a social or public responsibility for financing basic health care services. The Clinton proposal has a mixed score relative to this standard. It does conform to the basic tenet of social insurance by instituting community ratings so that health status or risk of illness does not correlate with increased cost. It would not, however, collectivize the financing of health care. Initially the Clinton administration considered imposing a consumption or new value-added tax (VAT) to finance health care reform. Many European countries rely on this type of national sales tax as a major source of income for social programs, including health care. However, after officials examined private polls showing that such a new tax would be unpopular, the administration opted instead for an employers' mandate as a major source of income.[42] Moreover, to avoid the onus of being accused of levying one of the largest tax increases in American history, employers' contributions are not being categorized as taxes. While this may be politically astute, it undermines acceptance of social or public responsibility for financing basic health care services.

C. The means by which the health care system is financed would need to be equitable and fair. There are several concerns related to the fairness of the proposed methods of financing health care. It is fundamentally inconsistent with the standards embodied in a human rights approach for health care primarily to benefit the middle class to be underwritten by savings in the health care services or costs available to the poor and elderly. Medicare is already underfunded, covering only about half of the potentially eligible population in most states, and paying fees unacceptable to many providers. There is also something seriously wrong with a proposal that increases costs for vulnerable and disadvantaged groups of persons, like the working poor, but refuses either to impose new broad taxes or increased levies on alcohol, guns, ammunition, or excess profits in the pharmaceutical industry. Justice considerations require a new broad-based form of taxation to finance the health care reform, such as an income tax increase or a value-added tax. Very stiff "sin taxes" on alcohol, tobacco, guns, and ammunition would at least underwrite a fairer percentage of the costs of treating the illnesses and injuries that their use produces. In a progressive system, costs would correlate with income or ability to pay, but not to the health care services received. This is why many countries utilize a value-added tax for funding health care. Under the three-tier system envisaged by the Health Security Act, however, benefits rather than contributions would reflect the ability to pay.

D. A formulation of the right to health care which links the scope of the entitlement to the resource levels available in a particular society also implies that the total cost of health care is affordable on a societal level. Controlling spiralling health costs is a justice issue because of the opportunity costs it imposes on other private and social investments and on potential opportunities for full-time employment with benefits. As health care has become more expensive, middle class Americans have also become more reluctant to underwrite the costs for low-income members of society. This study has linked cost reduction with a new paradigm for health care emphasizing preventive and primary health care services and utilizing family practitioner physicians, nurse practitioners, and other professionals in place of the current acute care paradigm which relies heavily on specialist physicians. Canadians and Europeans limit overall health spending by three means: (1) constraining the physical capacity of the system; (2) controlling prices; and (3) imposing something as close as possible to global monetary budgets on the entire system.[43] Many of these countries also impose limits on some high-tech medical interventions, such as renal dialysis or certain organ transplantations, if the attending physician judges the likely benefits to be low. High technology innovations are also introduced more cautiously on a more limited basis and only after undertaking careful benefit-cost analysis. In 1991, for example, there were fifteen M.R.I. scanners in all of Canada and 2,000 in the United States; the U.S. therefore had more than ten times more per person.[44] Within these constraints, however, Canadians and European health systems permit doctors considerable clinical freedom, trusting in the medical establishment's willingness and ability to use the resources made available properly.[45]

The Clinton health care reform plan unrealistically assumes that it is possible to control costs without adopting any of the approaches mentioned above, and therefore, if the proposal is implemented, it is unlikely to be able to achieve a cost-conscious standard of care or to reduce escalating health care expenditures. Nothing in the proposal fundamentally challenges the prevailing curative care paradigm. The plan backs off from advocating potentially unpopular measures necessary to constrain costs. Despite the belief, even among many of the proponents of managed competition, that global budgeting is necessary for health cost containment, the current version of the Health Security Act eliminates global budgets; the National Health Board is no longer responsible for developing a national or global budget for health care spending. Other measures considered once like instituting price controls to hold down on the cost of medicines, are also gone from the bill. Although the pharmaceuticals are the nation's most lucrative industry, with profit margins that average at least three times those of other Fortune 500 companies and, according to a congressional committee, "excess profits" of some $2 billion annually, the Clinton health care reform would not impose serious constraints on industry profits.[46] Nor does the bill address the problems of the proliferation of new technologies which some analysts argue is the main cost driver in the health care sector.[47] In contrast with other countries, the plan is likely to continue current practices of comanaging ongoing patient-doctor relationship, a uniquely American and also inefficient approach to attempting to hold down costs.

The bill relies on competition, cost awareness by consumers, and states enforcing limits for insurance premium increases as its major cost-containment measures, none of which are likely to be effective in doing so. The Clinton plan seeks to hold down health spending by inducing large numbers of participants to enroll in managed care plans. However, a four-year study by Mathematica Policy Research, a private consulting firm, concluded that the government does not save money on Medicare partients enrolled in health maintenance organizations. The General Accounting Office, the investigative arm of Congress, has also said that there is little empirical evidence of savings from HMOs. Part of the failure to reap potential savings through managed care is the difficulty in setting appropriate payment rates. If the government has not found a reliable way to adjust payments to HMOs to reflect the health needs of Medicare beneficiaries, health care alliances established under managed competition may not fare any better in determining their payments to networks of insurers, doctors, and hospitals to reflect the needs of alliance members.[48]

Just as Adam Smith hypothesized that there was an "invisible hand" that reconciles and harmonizes self-interest, managed competition proponents seem to assume that competition for market share by insurers will automatically reduce high administrative costs and eliminate other inefficiencies in the health care sector. However, competition in the health care sector has not necessarily held down costs. According to the principles of competition, a surplus should act to bring down costs. In contrast, pharmaceutical corporations and health care facilities are more likely to resort to additional advertising and marketing than to reduce prices. Medical specialists in overcrowded fields, rather than reducing fees so as to attract more patients, are more likely to compensate for seeing fewer patients by increasing rather than decreasing their fees. The establishment of regional and corporate health alliances may redress the balance of power between consumers and health insurance companies, but unless these alliances act as aggressive consumer-advocates, something which is far from assured, they may just introduce yet another level of expensive bureaucracy into an already complex, redundant, and fragmented system. Managed competition proponents also assume that encouraging consumers to make cost-conscious decisions will have a constraining effect on utilization patterns. Many economists, however, dispute that patients in need of medical care can or should act like "consumers" who are expected to shop around for cost-effective health care. While cost sharing by patients may have some constraining effects on utilization patterns for mild to semi-serious illness, it is unlikely to affect decision-making for the serious cases that appear to account for 50 to 70 percent of expenditures in a given year.[49] Thus Joseph Newhouse's assessment that managed competition alone (without global budgets) "will not, apart from a transitory period, slow the rate of increase in medical care costs"[50] seems on the mark.

7. A human rights approach underscores the importance of public participation in setting priorities and shaping health care reform as well as in assuring the accountability of health care institutions to citizens.

Both the process by which the Clinton proposal was developed and the proposed mechanisms for accountability are inadequate because they do not assure public participation or accountability.

A. Setting the agenda for health care reform cannot and should not be the prerogative of medical professionals, health care providers, or public policy elites. While the Clinton health care team widely consulted groups of citizens and professionals about problems with the current health care system through holding hearings and sponsoring town meetings, they have not invited participation from the public or consumer groups in setting the proposed framework for health care reform. The decision-making process has been confined to selected experts invited to serve on one of the policy task forces. Nor have they sought systematic evaluation from the public or specific groups to any aspects of the proposed plan. This drafting process by the policy wonks, with the policy wonks, and possibly for the policy wonks, compares unfavorably with the manner in which the Oregon state government proceeded with its reform. As described in Michael Garland's article in this volume, the Oregon task force used a wide array of approaches to consult with and involve the public in the design of the Oregon Plan, including hearings at various stages, telephone surveys, and consultations with special groups.[51]

B. A human rights approach also requires ongoing consultation and public participation in monitoring and oversight of the health care system. The National Health Board, which will be the primary oversight body vested with extensive powers, is envisaged as a quasi-governmental regulatory agency, created in the Executive branch, whose seven members will be appointed by the President with the advice and consent of the Senate. According to the bill, Board members will be selected on the basis of their experience and expertise in relevant subjects and not their ability to represent specific constituencies.[52]

Comparable to other regulatory bodies, provisions of the bill attempt to insulate the National Health Board, rather than to encourage it to engage in ongoing consultation and public participation. Because participating states are not required to establish new consultation or monitoring mechanisms to oversee the operation of constituent regional and corporate health alliances, there may not be opportunities for meaningful public participation in the monitoring process. In contrast, the Board of Directors of the Regional and Corporate Alliances are intended to have equal representation of employers and consumers. Half of the their members are to represent individuals who purchase coverage through the alliance.[53] Yet it is still difficult to know whether such boards will conceptualize their roles as consumer advocates or experts and whether they will establish effective consultative procedures for public participation.

C. A human rights approach further entails the accountability and transparency of major institutions in the health sector. As drafted, the Health Security Act focuses more on assuring free choice than accountability. To assist consumers/patients, the National Health Board will require quality measurement of all health plans in the form of a "report card" that all Health Alliances will publish annually and make available to consumers. Even so, many people will not be able to exercise consumer choice. Because subsidies will be set to the level of the lowest cost plan, low income groups will not have any real options. In addition, many people, perhaps up to 40 percent of the population, may be in areas which lack sufficient population density to support several competing plans. Moreover, quality assessment is more complicated than a short "report card" can reflect. Also, divergent outcomes can reflect differences in patient profiles; some plans may have positive ratings because they have a "gerrymandered" population base and do not have to serve numerous disadvantaged groups.[54]

There are few mechanisms to assure openness, accountability, and transparency. The National Health Board is to present an annual report to the President and Congress, not to the American people. This report is to contain information related to federal and state implementation; quality improvement; recommendations or changes in the administration, regulation, and laws related to health care and coverage; and finally, a full account of all actions taken during the previous year.[55] As such, it is likely to be more of a "state of the health care sector" than a rendering of the Board's governance. Aside from periodic audits by the General Accounting Office, the National Health Board will not have to take responsibility for its decision-making. Regional Health Alliance are responsible to the state, not to its members or to citizens. Nor are there adequate procedures, other than the fairly drastic one of superseding its authority, if it fails to execute its duties. Moreover, these provisions appear more relevant to financial irregularities than to neglect of other responsibilities, such as assuring nondiscrimination.

8. A rights formulation translates into a series of obligations on the part of federal and state governments.

In the case of a recognized legal right, the relevant governmental authorities assume major responsibility. The duty of governments has several distinct components, including to respect, to protect, and to fulfill. The Clinton proposal lacks a categorical acceptance of the duty of government to assure access to health care and implementation of the various components of the reform. Moreover, as indicated, many of the proposals to rectify structural problems are inadequate. It may also, perhaps inadvertently, introduce new forms of discrimination into the health care system.

A. The framework, priorities, and orientation of the health care system must be consistent with a human rights approach. A human rights perspective did not inform the shaping of the framework, priorities, and orientation of the proposed Clinton plan. The failure to propose recognition of any right to basic health care is indicative of an orientation that places economics ahead of equity considerations. The plan caters to security and improved coverage for the middle class ahead of, and in its financial provisions, at the expense of, low-income persons and vulnerable groups. The National Health Board, state governments, and regional and corporate alliances are assigned more responsibilities related to financial accounting than to assuring equality and nondiscrimination. Initiatives identified to address some structural barriers to access are not central to the plan either in its design or the proposed allocation of resources under the plan. While the Health Security Plan has many admirable features and would be an improvement on the current system, it cannot be given a ringing endorsement. If the Health Security Plan were being evaluated by professors at a human rights university, its would receive a C + grade.

B. The achievement of universal coverage has the highest priority and therefore should be achieved in the shortest possible time. As noted, the Health Security Act excludes coverage of undocumented aliens and postpones incorporating many of the nearly thirty-nine million Americans currently without insurance until 1998. Although there is no reason to question the sincerity of the commitment to achieving universal coverage, at best it is not a priority. Nor has the proposed health care plan been crafted in the manner most likely to be consistent with reaching this goal. Given the reluctance to levy new taxes to fund coverage for underserved and vulnerable groups, there is also the danger that the incorporation of additional low-income persons into the health care system will come at the expense of lowering still further the subsidies envisioned for these groups. If so, this will be a very nominal and inadequate form of universality.

C. With respect to health care, the duty to respect the equality of all persons is associated with a responsibility both not to discriminate and to prevent discrimination. Under the Health Security Act, anti-discrimination is a duty of the health alliances. Alliances are required to enroll all eligible members regardless of their background, employment status, or health risks and accord them equal status. Also in carrying out its activities a health alliance may not discriminate against health plans on the basis of race, gender, ethnicity, religion, mix of health professionals, location of the plan's headquarters, or organizational arrangement.[56] While states have the responsibility to certify and monitor the performance of regional alliances, they are not specifically assigned the task of assuring nondiscrimination. Given the Act's heavy stress on financial accountability, it is likely that states' audits will focus more on financial than equity or nondiscrimination issues.

As noted, there are inadequate protections against what may be a major form of discrimination, the gerrymandering of the boundaries of regional alliances. Drafters of the bill were aware of the possibilities of gerrymandering or redlining, particularly in relationship to urban areas, so as to exclude high risk and poorer participants. The bill states that "in establishing boundaries for alliance areas, the State may not discriminate on the basis of or otherwise take into account race, ethnicity, language, religion, national origin, socio-economic status, disability, or perceived health status.''[57] It also directs that the entire portion of a metropolitan statistical area located in a state shall be included in the same alliance, presumably to incorporate both inner cities and suburbs.[58] However, no effective mechanisms are envisaged to enforce these provisions. Also, by making undocumented residents ineligible for coverage the bill may itself give rise to a form of discrimination against foreigners and foreign-looking Americans.

D. The obligation of the governments has a positive component, to remove obstacles or barriers to access, a kind of affirmative action applied to the health sector. As noted above, the Working Group Draft recognizes the need to compensate for historical inequities in access to health care, but the Health Security Act backtracks in this regard. The mechanisms identified and the funding allocated are inadequate to the task. Efforts to develop and improve facilities in underserved areas are conceived more as discretionary than obligatory and more as providing financial incentives to the private sector rather than as imposing government mandates. Because such underserved communities do not have a right to access under the Clinton proposal, the plan does not accord a high priority to investments and measures to achieve coverage and reduce inequalities.

One of the structural impediments to equitable access not yet discussed is the composition of the health care workforce. There are currently three types of problems. Health care professionals are reluctant to locate in many underserved areas, both rural and urban. The current system relies too heavily on expensive specialists and does not train sufficient numbers of generalists or family practitioners. And nurse practitioners and physician assistants, who could perform many tasks related to primary care, are underutilized. Recognizing these problems, the Health Security Act proposes to shift the balance in the graduate training of physicians from specialties to primary care; after a five year phase-in period its goal is that at least fifty percent of new physicians will be trained in primary care. Without the retraining of current practitioners and incentives for them to enter primary care practice, neither of which is contained in the bill, it would take until 2045 for even fifty percent of physicians to be generalists or family practitioners.[59] The proposal also incorporates some much needed initiatives to recruit and support the education of health professionals from underrepresented population groups. The goal is to double the level of representatives of minority and disadvantaged groups in medical school to 3,000 by the year 2000 through financial assistance, increased support for recruitment and retention, and support programs.[60] What is missing from the mix are measures to assure that physicians receiving any form of government support in their education will serve a minimum period in underrepresented areas.

E. An explicit commitment to improving the public's health should be an explicit goal of all public policy formulation, and current policies inconsistent with this objective, such as subsidies to tobacco growers, should be changed. The section on public health initiatives in the Health Security Act, does not have a comprehensive approach to health protection. It does not propose a major redistribution of resources or public policy emphasis on prevention. Earlier plans to impose a series of stiff "sin taxes," both as revenue sources and to discourage consumption, were withdrawn, leaving only a cigarette tax on the table. Few voices have been raised about the inconsistency of subsidizing tobacco growers and then providing health care services for those suffering from smoking related disabilities. There is no apparent support from within the administration for Senator Patrick Moynihan's proposal to levy very high taxes on certain types of ammunition used with handguns or the call to tax handguns as a means to reduce violence and injuries.[61] Despite scattered references about the link between environmental quality and safety and health, there are no major initiatives contemplated in the bill to improve air or water standards or reduce exposure to toxic substances.

F. All government units require effective monitoring mechanisms whereby implementation of health care reform can be regularly evaluated and inadequacies that are identified can be rectified. In a country which currently lacks a data base and capacity to evaluate adequately access to health care services and health status of population groups, establishment of an information management system able to track the impact of features of health care reform is one the most positive innovations envisioned under the Health Security Act. Under provisions of the act, not later than two years after the date of enactment, the National Health Board, in consultation with federal agencies involved in the collection of relevant data and the provision of health care service, is to develop and implement a health information system by which the Board will collect, report, and regulate the collection and dissemination of health care information. As part of the health information system, the National Health Board is also to oversee the establishment of an electronic data network consisting of regional centers that collect, compile, and transmit information. It is specified that the health information system shall be developed and implemented in a manner consistent with privacy and security standards that respect confidentiality of patient data. Health care information shall include data on enrollment and disenrollment in health plans, clinical encounters, administrative and financial transactions, characteristics of regional alliances, including the number, and demographic characteristics of eligible individuals residing in each alliance area, the characteristic of corporate alliances, payment of benefits, terms of agreement between health plans and health providers, utilization management, and grievances filed.[62]

However, the purpose of this information system is not to monitor implementation of health care reform so as to assure universality and access to health care. Evaluation and reporting of quality performance is the major goal. The system is intended to assist consumers choose health plans and providers through reporting on such subjects as access to health care services by consumers, appropriateness of health care services provided, outcomes of health care services and procedures, health promotion, prevention of diseases, disorders, and other health conditions, and consumer satisfaction with care. Criteria to be used in developing and selecting national measures of quality performance are significance (of a disease, disorder, or other health condition), range of services, reliability and validity, variation, linkage to health outcome, provider control and risk adjustment, and public health.[63] These data can be helpful in evaluating the impact of the health care reform on specific groups, though this is not its primary purpose. Nor will the information system necessarily be designed in a manner that facilitates such analysis.

9. A rights approach provides potential recourse for those who experience violations.

On this subject, the proposal receives high marks. The intention is to provide an impartial, speedy, and simple to use mechanism for review of grievance and complaints. Each regional alliance must establish and maintain an office of an ombudsman to assist consumers in dealing with problems that arise with health plans and the alliance.[64] All health plans offering coverage through a regional or corporate alliance are required to establish a benefit claims dispute procedure. To reduce costs and increase the efficiency of the grievance process, the plan sets specific deadlines for resolution and provides for early review of disputes by neutral third parties. If the grievance procedure fails to resolve a complaint, consumers will have the option of pursuing the issue or pursuing other legal remedies. At the apex of the system, the Secretary of Labor is to establish by regulation a Federal Health Plan Review Board.[65]

10. The human rights approach advocated in this study balances individual needs with the common good thereby making the viability and effectiveness of the health care system a shared concern and responsibility.

By taking an individualistic approach, the Health Security Act neglects shared concern and responsibility for developing and sustaining the health care system. It neither promotes individual nor shared responsibility for the welfare of disadvantaged and vulnerable persons or for the viability and effectiveness of the health care system. By seeming to promise all things to all people, the Clinton plan forgoes the opportunity to appeal to Americans to sacrifice self-interest for the sake of the wider community, to make fundamental trade-offs between the security of an entitlement and limits on benefits, and to accept basic changes in health care delivery.

A. The claiming of rights implies associated responsibilities for all individuals and groups.   Just as the Health Security Act fails to vest individuals with clear rights, it does not articulate meaningful responsibilities. Although the bill does have a section on individual responsibilities, the duties listed are to enroll in an applicable health plan and to pay any premiums required.[66] For the most part, the bill associates individual responsibility with contributing to the cost of premiums and copayments, and not with duty to be sensitive to the health care needs of others or to carry a collective responsibility for the viability and effectiveness of the health care system. To win support, the Clinton administration does not link the security of the benefits promised by the new system with any proposed reduction in expectation or changes in behavior. Quite the contrary, for those who are already "haves" it seems to promise all things to all people, neglecting the opportunity to trade the promise of secure benefits for behavior and expectations more consistent with a cost conscious standard of health care. The bill also never mentions the collective responsibility of members of society for meeting the needs of the most vulnerable and disadvantaged members of society and for assuring the viability and coherence of the health care system.

B. There needs to be meaningful incentives for healthy life styles.   The proposed bill does not deal with this issue in a meaningful way. The bill fails to adopt either a punitive "good behavior model" of limiting health care benefits for those who engage in behavior harmful to one's health or positive incentives, such as lowering premiums. It should be noted though that a community rating system, such as the bill adopts, is difficult to combine with meaningful positive incentives. Nevertheless, the Health Security Act does not even articulate the principle that the individual is responsible to the community for adopting healthy life styles that will help prevent illness and reduce the need for medical interventions.

C. The primary goal of the health care system should be that of fostering the common good and collective health of society, not the particularized good of individuals.   Because the Health Security Act takes an individualistic approach to reform, it does not deal, at least explicitly, with collective responsibility for the common good and collective health of society. Proponents clearly believe that the managed competition system envisioned under the bill would improve the health of the members of society, and it is likely that it would. Nevertheless, it can be argued that fostering the collective health of society involves more than increasing individuals's access to health care. It requires instituting public policies that will create healthier conditions and protect the public's health. It is also related to the adoption of a new paradigm for health care that focuses more on prevention and less on curative care. It means setting more realistic expectations and clearer investment priorities so that the health sector does not absorb a constantly increasing investment of gross national product at the expense of other goals. In addition, there needs to be meaningful public discussion leading to the formulation of criteria that would reduce investments in futile care, particularly for terminally ill patients, that tend to prolong death rather than offer opportunities for living, often doing so contrary to the patient's directives. The Health Security Act does not even make an effort to address this sensitive and complex subject. Thus it misses the possibility of fostering a national consensus on a new cost-conscious standard of care in which no American would claim benefits that could not in principle be made available for all.

Conclusions

This analysis of the Health Security Act from a human rights perspective has been critical of many features of the bill. Of the ten criteria defining a human rights approach, the Health Security Act receives unqualified high marks only in regard to its proposed grievance procedures. Otherwise its scoring on the human rights report card was mixed, earning something equivalent to a C+. Since there was no attempt to comply with a human rights standard—in fact the bill refrains from recognizing any right to health care—the evaluation is not surprising. The single most problematic feature, however, is the cavalier disregard for the welfare of the poorest and most vulnerable groups. Despite the rhetoric of universality, the bill explicitly excludes undocumented aliens and questionably postpones coverage for most of the nearly thirty-nine million Americans who currently lack health insurance. Moreover, as noted, several of the proposed financial provisions would take resources away from low-income groups and illegal aliens so as to extend benefits for the middle class without imposing new taxes. If enacted, the managed competition system is likely to be an improvement over the present system, but it certainly misses a major historical opportunity to establish a truly just health care system that enshrines the principle of health care for all.

NOTES

1. "Health Security: Preliminary Plan Summary," (Washington, D.C.: U.S. Government Printing Office, 1993).

2. The New York Times, *The President's Health Security Act* (New York: Times Books, 1993).

3. Health Security Act, Bill to 103rd Congress (Washington, D.C.: U.S. Government Printing Office, 1993).

4. Dana Priest, "Health Plan May Let States Form 'Single-Payer' Systems," *The Washington Post,* October 23, 1993, A7.

5. Paul Starr and Walter A. Zehman, "Bridge to Compromise: Competition under a Budget," *Health Affairs* 12 (Supplement 1993): 9.

6. Starr and Zelman, 5–23.

7. Stuart H. Altman and Alan B. Cohen, "Commentary: The Need for a National Global Budget," *Health Affairs* 12 (Supplement 1993): 194–203.

8. Joseph P. Newhouse, "An Iconoclastic View of Health Cost Containment," *Health Affairs* 12 (Supplement 1993): 152–171.

9. The New York Times, p. 11.

10. President's Commission for the Study of Ethical Problems in Medicine and Biomedical Research, *Securing Access to Health Care: The Ethical Implications of Differences in the Availability of Health Services,* Vol. I (Washington, D.C.: U.S. Government Printing Office, 1983), p. 3.

11. Health Security Act, Title I, Sec. 1001, p. 13.

12. Sam Howe Verhovek, "Health Debate Stirs Concern in Boarder Town Over Aliens, *The New York Times,* October 25, 1993, pp. A1, A14.

13. Health Security Act, Title I, Subtitle B, pp. 32–33.

14. The New York Times, p. 91.

15. Health Security Act, Title I, Subtitle C, p. 94.

16. See Daniel Wikler's article in this volume.

17. Robert Pear, "Health Care Spending Is Found to Vary Greatly by State," *The New York Times,* October 7, 1993, A. 24.

18. *Ibid.,* pp. 44–45.

19. Health Security Act, Title I, Subtitle B, Part 3, pp. 73–82.

20. Lawrence O. Gostin, "Foreword: Health Care Reform in the United States—The Presidential Task Force," *The Journal of Law, Medicine & Ethics* 21 (Spring 1993): 8.

21. Health Security Act, p. 1.

22. The New York Times, p. 11.

23. Priest, p. A7.

24. Dana Priest, " 'Single-Payer' Health Plan Would Save U.S. $114 Billion a Year, CBO Says," *The Washington Post,* December 17, 1993, A10.

25. In addition to articles by Wikler and Baily in this volume, see Arnold S. Relman, M.D., "Shattuck Lecture—The Health Care Industry: Where Is It Taking Us," *The New England Journal of Medicine* 325 (September 1991): 854–859.

26. Health Security Act, Title III, subtitle D, p. 545.

27. Health Security Act, Title III, Subtitle D, p. 544.

28. Health Services Act, Title I, Subtitle B, p. 47.

29. The New York Times, pp. 205–215.

30. Health Security Act, Title III, Subtitle E, pp. 562–596.

31. Robert Pear, "Health Plan Leans on the Employers," *The New York Times,* December 16, 1993, p. A21.

32. *Idem.*

33. Dan Morgan, "Health Plan Assailed for Costs to Poor: Those Off Welfare Face Co-Payments," *The Washington Post,* November 21, 1993, p. A13.

34. *Idem.*

35.   Mary-Margaret Patterson, "A boost for the very disabled: But millions of other are deemed insufficiently impaired to get help," *AARP Bulletin*, November 2, 1993, p. 12.

36.   Tracy Thompson, "What If You Need Mental Health Care?" *The Washington Post Health Section*, November 2, 1993, pp. 17–18.

37.   *Idem.*

38.   Pear, "Health Plan Leans on Employers".

39.   Elliot Carlson, "President's plan gets high marks from AARP," *AARP Bulletin*, December 1993, pp. 1, 4,5.

40.   Robert Pear, "Influential Group Says Health Plan Slights the Aged: Two Tier System Is Feared," *The New York Times*, October 24, 1993, p. A1, A18.

41.   Robert Pear, "New Analysis Finds Higher Costs in Health Plan," *The New York Times*, December 9, 1993, A20.

42.   Richard L. Berke, "Clinton Aide Says Polls Had Role in Health Plan," *The New York Times*, December 9, 1993, A20.

43.   Uwe E. Reinhardt, "Reforming the Health Care System: The Universal Dilemmas", *American Journal of Law and Medicine* 19(1993)35.

44.   Elisabeth Rosenthal, "In Canada, A Government System that Provides Health Care to All," *The New York Times*, April 30, 1991, pp. A1, A11.

45.   Reinhardt, p. 35.

46.   Art Levine and Ken Silverstein, "How the Drug Lobby Cut Cost Controls," *The Nation*, December 13, 1993, pp. 713, 730, 731.

47.   Newhouse, p. 165.

48.   Robert Pear, "Medicare to Stop Pushing Patients to Enter HMOs" *The New York Times*, December 27, 1993, pp. A1, A14.

49.   Reinhardt, pp. 25–26.

50.   Newhouse, p. 152.

51.   See Michael Garland's article in this volume.

52.   Health Security Act, Title I, Subtitle F, p. 254.

53.   Health Security Act, Title I, Subtitle D, pp. 115–116.

54.   Gostin, 121.

55.   Health Security Act, Title I, Subtitle F, p. 258.

56.   Health Security Act, Title I, Subtitle D, p. 148.

57.   Health Security Act, Title I, Subtitle C, p. 95.

58.   *Idem.*

59.   This date is extrapolated from the calculations in Fitzhugh Mullan, Marc L. Rivo, and Robert M. Politzer, "Doctors, Dollars, and Determination: Work-Force Policy," *Health Affairs* 12 (Supplement 1993) 148.

60.   The New York Times, p. 139.

61.   Daniel Patrick Moynihan, "Guns Don't Kill People. Bullets Do." *The New York Times*, December 12, 1993, p. E15.

62.   Health Security Act, Title V, Subtitle B, pp. 845–848.

63.   Health Security Act, Title V, Subtitle A, pp. 826–831.

64.   Health Security Act, Title I, Subtitle D, p. 147.

65.   Health Security Act, Title V, Subtitle C, pp. 872–917.

66.   Health Security Act, Title I, Subtitle A, pp. 114 and a5.

Audrey R. Chapman

Policy Recommendations for Health Care Reform

The United States is on the threshold of national health care reform. For the sixth time in this century, policymakers are considering major changes in the manner in which health care is financed. This may be the final opportunity to end the national disgrace of being the only major industrialized country that does not recognize the right of its citizens and residents to basic health care. If the health care system is not made more equitable now, it is unlikely to become more so in the future. More than any other policy initiative, failure to achieve meaningful health care reform will confirm the sense that it is not possible for the government to resolve national problems. Moreover, nothing less than the national covenant between the government and its citizens is at stake. Very likely, the manner in which the reform addresses the needs of the nearly 39 million Americans who currently lack health care insurance will also play a major role defining what kind of country this will be in the twenty-first century.

Of the various health care reform plans under consideration by Congress, the "single-payer" system introduced by Rep. Jim McDermott (D-WA) and Sen Paul Wellstone (D-MN), is the most consistent with human rights criteria. The single-payer plan would establish a health care system similar to Canada's in which all citizens and legal residents would have immediate guaranteed access to a comprehensive standard benefits package. As noted in the previous chapter, a single-payer system would be more capable of achieving and sustaining universality, assuring social equity, and holding down health costs than managed competition. Under the proposed single-payer plan, a national health security board would set pricing standards for covered services but delivery would basically be unchanged. The government would also establish annual national health budgets to control costs. To finance health care, substantial payroll taxes would be imposed on employers, replacing the cost of insurance that most employers now pay. Individuals would pay nothing.

Four other major health reform proposals, variously put forward by Senators John Chafee (R-RI), Phil Gramm ((R-TX), George Michel ((D-ME), and Rep. Jim Cooper ((D-TN), are even more problematic from a human rights perspective than the Clinton Health Security Plan. Although universal health insurance coverage is an ostensible goal, they lack a strong commitment to universality and an effective means to cover those currently without health insurance. These proposals rely on private insurance arrangements financed by individuals rather than employer mandates. The Cooper plan proposes to finance insurance premiums for individuals below the poverty line from accrued savings that may never materialize. In contrast with the Health Security Act, these more conservative alternatives lack controls on premium payments, copayments, and deductibles and therefore are even less likely to limit health care spending.[1]

Despite criticisms and reservations, such as those expressed in the previous chapter, managed competition is likely to provide the framework for health care reform. It is the basis for the Cooper plan as well as the Clinton proposal. While the American Health Security Act, the bill establishing a single-payer system has gained popularity with some 90 members of Congress and about one-third of the American public, it also has very strong opposition from the health insurance lobby, whose role would be virtually eliminated, and health care providers, whose fees and profits would be reduced. With these groups mobilizing to defeat the single-payer plan, a modified version of the Clinton administration's Health Security Act may be the compromise between the more progressive American Health Security Act and the group of more conservative alternatives.

Assuming then that a revised version of the Health Security Act is likely to be adopted, how can it be made more consistent with human rights concerns? This chapter turns to the task of making specific recommendations to correct some of the deficiencies in the current proposal. While the incorporation of these recommendations would not completely eliminate the problems noted in the previous chapter, since the managed competition model itself is the source of fundamental reservations, it would considerably improve the plan from a human rights perspective.

(1) Recognize the right of all citizens and residents to basic and adequate health care, with coverage for those currently without health insurance to be phased in within eighteen months of the passage of a health care reform bill.

As noted many times in the volume, legal recognition provides a more secure grounding for universal coverage. It establishes universality as the norm rather than an option which is dependent on the outcome of an election or the achievement of cost savings. While the provision of a legal entitlement does not in and of itself assure access to health care, it creates an obligation for federal and state governments to establish a broad framework and enact specific policies to promote that goal. The recognition of a right would also provide individuals and communities with potential recourse if regional health alliances, states, or the federal government did not adopt or implement policies to address current financial and nonfinancial barriers to health care. A truly universal health care system would not distinguish between legal and undocumented residents, but it is probably politically unrealistic to expect the United States Congress to be so inclusive.

(2) To promote equality and reduce stratification in the proposed three-tier health care system, limit the price differentials that can be charged between the highest and lowest cost plans in any regional or corporate health care alliance to no more than thirty percent.[2]

Limiting price differentials would promote equity and would have two additional benefits. It would very likely improve the quality of the benchmark or lowest cost plan and inhibit the development of "Medicaid mills" achieving significant cost savings through providing inadequate services and care to the poor. It would also limit the types of "extras" that the highest cost plans could offer.

(3) Develop stronger regulations and require ongoing monitoring to prevent "gerrymandering" of geographic catchment areas to avoid certain populations because of their risk profiles or special health care needs and to assure diversified bases.

One way to discourage regional and corporate alliances from "skimming" off lower insurance risks is requiring all health alliances to incorporate a minimum percentage of disadvantaged persons, low income residents, and persons with special health care needs reflecting the approximate distribution of these groups within the population of each state. State governments should also monitor regional health alliances so as to assure that they do not impose obstacles to the full participation of these groups and that providers offer appropriate services.

(4) Incorporate older Americans into the regional health alliances so that they are eligible for the same benefits as those under 65 years of age.

Principles of universality and equality preclude any form of age discrimination. Benefits should not be the same for all age groups.

(5) Place greater emphasis on health protection and prevention of disease and provide greater resources for these objectives.

An important component of health care reform is shifting from the curative health care paradigm to a new model which emphasizes protecting and improving the public's health status. Relevant measures not contemplated in the Health Security Act include major initiatives to reduce exposure to toxic substances, improving the quality of air and water, providing incentives to health lifestyles, ending subsidies for the growing of tobacco, and discouraging the use of alcohol, cigarettes, and guns through imposing significantly higher taxes.

(6) Facilitate states adopting single-payer systems.

States should be able to adopt a single-payer system for the whole state or a portion of it. To enable states to do so, bureaucratic and legal obstacles should be eliminated. It is appropriate to require states to guarantee that the standard benefits available to state residents under a single payer system will be at least comparable to those provided for in the Health Security Act. Other restrictions on single payer systems in the Health Security Act, however, are not defensible. Current requirements in the Health Security Act precluding state-run health alliances to pay more for coverage of low-wage workers than it would otherwise, for example, should be eliminated. States should not be penalized for attempting to provide greater equity.

(7) Vest regional and corporate health alliances with the responsibility of providing health care services to underserved areas and populations and either provide sufficient federal subsidies to enable them to fulfill this obligation or have them tax all consumers in the regional alliance so as to offset the costs of extending services.

Initiatives to address the uneven distribution of health care providers and facilities, particularly the lack of quality health care in urban centers and rural areas, should be a requirement not an option. Rectifying historical and structural inequities requires planned initiatives with specific goals and timetables. Merely offering incentives to the private sector is an insufficient approach.

(8) Reallocate financial resources so that the provision of adequate and meaningful subsidies and grants to underwrite the health care needs of low income persons and persons with disabilities and special needs has the highest priority.

A human rights approach requires a pattern of distribution that confers priority on the disadvantaged and those with greatest need. Hence improved security and comprehensive benefits for the middle class should not be financed at the expense of the poor. More equitable budgeting would provide subsidies to cover the full cost of premiums, copayments, and fees for persons below the poverty line and offset the increased costs of participation in regional alliances to the working poor. Nor should funding be reduced to hospitals that currently serve large Medicaid populations in advance of incorporating their clients into regional health alliances. If undocumented aliens remain ineligible for membership in a regional health alliance, then the hospitals and clinics that currently provide services should be adequately funded so as to be able to offer basic and adequate health care to them. It is also important to allocate sufficient funding to enable all disabled persons who are eligible, based on a needs assessment, to receive services.

(9) Make the financing of health care reform more progressive by adding to the proposed seventy five percent increase in the federal excise tax on cigarettes, substantial "sin" taxes on the sale of alcohol and on guns and ammunition and use these taxes to provide more generous subsidies to underwrite the costs of low income groups.

Health care reform requires equitable and fair means of financing. These proposed taxes are equitable because they would more adequately offset the actual costs of smoking, drinking, and gun use on the health care system.

(10) To control health care costs, establish global budgets that set expenditure limits identify funding priorities, and impose price

controls on pharmaceuticals, physicians's fees, and high cost medical procedures.

This proposal would restore the Clinton administration's initial assessment that managed competition and global budgets were required to hold down health care costs. Global budgets could also restrain the introduction of new technologies and encourage providers to ration organ transplants and other costly procedures.

(11) To promote public participation in shaping health care reform, as well as assuring accountability of health care institutions to citizens, add public interest representatives or consumer advocates to the composition of the National Health Board and require the National Health Board to establish effective consultative procedures for public participation, including an annual hearing process evaluating major components of the health care system.

The legitimacy of both the process and specific decisions will depend on the broadest possible citizen involvement. Oversight and control are not the prerogatives solely of health care professionals and experts. To assure public participation, all national, state, and regional corporate health alliances should be required to have public and/or consumer representatives.

(12) Develop an effective monitoring system that will be able to assess the impact of health care reform on an ongoing basis, particularly the ability of the new system to provide disadvantaged and currently underserved communities with basic and adequate health care.

This will require the development of a national health information system. Effective monitoring entails more than quality evaluation of insurance plans. It includes the formulation of appropriate indicators and standards, the development of new instruments capable of collecting relevant data, disaggregation of data into appropriate categories, and regular evaluation.

NOTES

1. "Health Care: Clinton's Plan and the Alternatives," *The New York Times*, October 17, 1993, A12.

2.   This recommendation is based on Larry Gostin's suggestion that the highest cost plan be prohibited from charging people more than twenty percent over the benchmark plan. See Lawrence O. Gostin, "Editorial: Health Care Reform in the United States," *The Journal of Law, Medicine & Ethics* 21 (Spring 1993): 8.